CLINICAL PSYCHIATRY • EMIL KRAEPELIN

Publisher's Note

The book descriptions we ask booksellers to display prominently warn that the book may have numerous typos, missing text, images and indexes.

We scanned this book using character recognition software that includes an automated spell check. Our software is 99 percent accurate if the book is in good condition. However, we do understand that even one percent can be a very annoying number of typos! And sometimes all or part of a page is missing from our copy of a book. Or the paper may be so discolored from age that you can no longer read the type. Please accept our sincere apologies.

After we re-typeset and design a book, the page numbers change so the old index and table of contents no longer work. Therefore, we often remove them.

We would like to manually proof read and fix the typos and indexes, manually scan and add any illustrations, and track down another copy of the book to add any missing text. But our books sell so few copies, you would have to pay up to a thousand dollars for the book as a result.

Therefore, whenever possible, we let our customers download a free copy of the original typo-free scanned book. Simply enter the barcode number from the back cover of the paperback in the Free Book form at www.general-books. net. You may also qualify for a free trial membership in our book club to download up to four books for free. Simply enter the barcode number from the back cover onto the membership form on the same page. The book club entitles you to select from more than a million books at no additional charge. Simply enter the title or subject onto the search form to find the books.

If you have any questions, could you please be so kind as to consult our Frequently Asked Questions page at www. general-books.net/faqs.cfm? You are also welcome to contact us there.

General Books LLC®, Memphis, USA, 2012. ISBN: 9780217823999.

❖ ❖ ❖ ❖ ❖ ❖ ❖ ❖

PKEFACE TO THE FIRST EDITION

The motive for this work was to make the teachings of Kraepelin in psychiatry accessible to American medical students and general practitioners, and, at the same time, to provide a full, but concise, text-book, not only for the writer's own classes in psychiatry in the Medical Department of Yale University, but as well for other American teachers who follow Kraepelin's views. Urged by the rapidly increasing interest in Professor Kraepelin's teaching during the past five years in this country and the constantly growing number of his disciples, it was the writer's first intention to publish a complete translation of the sixth edition of Kraepelin's "Lehrbuch der Psychiatrie." It was feared, however, that a full translation would be too large to best subserve the function of a text-book, and would have rendered impossible the adaptation of the Kraepelin psychiatry to our peculiar American needs.

The classification, terminology, and, wherever possible, the phraseology of this work are Kraepelinian, but the writer has taken the liberty of abbreviating disproportionately the description of some psychoses which are of less importance to the American physician, especially the constitutional psychopathic states and thyroigenous insanity, and of laying more stress upon other more important forms, the description of acquired neurasthenia, traumatic neuroses, also the treatment in epileptic and hysterical insanity and acquired neurasthenia.

V 104060

The only omissions are the general etiology, diagnosis, and treatment in the first volume of Kraepelin, but such points as are of most importance have been added to the etiology, diagnosis, and treatment of the different diseases.

The work has been done in the pres-sure of routine duties as Assistant Physician and Pathologist of the Connecticut Hospital for the Insane, and the writer begs leave to express in this place his grateful appreciation of the generous advice and help of his colleagues in the hospital, especially Dr. Charles W. Page. He is particularly indebted to Dr. J. M. Keniston for a general revision of the text as well as for the arrangement of the chapter on Epileptic Insanity, to Professor Raymond Dodge, Ph.D. , of Wesleyan University, for criticism and suggestion with regard to the general symptomatology, and to Dr. August Hoch and Adolf Meyer for their continued inspiration and critical assistance.

A. BOSS DIEFENDOEF.

MIDDLETOWN, CONNECTICUT, January 15, 1902.

PEEFACE TO THE SECOND EDITION

The favorable reception of the first editions of Clinical Psychiatry and its constantly increasing use as a text-book encouraged the writer to undertake a thorough revision based on the seventh edition of Kraepelin's "Lehrbuch der Psychiatric" In accord with the present views of Professor Kraepelin there are introduced many important changes, both in the general symptomatology and in the description of the forms of mental disease. For the convenience of students the chapter on Methods of Examination is amplified by explicit practical suggestions adapted to the circumstances under which most of them will be compelled to work, while the more elaborate procedure of the modern experimental laboratory has been omitted. In response to a general demand, an abridgment of the chapter on the Classification of Mental Diseases is added to the present edition. Less hampered by restrictions as to size, the present edition follows more closely the context of the "Lehrbuch." The description of the more important forms of insanity is less curtailed, while the psychogenic neuroses and the psychopathic states which received scant attention are now given fuller consideration. The chapter on Psychopathic Personalities did not appear in Kraepelin's earlier edition. The writer has tried to make it clear by references wherever additions of his own have been made. The most important additions without explicit references occur under the head of Treatment.

As in the preparation of the first edition, the work has been done under pressure of routine duties as Assistant Physician and Pathologist of the Connecticut Hospital for the Insane, and the writer desires to express to his colleagues his appreciation of their help, and especially to Dr. Henry S. Noble, Superintendent, his grateful obligation for placing at his disposal the time and much of the material for the work. He is under special obligations to Dr. J. M. Keniston for help in reading proof and the arrangement of the chapter on Epileptic Insanity, and to Professor Raymond Dodge, Ph.D., of Wesleyan University, for criticism and suggestions with regard to the general symptomatology and the Psychopathic Personalities.

A. KOSS DIEFENDOEF.

MIDDLETOWK, COIWICTICUT,

April 6, 1907.

ILLUSTRATIONS

Faoiho Paok

GENERAL SYMPTOMATOLOGY A. DISTURBANCES OF THE PROCESS OF PERCEPTION

The perception of external sensory stimuli depends upon two conditions: the adequate stimulation of the sensory end organ; and the elaboration of this stimulation by the central nervous system.

The loss of one or more of the senses modifies mental development in proportion to the importance of the sensory material lost and the possibility of substituting other sensory experience. Loss of sight is relatively unimportant, but loss of hearing, on account of its relation to language, is of great importance; indeed, unless specially trained, deaf mutes remain mentally weak through life.

Illusions and Hallucinations. — More important than the mere absence of sensory experience is its falsification.

Inadequate stimulation of the sense organ produces impressions corresponding to the "specific energy" of that sense; for instance, an electric current may produce a sound, a taste, a tactual or a visual sensation, according as it stimulates the corresponding sense organ. Such sensations are real illusions, but they do no harm because they are immediately recognized as illusions. In conditions of mental disturbance, on the contrary, especially where there is great clouding of consciousness, the subjective sensations of light as the result of congestion of the eye, or a roaring in the ear, may be interpreted as fire or torrents of water, giving rise to genuine deceptions which are not corrected. This sort of peripherally conditioned sense deception has been called *elementary,* on account of its origin in that part of the sensory apparatus which receives the stimulus.

States of consciousness similar to sensory perceptions may be produced by the excitation of the so-called cortical sensory areas. This is naturally referred to an external object, and results in an illusion as to the real source of the stimulus. This group of hallucinations may be called *perception phantasms.* They may occur in normal individuals, particularly at the onset of sleep, as hypnogogic hallucinations. In abnormal conditions, they are often extremely vivid and misleading. They usually bear no relation to the content of thought, and, consequently, seem to the patient to belong to the external world. They have a fairly uniform content, subject only to slight modification (stable hallucinations of Kahlbaum), and consist of senseless words, noises, figures, and the like, which are repeated over and over again. Because of their central origin, they may occur after destruction both of the peripheral sense organ and the afferent nerve. The cases of hemilateral disturbance of the field of vision, in which the gaps produced by the disordered perception are filled out by the patient, point clearly to central origin in that portion of the cortex which has to do with visual perception. There are some cases in which sense deceptions have prevailed in the normal half of the field of vision, where the cortex in both occipital lobes has been diseased. Again, coincident with the rapid development of the bilateral cortical blindness there has been observed sudden development of active perception of light. *Peripheral influences* may also produce, directly or indirectly, conditions of excitation in the higher portions of the sensory tracts, which lead to sense deceptions, particularly if the general irritability of these parts is increased. In morbid conditions, ordinary organic stimuli suffice to produce such falsification. In other cases, these hallucinations may appear if attention is merely directed to that sensory field, or if an emotional condition temporarily increases the general susceptibility to stimulation. It disappears, on the other hand, as soon as the patient becomes quiet or directs his attention elsewhere, as in conversation, manual or mental employment, change of environment, etc. Further evidence of cooperation of conditions of stimulation in the sense organ is found in the occasional occurrence of one-sided hallucinations, the frequent association of chronic middle ear disease with hallucinations of long standing, and the production of hallucinations of sight in alcoholic delirium by gentle pressure on the eyeball. Usually these sense deceptions appear only in a single sensory field, and are most frequent in the fields of hearing and sight.

Sense deceptions are divided clinically into *hallucinations and illusions. In the former there are no recognizable external stimuli; the latter are falsifications of real percepts.* In some cases this distinction may be difficult to carry out on account of internal stimulation of the sense organs, such as occurs in phosphenes, entotic noises, etc. In other cases the distinction is clear. The perception of ghosts in moving clouds and limbs of trees, curses and threats in ringing bells, are evidently illusions. But the well-known visual disturbance of the alcoholic, and the voices which torture the condemned in his prison, when everything is quiet, are pure hallucinations.

The universal characteristic of the entire group of sense deceptions is their *sensory vividness.* They depend on the same sort of cerebral processes as does normal perception, and the false perception takes its place in consciousness among the normal sensory impressions without any distinguishing characteristic. The patients do not merely believe that they see, hear, and feel, but they really *see, hear, and feel.*

In morbid conditions *very vivid ideas* or *memory images* may assume the form of hallucinations, being regarded by the patients as real perceptions of a peculiar kind. Many investigators hold that all false perceptions should be regarded as ideas of imagination of extraordinary sensory vividness. But in order that an idea attain the clearness of a perception, some special cause must be present. This is indicated by the fact that in patients suffering from hallucinations, not all, but only certain groups of ideas seem to play a role in the sense deceptions, and besides these there are usually ideas of the ordinary, faded, and formless type. The element which makes a hallucination out of a vivid idea is probably a reflex excitation of those central sensory tracts, through which alone normal stimuli come to consciousness (the so-called "reperception" of Kahlbaum). If it is really these areas of the brain through whose excitation perception acquires its peculiar sensory marks, it is easy to see how they may participate in varying degrees in the active process of renewing previous impressions. A view of this sort would explain the fact that there lies between the sense deception of pronounced sensory vividness and the most faded memory image an unbroken series of transition stages. It is possible that during the ordinarythought processes this *reflex excitation* or *reperception* is always present in a very slight degree, but that only when the process becomes morbid, or the sensory areas themselves are in a condition of increased excitability, does the vividness of the memory picture approach that of true sense perception. Probably there is, moreover, a definite relation between the strength of the *reperception* and the irritability of the sensory areas; the greater their irritability, the more easily will the memory images attain sensory vividness, the lighter the reflex excitation need be to release them, and the more independent they are of the current of thought. The extreme case would be found in the sense deceptions depending upon local excitation, which seem to the patient to be something quite foreign and external. The extreme case in the other direction

would be those instances which are not true sense deceptions at all, but merely ideas of great sensory vividness. By careful investigation it is often possible to analyze the data given by the patient, which apparently indicated hallucinations, and to discover that the patient does not regard the impression as objectively real, but merely differentiates it from his ordinary ideas on account of its forceful vividness. In these cases it is probable that the reperception is strongly developed, while irritability of special sensor'-tracts is not increased. This seems to be borne out by the fact that this group of hallucinations, which has been variously designated as psychic hallucinations (Baillarger), pseudohallucinations (Hagen), and apprehension hallucinations (Kahlbaum), involves several or all of the sensory fields, and that it always stands in close relation to the other contents of consciousness; while the true falsifications of perception, on the other hand, usually belong to a single sensory tract, and are independent of the train of thought.

A striking illustration of this type of hallucinations is found in a condition called "double thought." Immediately upon the appearance of any idea, the patient has another distinctly subsequent idea of the same thing; *i.e.* every idea is followed by a distinct sensory after-image. This double thought occurs most frequently when the patients are reading, sometimes when writing, and occasionally, also, when linguistic ideas come vividly to consciousness. The sensory after-image disappears if the words are actually spoken. Other hallucinations of hearing universally accompany this condition.

Apperceptive illusions are those in which subjective elements unite with the objective sensory data, giving rise to a distorted and falsified impression. They are of very frequent occurrence in normal life; prejudice, expectation, and the emotions continually influence our perceptions even in spite of our earnest effort to be neutral. Even the most tranquil scientific observer is never quite certain that his perceptions do not unconsciously suit themselves to the views with which he approaches his investigation; while in reading we all unconsciously correct the errors of the type-setter from the residua of our experience. In mental disturbances the conditions are often extraordinarily favorable for this falsification of apprehension. Marked emotional excitement, great activity of the imagination, and finally, the inability to sift and correct experience by reason, — all are favorable to its development. Thus, it frequently happens that the sensory impressions of patients take on fantastic forms and become the basis of a thoroughly falsified apprehension of the external world, even when there are no true hallucinations. This phenomenon naturally occurs most frequently, both in normal and abnormal states, when the sensory impressions are confused and indefinite, and not readily differentiated.

There is an allied group of disturbances which consists in the release of a false perception in one sensory field through a real impression received by another, constituting the so-called *"reflex hallucinations of Kahlbaum."* A sensory stimulus may produce conditions of excitation, which, transferred to an overexcited sensory area, occasion the development of an hallucination. Similar conditions are daily encountered in the so-called sympathetic sensations, like the unpleasant sensation of an inexperienced onlooker at a painful surgical operation. In morbid conditions these may be very marked. Especially sensations of movement which frequently accompany sense impressions seem to rise in this way. There are patients who feel on their tongues the words spoken by others; a glance from some one may excite a sensation of strain.

A very important characteristic of sense deceptions, which in one way points to their origin and in another to their importance as a disease symptom, is the *powerful and irresistible influence* which they exert over the *entire thought and activity* of the patient. It is true that occasionally a pronounced illusion appears in persons mentally sound; and, also, that at the beginning, as well as at the end, of a mental disease the illusions

are often recognized as such, because of their improbable content, but usually persistent illusions and hallucinations overpower the judgment, and ultimately the patients invent the most foolish and fantastic explanations to account for them.

The basis for this irresistible influence is not to be found in the sensory vividness of the illusion, since real sensations and definite evidence are useless as correctives. Its explanation is found rather in the *intimate connection between the illusions and the patient's innermost thought, morbid fears, and desires.* The emotional states and the feelings color the illusions in a peculiarly high degree, as one might expect from their influence in normal life. It is frequentlyobserved, especially in the end stages of dementia praecox, that illusions appear only in connection with the periodical vacillations of the emotional state, while they completely disappear in the interval. This influence of the emotional life upon the thought and actions only disappears with recovery, or when progressive deterioration obliterates emotional activity. In both cases the illusions may continue, but the patients do not react upon them.

These facts manifestly disprove the general view that sense deceptions regularly, or even frequently, act as the real causes of delusions. To be sure, patients point to their hallucinations as the basis of their symptoms, but there can be no doubt that the *sense deceptions have a common source of origin vrith the other disturbances of the mental equilibrium.* In reality the patient's attitude toward his illusions and hallucinations is not the same as his attitude toward his actual perceptions. No healthy individual would refer to himself such words as "That is the president," and then immediately believe he must be the president. But when these words form the keystone of a long chain of secret misgivings, an hallucination of that sort makes the most profound impression, and immediately there arises a firm conviction, not only that the words were really spoken, but that they express the truth.

In view of these facts we see no spe-

cial practical value in distinguishing in single cases whether the delusion, the emotional state, or the corresponding sense deceptions appear first. In the vast majority of cases, and especially where the sense deceptions appear with persistent delusions, all of these disease symptoms are certainly only the result of one and the same common cause.

Illusions and hallucinations present a large number of clinical types in the different sensory fields. The most frequent sense deceptions of *sight* are those which occur at night, the so-called visions; God, angels, dead persons, distorted figures, wild animals, and the like. The less common sense deceptions of sight which appear in daylight along with the normal impressions are much more like normal perceptions and consequently more deceptive. The sense deceptions of the alcoholics are of this type (see p. 176). The objects of the surroundings may take on an entirely different appearance; patients mistake strangers for relatives and *vice versa,* and believe that the same persons are taking on different forms and faces, are making grimaces, etc.

The most important sense deceptions of *hearing* are the so-called *voices,* a term which is usually well understood by the patient. The basis for their importance lies in the fundamental significance of language in our psychic life. The voices usually have an intimate relation to the content of consciousness; in fact, they are the linguistic expressions of the patient's inmost thought, and for this reason have for him a far greater convincing power than all other sense deceptions, more even than real speech. The voices mock the patient, threaten him, and tell his secrets. They are heard in the scratching of a pen, in the barking of dogs, etc. Sometimes there are several distinct "voices" with characteristic differences. Usually they are low, as if coming from a distance, though occasionally they are loud enough to drown all other noises. It rarely happens that the "voices" speak long sentences. Usually they consist of short, interrupted remarks. The hallucinations in fever delirium and in greatly bewildered patients are changeable and confused.

Auditory sense deceptions are seldom indifferent to the patients, but are almost always accompanied by strong emotional disturbances and wield a powerful influence over the patients' actions. They make them distrustful, excited, and even drive them to angry attacks on their imaginary tormentors.

The so-called *"internal voices,"* "suggestions," "telephoning," "telegraphing," etc., form a special group of hallucinations of hearing. These naturally are not regarded by the patients as sensory in their origin. They may occur as a kind of monologue or as a conversation with distant persons; sometimes the voices of conscience seem to criticise the patient or spur him on. In all these cases the patient develops the delusion that his thoughts are known to every one, or that they are produced and influenced by outside forces.

Sense deceptions in the other senses are of much less importance. False perceptions of taste, smell, dermal, muscular, and general senses, so far as they derive their origin from the thoughts of the patient, and not from the disturbance of the sense organs, point to a profound change of the whole psychical personality.

Where delusions of electrical influence, of position, of incasement of different organs of the body, the disappearance of the ears, mouth, etc., are present we no longer have simple illusions and hallucinations, but almost always a severe disturbance of the higher psychical processes.

Hallucinations develop differently. One might judge this from their great variety. The type of the hallucination may be determined in a measure by the form of the mental disease. In fever delirium and infection psychoses the hallucinations and illusions are variable and dreamlike, occurring in all the different fields of sensation and producing a most confused and fantastic experience. Similar hallucinations and illusions exist in the alcoholic delirium, but here they present a *peculiar sensory vividness* and they combine so that the separate experiences are much more

definite. Indeed, they combine so intimately with each other that they offer a good foundation for the development of an "occupation delirium." Another characteristic of these alcoholic hallucinations and illusions is that they are very numerous and change rapidly. These sense deceptions, originating as they do from imperfectly perceived impressions, can even be created and influenced by mere suggestion. The hallucinations in cocainism which appear in the visual and auditory fields and in the field of general sensibility are closely related. The "microscopic" hallucinations of sight are particularly characteristic; *i.e.* the perception of numerous minute objects, little animals, or holes in the wall or little points. On the other hand in the epileptic delirium the hallucinations are accompanied by a peculiarly intense tone of feeling; for instance, the sight of blood, of fire, objects of fear, the hearing of threats, the noise of shooting, or the music of angels. In all of these conditions it is probable that there is an extensive involvement of the cortex by the disease process. This seems the more probable as clouding of consciousness regularly accompanies these states. Other disease processes present even more transitory delirious states with hallucinations involving the different senses: such as manic-depressive insanity, senile dementia, dementia praecox, and occasionally paresis. In the bewildered and excited stages of dementia praecox hallucinations of hearing predominate, while in similar states in manic-depressive insanity hallucinations of sight are more prominent, and particularly hallucinations of the general sensibility. In paresis illusions are much more evident than hallucinations, although both are comparatively infrequent. There is only a small group of cases in which the sense deceptions involve only a single sensation; as, for instance, in most cases of acute alcoholic hallucinosis, and some cases of alcoholic hallucinatory dementia, in which there are very striking hallucinations of hearing. Also in some epileptic states, hallucinations of hearing only appear. Hallucinations of

hearing alone are by far most frequent in dementia precox. They are rarely absent long. Usually they represent one of the first symptoms and often they continue as the only symptom for some time. In the delirious states of dementia praecox they are usually associated with hallucinations and illusions of the other senses. It is also in dementia praecox that the peculiar disturbance called "double thought" mostly occurs. The content of the hallucinations is of a fearful or disturbing nature only at the beginning, while later it becomes more or less indifferent and senseless, which is in marked contrast to the other forms of mental diseases mentioned above.

Clouding of Consciousness. — External stimuli occasion within us characteristic mental phenomena which we apprehend immediately and distinguish as presentations, feelings, and volitions. This experience is designated as consciousness, which is present whenever physiological stimuli are converted into psychic processes. The nature of consciousness is obscure, yet we know not only that it in general depends upon the functioning of the cerebral cortex, but also that its individual phenomena are connected with definite, but as yet undetermined, physiological processes in the nervous system. Just as the transition of the external stimuli into sensory excitations depends upon the nature of the sensory organ, so the condition of the cerebral cortex is the determining factor in the transformation of physiological into conscious processes. Whether such transformation takes place in individual cases is often very difficult to determine, since we have no immediate insight into the inner experience of others and are compelled to draw our conclusions from their behavior.

The condition in which the transformation of physiological into psychical processes is completely suspended, is designated *unconsciousness*. Every stimulus which crosses the threshold of consciousness, thereby arousing a psychic process, must possess a certain intensity which cannot sink below a definite limit. This limit is called the threshold value and varies greatly according to the condition of the cortex. While it is lowest in strained attention, the threshold value reaches infinity in the deepest coma. It is thus possible to distinguish different degrees of the *clearness of consciousness* according to the character of the threshold value. But even when conscious processes are no longer aroused by external stimuli, consciousness in the form of obscure presentations and general feelings may still exist.

If the clearness of consciousness decreases sufficiently, befogged consciousness results *(Dammerzustand)*, during which neither the external nor internal stimuli can create clear and distinct presentations. These *befogged states* are encountered in epileptic and hysterical insanities, as transitory states contrasting sharply with the normal life of the individual. Prolonged befogged states are also found in which mental processes are rendered difficult and the psychophysical threshold is considerably raised. Sometimes the threshold value may be so altered that it is different for external and internal stimuli; that is, while external stimuli have little effect, internal stimuli produce vivid conscious processes. This is what occurs in delirious states. The opposite condition obtains in demented states, where not infrequently external stimuli easily produce sensations, while internal have little effect in consciousness. What occurs here is not an increase of the threshold value, but a prolonged sinking of the psychophysical excitation. Indeed, this is the distinction between dementia and the befogged states.

Disturbance of Apprehension. — The full effect of an external stimulus takes time. Experiment demonstrates that our sense perceptions reach the point of greatest clearness only after a period of some seconds. Under some circumstances this process may be retarded. Stimuli of short duration are either not apprehended at all, or only incompletely, although no real difficulty of apprehension is present. If the retardation in the development of sensory impressions is considerable, the impressions fade

away before they are really perceived. Some very strong impressions may be apprehended, but they are more or less incoherent because the connecting links and the accompanying events reach consciousness only in an incoherent and confused form. This disturbance of apprehension in its pronounced form is encountered in senile dementia (presbyophrenia) and Korrsakow's psychosis, but exists in a much less marked degree in many other psychoses, particularly of the delirious type.

The apprehension of external impression requires not only the development of a percept of sufficient strength, but also its absorption into the systematic interconnections of our experience. The vast majority of our impressions at any given moment are obscure and confused. Presentations only become clear and distinct when they find residua of past experience in the memory, "resonators," as it were, through whose sympathetic vibration the sensory stimulation is intensified. It is through this process, which Wundt calls "apperception," that each percept becomes united with our past experience, through which alone it can be understood. This supplementing the given impression by memory images greatly increases the delicacy of our apprehension, but brings with it the danger of a *falsification of perception.*

The most frequent type of the disturbance of apprehension is the increase of the threshold value for external stimuli. The more intense the stimuli must be in order to produce an impression, the more confused and defective will be the picture of the external world. The patients apprehend only a small part of the impressions which they receive. They fail to note and to understand their environment. We call this *diminished sensibility.* The gradual development of this disturbance of apprehension is found in simple fatigue and its transitions into sleep, but also in the morbid states of extreme mental exhaustion. Ether and chloroform isolate our consciousness from the external world most completely and rapidly, but a number of narcotics act in a similar way; such as, alcohol, paraldehyde, and trional. Dimin-

ished sensibility is also found in fever, and intoxication deleria, as well as in the clouded consciousness of epilepsy and hysteria. Oftentimes it is also found in the various phases of manic-depressive insanity, especially in the depressive and manic stupor, but also in the more intense maniacal excitement.

The entire sensory experience in the first stages of mental development remains on the plain of simple perception. As long as the impressions of the external world have left no memory residue there is no network of psychological associations through which new experience may be related to the past. In the severest forms of arrested mental development this condition persists, and there is no possibility of the gradual clearing of the clouded consciousness. It remains forever a confused medley of vague isolated presentations and feelings, in which there is no clear apprehension or order.

Disturbances of Attention. — At any one moment there is present in our inner field of view only a limited number of mental phenomena. This limitation of consciousness is called the "span of consciousness." Since the entire chain of our psychical life must pass under the limitations of this span, our inner life presents a constant coming and going of mental processes. One experience after another appears and disappears; each approaches from the darkness of the unconscious, at first being indistinct and weak, after a short time reaching the climax of its clearness and strength, and then sinking from sight to give place to another. This development of a mental phenomenon within the field of consciousness is coincident with that inner activity of the will which we call *attention.* Our sense organs turn to the forceful impressions, and those presentations appear which strengthen the process that claims our attention. The strain of attention may have various degrees and directions. It is accompanied by certain physical phenomena; such as, movements of the body, alterations in breathing, pulse, and blood pressure.

Attention not only strengthens a developing impression, but without doubt it retards its fading. In this way each impression exerts an influence on its successors. Their relation to their predecessor inhibits or promotes their development. In this manner the primitive *passive* and aimless attention becomes *active* and selective. It is not the force of the external impressions, but rather the attention, which determines our inner experience. Experience is determined not so much by the strength of external impressions as by the favoring or inhibiting effect of attention. In a child the content of consciousness is helplessly dependent upon accidental circumstances; it perceives only the most striking stimuli. In adults, on the other hand, the process of perception is more and more dominated by personal tendencies which gradually develop out of the experiences of the individual. We train ourselves to notice certain impressions in preference to others, so that some stimuli, however faint, have decided advantage over others. On the other hand, we accustom ourselves to be *inattentive* to regularly recurring stimuli, yielding them no influence over our psychic processes. This development of definite "points of view," definite directions of interest, leads to an extraordinary variability of the threshold of consciousness, so that at the same moment when strong stimuli pass quite unnoticed, we apprehend with greatest acuteness the slightest alterations in some special object.

The attention is variously affected in different psychoses. In the first place, in all conditions of advancing dementia there is a *blunting of attention.* Perceptions arouse no corresponding memory images. They are not united with the patient's past experience and they fail to incite him to pursue them further on his own initiative. In the case of a deteriorated paretic the most striking occurrences may take place without creating any impression, although he may be able to comprehend questions. In dementia praecox a striking disorder of the attention is present from almost the inception of the disease. Particularly in the stuporous states, all attempts to arouse the attention are unsuccessful, even prodding with a needle, or touching the cornea, fails to create any voluntary movement. This is not a blunting of the attention but a *suppression of the attention.* The patients perceive well enough what takes place about them, but they involuntarily prevent the perception influencing their thought or action. Even all the external expressions that accompany attention, such as the turning of the head and eyes, and apparently also the alteration of the pulse and breathing, are absent. This disorder corresponds with the negativistic processes found in disturbances of volition and may be called a *blocking* (Sperrung) *of the attention.*

In some stuporous states of manic-depressive insanity a *retardation of the attention* occurs. Here also it is difficult to get into touch with the patient, but only because he lacks that internal process which connects his external impressions and his past experience, and incites the selective activity of the attention. The development of ideas is rendered difficult, not on account of deterioration in the mental life, but through the process of retardation which prevents the perceptions from gaining any extensive influence over the internal life. In manic-depressive insanity the external expressions accompanying attention are usually preserved, the patients look around inquiringly, although not understandingly. They look at objects placed before them and turn the head at a noise.

An immediate result of these disturbances of attention, both blunting and retardation, is the loss of their determining influence upon new perceptions. A single impression may be able to arouse the attention and be strengthened by it, but the persistent continuance of this psychical process, with its resulting choice of the incoming perceptions, is lacking. An impression once aroused may last some time, but it can always be displaced by a new stimulus, provided only the latter is strong enough. This is *passivity of the attention* which is observed particularly in paresis and senile dementia. It also occurs in the stuporous forms of manicdepressive insanity and in many of the demented states following infectious diseases.

The patients resemble children who have never had experience, therefore have no ideas or memory pictures that can be awakened to direct the attention. In those forms of mental weakness, in which mentality does not develop beyond the grade of childhood, the attention throughout life remains passive and lacks independence.

Distractibiiity of attention is the domination of the attention by accidental, external, and internal influences. Limitation of the attention arises through the want of ideas that have strength enough to influence the process of apprehension; in distractibility there is a greater flightiness of the mental processes. The attention leaps from one impression to another, in spite of the fact that an endeavor is made to direct the attention. This disturbance regularly accompanies those mental states that exhibit increased irritability. It is probable that in increased distractibility of the attention the separate impressions fade so rapidly that they have no dominating influence upon the incoming perceptions. Details are apprehended without a comprehensive view of their relations, and the entire apprehension is superficial.

The lightest form of distractibility is found in the absentmindedness of fatigue. In chronic nervous exhaustion it is more persistent, as is also the case in convalescence from severe physical or mental disease. It appears to a marked degree in the excited stages of paresis, sometimes also in catatonia, collapse delirium, and in the infection psychoses, but particularly in the manic forms of manic-depressive insanity. In these conditions a single word or the most casual stimuli suffice to distract the attention.

Distractibility of attention is continuously present in some forms of constitutional psychopathic states, where it exerts a very powerful influence upon the mental development. The more distractible a man is, the less perception is controlled by inner motives arising from experience, and the less coherent and uniform is the conception of the external world. Distractibility is not to be confounded with *hyperprosexia,* which consists in the total absorption of the attention by a single process, examples of which are found in the so-called absent-mindedness of scholars and the complete absorption of the melancholiac in his sad ideas.

B. DISTURBANCES OF MENTAL ELABORATION

The material of experience, received through the different senses and clarified by attention, forms a basis for all further mental elaboration, and it is self-evident that both disturbances of apprehension, and the inability to make a systematic choice in the impressions, must affect to a marked degree the character of all intellectual processes.

Disturbances of Memory. — All higher mental activity depends largely upon memory. Every impression which has once entered consciousness leaves behind it a gradually fading "disposition" to its recall, which may be accomplished either through an accidental association of ideas or through an exertion of the will. This disposition to recollection is really identical with the residua which each new perception contributes to the store of experience and to the resources of memory. The residua are strong and permanent in direct proportion to the clearness of the original impression, and to the multiplicity of its relations to other processes, *i.e.* to the interest it arouses and to the frequency of its repetition. The vast majority of our ideas and the greater part of the association complexes with which we have to do daily, are so accessible to us that they appear of themselves under the least provocation and without any effort.

Memory is really a dual process dependent on *impressibility* and on *retentiveness,* each of which may be disturbed independently of the other.

Impressibility is the faculty for receiving a more or less permanent impression made by new experience. The clear apprehension of events, especially when aided by active attention, increases this impressibility, while it is lessened by difficulty of apprehension, by dis-

tractibility and indifference. It, therefore, is diminished wherever there is cloudiness of consciousness, as in amentia, to a less extent in the absent-mindedness of fatigue, and in the states of deterioration in dementia praecox, paresis, and in epileptic insanity, which are characterized by stupid indifference to the environment. The most marked disturbance of impressibility occurs in Korssakow's psychosis and senile dementia, especially presbyophrenia, although the moment impressions are well apprehended and assimilated. In these patients the process of perception develops very slowly, so that with those stimuli which act quickly the process of apprehension becomes distinctly impaired and at the same time the processes of consciousness fade very quickly.

In normal life it is the greatly diminished impressibility which renders it difficult to recall our dreams. This demonstrates that psychic life, and therefore consciousness, can exist without memory. Similar conditions of clouded consciousness, with undoubted evidences of a psychic activity, but yet without memory, occur in epilepsy, many delirious conditions, profound intoxications, and hypnotism. "Retrograde amnesia," in which memory is more or less permanently destroyed without clouding of consciousness, occurs in epileptic, hysterical, and paralytic attacks, head injury, and some attempts at suicide, in which patients cannot remember the events which immediately precede the attack. Memory for this period may return.

Retentiveness of memory for past events depends upon the previous impressibility, upon repetition and the native tenacity of the individual memory. Its disturbance is manifested by an inability to accurately recall former knowledge and important personal events. Lack of impressibility usually accompanies lack of retentiveness, but the converse is not necessarily true, as impressibility is affected by clouding of consciousness, while retentiveness is not. In senility the former is far more disturbed than the latter; recent events leave no residua, while remote events

recur in memory with ease and accuracy. This is even more striking in senile dementia and may occur in paresis. In Korssakow's psychosis the weakness of memory may extend back to cover a definite period of the life.

The *accuracy of memory* may be disturbed. Even in normal conditions, accuracy is only relative. In morbid change of personality or the emotions, and in the development of delusions, the past is always more or less falsified. Vivid imagination and pronounced egoism imperceptibly modify the memory of past experience even in normal life; stories are embellished with interesting details, while the self becomes a more and more important factor. This is always exaggerated in disease, while in melancholia, persecutory and expansive delusions often color the memory of the past until it seems like pure invention.

A mixture of invention and real experience is called *paramnesia.* There also exist "hallucinations of memory" (Sully), which consist of pure *fabrications,* being found especially in paresis, paranoid dementia, and sometimes also in maniacal forms of manic-depressive insanity. It also occasionally occurs in epileptic and hysterical befogged states. But fabrications are particularly characteristic of Korssakow's psychosis, and presbyophrenia, in which states the gaps produced by disordered perception are filled in with falsifications of memory, including even incidents of youth. These are often fantastic accounts of wonderful adventures; they may be modified by suggestion and are frequently selfcontradictory (see p. 186). The delusion of a double existence may be produced by confusing present experience with indistinct memory images of the past, so that every event seems like a duplicate of a former experience. This sometimes occurs transiently in normal life; in disease it may last for months, and is found particularly in epilepsy.

Disturbances of Orientation. — Orientation is the clear comprehension of the environment in its temporal, spacial, and personal relations. Our present is related to our past experience in a temporal series through the function of memory. Only recent events are remembered with the greatest distinctness; while the rest is grouped around more or less isolated points, which form the basis for the general chronological arrangement of our experience.

Spacial orientation is partly dependent on memory. In the first place, memory enables us to recognize immediately parts of our present environment, while even an unknown environment may be comprehended through our experience when the latter includes the motives or conditions for the former. But apprehension may also play an essential rôle in place orientation. In any unknown environment into which one happens to be placed, the process of perception regularly clears up the real situation by bringing about a connection between the immediate impressions and our past experience. This often involves more than a mere identification of the present with the past. It may result from a more or less complicated process of reflection and reasoning. In the same manner, orientation as to persons arises from the cooperation of memory, perception, and judgment.

Thus it becomes apparent that lack of orientation or *disorientation* may arise from disorder of memory, from disorder of apprehension, and from disorder of judgment. In many cases two or more of these causes are combined. Further, the disorder may involve all the fields of orientation or it may be limited to a single field, so we may differentiate between total and partial disorientation. The apprehension of the environment may be prevented by the fact that the patients cannot elaborate their external impressions, or by an inhibition of thought, or by a clouding of consciousness with or without falsification of perception. The first case is very common in dementia praecox, where the disorientation usually results from the lack of mental activity, and may be called an *apathetic disorientation*. There is no difficulty in perception. The patients simply lack the inclination to understand the meaning of what they see and hear, so that for weeks at a time they may give themselves no concern as to

where they are, how long they have been there, or whom they see. In the depressive phases of manic-depressive insanity the apprehension of the environment is rendered difficult through the presence of retardation and there develops a condition of *perplexity.* The patients perceive details well enough, but they fail to synthesize them. The disorientation in the most pronounced manic states may perhaps be similarly accounted for, as there accompanies it a marked difficulty in the apprehension and elaboration of external impressions. The different forms of clouding of consciousness in focal lesions of the brain, in epilepsy, and in alcoholics cause a more or less pronounced disorder of orientation. In the delirious states found in infection and intoxication psychoses, also in hysteria and epilepsy, there exist, besides the lack of clearness of apprehension, also sense deceptions, both of which cloud and falsify the picture of the environment.

In Korssakow's psychosis there is an *amnesic disorientation* which depends neither upon disturbances of apprehension nor of perception. While in this condition place orientation is usually well retained, the patients are absolutely helpless as regards time. They do not know when they came into the institution, when they were last visited by relatives, when they last dined, etc. Events of a month ago may be referred to as occurring yesterday, and again an occurrence of yesterday may be mentioned as happening months ago.

This amnesic form of disorientation may occur even more strikingly in presbyophrenia, where on account of the marked disturbance of perception in connection with the difficulty of apprehension, mental elaboration of external impressions is almost impossible, hence patients fail to get any idea of their environment, although details are understood without difficulty. The amnesic form of disorientation also occurs in paresis, where time orientation is most often at fault. Amnesic disorientation occurs in other psychoses, indeed, wherever the disorder arises from faults of memory. One's own experience in

orienting himself upon awakening from a sleep or after fainting indicates how difficult it is to regain time orientation after a severe clouding of consciousness.

The *delusional form of disorientation* is quite different. Here we have to do with a faulty mental elaboration of impressions which are correctly perceived and apprehended, leading to a false opinion as to the environment in its temporal and spacial relations. The patients are not clouded, but they maintain delusional ideas as to the time, place, and persons. Illusions or hallucinations may be the basis for such beliefs, as in mistaken personalities and the assertions of paranoid patients that they are in prison, in a bad house, etc.

Disturbances of the Formation of Ideas and Concepts. —

Most of the complex ideas of normal life are composed of heterogeneous elements, furnished by the various senses. In these complexes the importance of the material furnished by any one sense depends upon the peculiarities of the individual. For some, vision is the most important sense, for others audition; but both of these senses may be entirely lacking without preventing a high development of ideation. On the other hand, lack of permanence of sensory impressions and imperfect assimilation always interfere with the formation of complex ideas. This is illustrated in congenital and acquired imbecility.

The *formation of concepts* is the necessary condition for the fullest development of ideation. In normal life those elements of experience which are often repeated impress themselves more and more strongly, while the accidental variations of each individual experience are driven more and more into the background. The concepts thus developed are a sort of composite photograph or generalization of experience.

These concepts are the most permanent and most easily reproduced of all our ideational processes. But even these may not be reproduced in totality. More and more in the developed consciousness single elements of these concepts are made to stand for the whole. The exact form of this abbreviation of thought is often accidental, as when some single image comes to stand for the total concept. The highest form of this development is found in the abbreviation of thought by the use of linguistic symbols, *i.e.* when a word stands for the idea.

In morbid conditions, especially in congenital imbecility, this development may stop at any point. The patients may cling to individual experience without being able to sift out the general characteristics of different impressions of a similar nature. They are unable to find concise expressions for more extended experience; the essential is not distinguished from the unessential, the general from the particular.

This not only prevents the development of thought, but it also retards the assimilation of new material. New impressions find no point of attachment in the mental life; they cannot be arranged or systematized, and pass rapidly into oblivion. In acquired imbecility the residua of earlier experience may partly conceal the inability to receive new impressions and to form new ideas. Later, however, this defect gradually becomes more evident. Similarly in paresis, dementia praecox, and senile dementia, the circle of ideas narrows, and general ideas and concepts are gradually replaced by the specific, the immediate, and the tangible. New impressions are no longer elaborated and the most recent experience is quickly forgotten, while the memory of the past is still fairly constant.

In direct contrast to this is the disturbance produced by *morbid excitability of the imagination,* which correlates dissimilar and even contradictory ideas. Such forced and arbitrary combinations naturally interfere with the normal development of concepts. Thus the foundation of all higher mental activity becomes a mass of confused and indistinct psychic structures, which can give rise only to one-sided and mistaken judgments as soon as the patients leave the region of immediate sensory experience. The tendency to reveries and dreams, lack of appreciation of facts,

impossible plans and chimeras, so often found in imbecility, paresis, and paranoid dementia, are clinical forms of this disturbance.

Disturbances of the Train of Thought. —The association of ideas may be divided into two groups: *external* and *internal associations,* the former being effected by purely external or accidental relations, while the latter arise from a real coherence in the content of the ideas.

External associations usually arise through the customary connection of ideas in time or space, of which thunder and lightning is an example; or through habits of speech, in which a definite association of words becomes so fixed by frequent repetition that one word always calls up the others, as in quotations and stereotyped phrases. Sound associations, an important and extreme form of this type, are based either upon similarity of sound or of the movements of the vocal organs, as seen, for example, in a morbid tendency to rhyme. This disturbance may be so marked that the associated sounds are altogether meaningless. *Internal associations* depend upon the logical arrangement of our ideas according to their meaning. The association between different individuals of the same species, or different species of the same class, is of this kind; for instance, the association of boy with man and man with animal, etc. The special form of internal associations, which emphasize some particular characteristics of a concept, usually attributes, states of being, or activities, by means of which a preceding idea is more closely defined, is called *predicative* association. That the dog is an animal belongs to the first class of internal associations; that he is dark-colored, or that he runs, belongs to the second. *Paralysis of thought,* the simplest form of disturbance of the train of thought, is characterized by complete absence of all associations. It begins as a more or less marked retardation, and develops into characteristic monotony and distractibility of thought. It occurs in a moderate degree in fatigue. Narcotic poisoning presents severer forms. It is a

fundamental symptom in the psychoses accompanied by deterioration: paresis, dementia praecox, and senile dementia. *Retardation of thought* is manifested by difficulty in the elaboration of external impressions; the train of thought is markedly retarded, and the control of the store of ideas is incomplete. It may bring the train of thought to a complete standstill. In contrast to the paralysis of thought, to which it presents a superficial similarity, this inhibition may suddenly disappear under certain conditions, as fear. The patients do not lack mental ability; they are not, like the weak-minded or deteriorated, obtuse and indifferent, but they are unable to overcome this restraint which they themselves very often realize. The most pronounced form of this disturbance is seen in the depressed and mixed forms of manic-depressive insanity, and perhaps, also, in the disturbance of thought in epileptic stupor.

The *disturbances of the content of thought* are best understood as a faulty arrangement of the individual links of our thought with relation to the goal ideas. Normal thought is usually directed by definite goal ideas, and of the ideas which appear in consciousness, those elements are specially favored which stand in closest relation to these controlling goal ideas. Out of the large number of possible associations those only really occur which he in the direction determined by the general goal of the thought process.

In morbid conditions the train of thought may be interrupted by individual ideas, or other trains of thought with an especially prominent emotional tone (cf. Melancholia, p. 355). The memory of some sad experience or a fright may so dominate us that our thoughts in spite of all effort return to the same channel. *Compulsive ideas* are those ideas which irresistibly force themselves into consciousness. These are usually accompanied by a disagreeable feeling of subjection to some overwhelming external compulsion. The mere fear of their recurrence is often sufficient to bring them into consciousness. They usually develop on a basis of emotional disturbance, and, therefore, accompany melancholia and depressed phases of manic-depressive insanity, also sometimes the depressive states of dementia praecox. The content of these impulsive ideas is unpleasant and harassing. The patients are compelled to think constantly of some shocking experience, which they have had, or to depict some misfortune, which may befall them. The profound emotional despondency which serves as a basis for these thoughts and at the same time furnishes a good soil for their development has associated with it a feeling of compulsion. As the disease develops, despondency becomes more predominant, particularly if the resistance of the patient to the ideas is gradually weakened, so that the feeling of subjection vanishes. In this way the original compulsive ideas are transformed into delusions.

If the fundamental emotional state is independent of morbid changes of the emotions, as encountered in various psychoses, the disturbing factor in the compulsive ideas does not reside so much in their content as in the fact of their constant recurrence. The most striking forms of these compulsive ideas develop in the states of hereditary degeneracy (cf. Compulsive Insanity, p. 498). Increased emotional susceptibility, as well as a tendency to morbid introspection, are the fundamental states from which these compulsive ideas develop. In the very lightest forms there develop ideas which are unpleasant.

There is still another group of cases in which some simple common ideas interfere with the development of every train of thought, later gaining mastery; such as the compulsion to recall the name of some one, which may become so prominent that the patient makes out a long list of names, and finally indexes the names of every person whom he meets. The compulsion to count is of the same sort and again there is the compulsion to ask of themselves all sorts of questions (Gruebelsucht) (cf. p. 500). There is here a feeling of uncertainty which incites the patient to a distinct effort, which feeling can never be quite satisfied, because every sugges-

tion leads to still another series. There is no end to the names, the numbers, and the questions to be asked. The real basis for these ideas is, therefore, a feeling of discomfort, identical with that which incites all of us to seek for clearness and truth; but in the case of the patient these ideas are no longer the servants, but are masters of the psychical personality, because he has not the power to suppress them when they hinder the train of thought.

Distinguished from the compulsive ideas are the *simple persistent ideas,* unaccompanied by marked unpleasant feelings of compulsion. This phenomenon is probably due to the absence of definite or fixed goals in the train of thought — a view which is borne out by our experience with the persistence of some of our own ideas, whenever we give free rein to our thoughts. Rhyme, verses, and melodies sometimes cling to us even in spite of our efforts to throw them off.

In gross brain lesions there is often found a peculiar persistency of linguistic expressions. Words and phrases used shortly before are repeated by mistake. Patients in naming objects use words which they have just heard or spoken. Fatigue may so aggravate this disorder that it is impossible to secure a correct answer, as one gets only a monotonous repetition of previous statements.

In another phase of the disorder, more or less motor to be sure, patients use an indicated object in the same way they have just previously and correctly used another. Neisser happily names this disturbance *perseveration.* In some cases of senile dementia with pronounced persistency of ideas, Schneider has pointed out that ideas once aroused develop very slowly. In fact, in perseveration, one often has the impression that the patients fail to understand the new perceptions and when forced simply repeat themselves. Patients only named a picture right after one or two other pictures had been shown. If this hypothesis is correct, the disorder is conditioned not so much by the peculiar stubbornness of a particular idea, but rather by the difficulty of releasing oth-

er ideas to displace it.

One should distinguish carefully from perseveration the tendency "to run to death the same ideas" so often occurring in dementia praecox in a pronounced form. It is but another expression of stereotypy of the will. Examples of this condition may occasionally be encountered in children. It consists of an impulsive, often limitless repetition of similar expressions, sometimes alone and sometimes interwoven in other more or less incoherent trains of thought. The content of these stereotyped ideas is quite accidental and is not, as in simple persistent ideas, determined by that which has preceded.

In morbid conditions, even when the collection and elaboration of new impressions is prevented by mental disease, there remain some residual ideas of the normal state, fixed by constant repetition. This results in a monotonous content of consciousness with a marked impoverishment of the store of ideas. This occurs in senility, paresis, and other deterioration processes, in which the train of ideas may shrink down to a few phrases, or even a few words which are repeated over and over. These phrases, in contrast to the persistent ideas of the catatonic, are not senseless, but actually express the content of the patient's consciousness. The following is an example:—

"Frazier went away this morning, will be back soon. Didn't ask him what time he'd come home. Frazier is working up in the lot at something. I was up in the lot yesterday. I forget what I went for. Frazier is talking of selling the place. He asked me what I cared about it. Father is going over there today. Father don't care for the farm. He didn't speak to me; he is downhearted. He should bring up his boys to work upon it. Frazier don't have time to work. He don't stay home much. I would advise them to have a place and keep it. If I get well I will keep it, if I can. The boys would like to have some farm. They won't stay in a place. Frazier don't like to work on the farm. Patient hears a woman coming up the hall. Some woman I hear coming. If she was on a farm, she wouldn't handle much money. If they sell the place, the children will starve for hunger. Patient looks at her hand. I am all blacked up. I have been out on the farm a good deal. If he sells the place, the little children will starve for hunger," etc.

Circumstantiality is the interruption of the course of ideas by the introduction of a great multitude of nonessential accessory ideas, which both obscure and delay the train of thought. The disturbance depends upon a defective estimation of the importance of the individual ideas in relation to the goal ideas. The goal may, indeed, be ultimately obtained, showing some real coherence, but only after many detours. The simplest form of circumstantiality appears in the prolixity of the uneducated, who are unable to arrange their general ideas in accordance with their importance, and show a tendency to adhere to details. Some even have difficulty in distinguishing sharply what is actually seen from what is simply imagined. The circumstantiality of the senile is probably due to the disappearance of the general ideas and concepts. Circumstantiality is also present to a marked degree in epileptic insanity, of which the following passage taken from the bibliography of an epileptic is an example: —

"Before one believes what others have told him or what he has read in the almanacs he must be convinced and examine himself before one can say and believe that a thing is beautiful or that a thing is not beautiful; first investigate, go through it yourself, and examine it, and then, when man has investigated everything and has gone through it himself and examined it, then man can at once say the thing is beautiful or is not beautiful or not good; therefore, I myself say, if one will make a statement about a thing, or will sufficiently establish something or will speak in conformity with the truth, the thing is right or is not right, so must every man likewise examine the thing as he believes himself responsible before the tribune God, and before his Majesty the King of Prussia, William the Second, and the Emperor. of Germany. I will now relate further

what the soldiers have done to me."

The absence or incomplete development of goal ideas gives rise clinically to two important forms of disturbance of the train of thought: (1) flight of ideas, (2) desultoriness. The first effect of a defective control over the train of ideas is a frequent and abrupt change of direction. The train of thought will not proceed systematically to a definite aim, but constantly falls into new pathways which are immediately abandoned again. The impetus for such changes of direction can arise from both external stimuli and from internal processes.

In *flight of ideas* the instability of goal ideas produces a condition in which the successive links of the chain of thought stand in fairly definite connection with each other, but the whole course of thought presents a most varied change of direction. The patient is unable to give long answers to questions, and cannot be held to a problem requiring much mental work, because ideas once aroused are immediately forced into the background by others. This is a fundamental symptom of the manic form of manic-depressive insanity, and also occurs in acute exhaustion psychoses, infection deliria, paresis, occasionally also in fatigue of normal life and especially in dreams. It may appear in alcoholic intoxication. There is no great wealth of ideas, but on the contrary it is often accompanied by a conspicuous poverty of thought. Moreover, the rapidity of the association of ideas is not at all increased, but on the other hand is usually diminished. The patient's incoherence, therefore, depends simply on the lack of that unitary control of the association of ideas which represses all secondary ideas and permits progress only in a definite direction. As the result of this, any accidental idea which would normally inhibit the goal idea may assume importance. It is not, then, the rapid succession of ideas which warrants the designation of a flight of ideas, but the instability of single ideas which are unable to exert any influence over the course of the train of thought.

In flight of ideas the direction of the

train of thought is determined by external impressions, chance ideas, or finally by simple associations, external or internal. The influence of chance ideas is well demonstrated in intoxication deliria, and especially in opium intoxication, in which vivid ideas of the imagination follow each other in a variegated series, giving rise to an incoherent progression of unrelated fancies, to which experience offers no key. This might be called the *delirious form of flight of ideas.*

The *rambling thought* of the hypomaniacal patient is another form of the flight of ideas in which the patients are diverted by unimportant ideas, reminiscences, and incidents, and need to be frequently led back to their subject. The following is an example (the patient being asked when she left the Hartford Retreat): —

"My mother came for me in January. She had on a black bombazine of Aunt Jane's. One shoestring of her own and got another from neighbor Jenkins. She lives in a little white house kitty corner of our'n. Come up with an old green umbrella 'cause it rained. You know it can rain in January when there is a thaw. Snow wasn't more than half an inch deep, hog killing time, they butchered eight that winter, made their own sausages, cured hams, and tried out their lard. They had a smoke house. But how about your leaving Hartford? She got up to Hartford on the half-past eleven train and it was raining like all get out. Dr. Butler was having dinner, codfish, twasn't Friday, he ain't no Catholic, just sat with his back to the door and talked and laughed and talked."

Here, in spite of many diversions, we see a fairly good sequence in the content of thought which centers around a visit of the patient's mother.

In the following example, on the other hand, the predominance of motor speech ideas has led to a massing of habitual speech associations, combinations of common words, and finally to simple sound associations. It might be called an external flight of ideas in contrast to an internal flight of ideas characterized by internal associations.

"I was looking at you, the sweet boy, that does not want sweet soap. You always work Harvard for the hardware store. Neatness of feet don't win feet, but feet win the neatness of men. Run don't run west, but west runs east. I like west strawberries best. Rebels don't shoot devils at night."

The train of thought is supplanted by fixed and familiar phrases, in which the influence of linguistic ideas clearly outweighs that of the content of thought; while sound associations, rhymes, and quotations, etc., stifle all internal associations. The most favorable condition for the appearance of £this form is an increased motor excitability and alcoholic intoxication.

DesvMoriness, the second form of this type of incoherent speech, is more difficult to characterize, as it is not well understood. In it the external form of speech is fairly well retained, but there seems to be a complete loss of goal ideas, while an incoordinate mass of ideas follow each other aimlessly and abruptly. In the flight of ideas we were able to discover some connection, if only the most external, between the separate links of ideas, which gradually led to a new chain, until the original standpoint was entirely lost sight of. In desultoriness there is no recognizable association between the successive ideas, while the trains of thought often move along for some time in similar phrases. They are confused and contradictory. In flight of ideas the course always tends toward changing and hence never attained goals, and is, therefore, always entering new circles; in this form, on the other hand, the train of thought does not progress at all in any one direction, but only wanders with numerous and bewildering digressions in the same general paths, the following of which is an example: —

Middletown, Dec. 15,1901. Dear Sister:—

I received your box in perfect shape and money as well. Do you wish to see me. If you care or somebody else will. Do. Awful lonesome. A new suit and fair words. This time give me a little money if you will (tell her to use slang my front yard). Give me a punch for fun. You are read that way) leave (Give her a drop of your poison). Latest song attendant. (Give her a wife she is lonesome). Hill St. I suppose Tom Kellhams Pete whair Fitch. Right tell me give over Pa Ma Nell Har. Will Eddy. I strong don't you know he passed it to the other young from Newark but he could not start it. He did not know where it came from. He sleeps under. I got McKingleys Son over me at times he works on the stylish horse. He is a black strong. I am a red. You know the Pres. Brokerage and drink cigars and walks, speeches. He is 37 Port Rhoda he served 10 years at his trade he is working 14 good mack. Tell Burnie he is liked by him but not strong enough they live 9,000 miles in the air over the three miles you read in school.... Pa Pa you know the stove he carried. 1,700 lb. trunk strong nature, hard life when I got to let him know how on pipe here through the converser the head electro gave me a dime for sense and they don't speak and it was a corn sense. I am bed now good by. Yours Aff.

Distractibility through internal and external influences may also be present to a marked degree, but the newly aroused ideas do not serve as bases for others, but simply intrude into the desultory train of thought in an incoherent manner. In this way it is often possible, in the midst of their incoherent jumble, to obtain coherent replies to questions. The following is an example of this (the physician's questions are enclosed in brackets): —

"Why are you here? Because I am the empress. The dear parents were already there and everything was already there and had given me permission. I have also learned stenography. Why, David, how are you? Even a member of the reserve, megalomania, empress. Do you feel well? Oh, thanks, very well, since the government has given me permission we will be good friends. Oh, God! my brother Carl David the first and Olga. Ah, let me write something. Why are you here?j Insane. Megalomania. What is that? Nothing, nothing, at all. How old are you? 22-7-1872. Will you come again? I do not know. When he comes I will not run after him (laughs). I must always be close (clasps her hands). I have nothing (grasps at the watch chain. But the chain is nothing. How I will at once see what time it is."

This example does not show, however, the repetition of single words or phrases which so frequently occur in the catatonic productions, and is shown in the following: —

"You don't own this building, I know that. The Hartford pigpen never supported, never confirmed food, therefore are not supported and this building will pay for that and food which confirmed it. White immortal eternal receipt for that food. The war planet Mars. I have the white immortal eternal receipt. Mars war planet, or war world Mars. The war world or the war planet Mars. White immortal eternal receipt for its existence and confirmation receipt. The Hartford pigpen is not supported or has not confirmed food or the laws of food, therefore will not be supported by those who have confirmed food. The white immortal eternal receipt."

In extreme desultoriness the speech consists of a mere series of letters, syllables, or sounds, while in the severest forms of flight of ideas there is always some goal idea even though it rapidly changes, and the majority of the expressions consist of actual words; here there is a perfectly senseless repetition of the same sounds with only insignificant modifications, like the following: —

"Ellio, ellio, ellio altomellio-altomellio, — selo, eloo, devo, heloo

— f. f. f. dear father, f. f. f. dear father, e. e. f. old and new — f. f. f.

— f. f. —Catholic Church," and so on in monotonous repetition. Sound associations seem to play an important role here, but the train of thought does not advance through it to new ideas.

These disturbances which destroy or interrupt the internal coherence of thought gives rise to what is called *confusion* of thought, which is a prominent symptom of mental disease. This symptom develops variously. If the interference with the coherence of thought arises from flightiness of the goal ideas, then we have a form of *confusion charaeterized by flight of ideas* with its tendency to external and verbal associations. The abrupt development of many different ideas without order, and not leading to any definite goal idea, gives rise to the *desultory confusion.* There may also be differentiated still another form of confusion, *dreamy confusion,* which is characteristic of delirious states. In this type there exists besides the disturbance of apprehension and the rapid fading away of the perceptions, a marked prominence of sensory elements in thought. There is also a *combined form of confusion,* in which there is a transitory appearance of abundant, new trains of thought following each other incoherently. The head fairly swims because there is not an opportunity to marshal or survey the rapidly appearing ideas. This type of confusion characterizes those forms of mental disease in which the rapidly appearing thoughts are elaborated into a permanent delusion formation, in the same way that in normal life a person gradually works into his train of thought a new idea that at first was confused. Also the presence of many hallucinations may be regarded as a cause of an *hallucinatory confusion,* just as a normal person sometimes loses his orientation if he is suddenly placed in an inextricable environment with new and puzzling impressions.

Mental retardation can also produce a form of confusion of thought, through the slowing of the process of comprehension and mental elaboration. This has been designated *stuporous confusion.* In it one sometimes encounters a combination with a genuine flight of ideas. Finally the emotional attitude may play a very important role in the development of different forms of confusion of thought. In some diseased mental states with marked disturbances of the emotions, this element is of great importance.

Disturbances of Imagination. — The fund of our earlier experience becomes of most value to us when we are able to bring from it into consciousness voluntary ideas and memory images. This

ability is provisionally named *imagination.* It requires on the one hand reproducible residua of former mental processes, and on the other hand that process which enables us to formulate new mental pictures out of the simple residua of memory and make it possible to elevate ourselves above our simple sensory experience and perform original mental work.

The power of imagination may be seriously disturbed in disease. In some degree this is observed in simple mental fatigue, also in poisoning with narcotic and hypnotic drugs, but more especially in the severe grades of deterioration found in paresis, senile dementia, and other mental diseases. In these latter disturbances the atrophy of the imagination is usually combined with defective memory. The ideas are not only not at one's disposal, but they may also in large numbers disappear. Where this loss is less extensive, as, for instance, often in epileptic insanity, there develops a *simple sluggishness* (Schwerfalligkeit). These patients still have some command of their store of ideas, but they require a very long time and considerable stimulation.

The retardation which is encountered in the depressive and mixed phases of manic-depressive insanity is to all external appearances similar to sluggishness. The disturbance of thought processes of the befogged states of epileptic and hysterical insanities probably also belong here. Retardation differs from sluggishness in that it is a transitory state, while the latter is a permanent one. Retardation is usually accompanied by alterations in the emotional background which exert some influence over the function of imagination even in normal life. In it one finds that the elaboration of external impressions is rendered difficult; indeed, it may even be so much impaired as to cause complete perplexity, owing to the lack of memory pictures; the patients cannot think of anything, they lose all connection with their earlier experience, and sometimes cannot even give the names of their nearest relatives. Nothing occurs to them. Thought seems to come to

a standstill. Such patients may present the external appearance of profound dementia; but the fact that all of these severe disturbances suddenly disappear indicates retardation, moreover the patients suffering with retardation themselves recognize the resistance against which they have to struggle. They are not stupid or indifferent as demented patients are; they are simply unable, in spite of great effort, to overcome the constraint of thought.

In the *indifference* so characteristic of dementia praecox there is no resistance offered to the activity of thought, but there is a more or less complete lack of motive for mental work. If these patients are sufficiently stimulated, they are able to call up some of their favorite ideas, but they are never forced to mental work of their own accord. They take no account of what happens to them, and they have no thought of the future. Mental activity stagnates more and more, and there gradually develops a shrinking of the store of ideas—a sort of atrophy from disuse. In contrast to the paretic they often surprise one by the occasional display of a much greater wealth of ideas than it was supposed they actually possessed. This very rarely happens in the deteriorated stages of dementia paralytica. This observation confirms the belief that in dementia precox there is a real loss of mental activity.

Morbid excitation of the imagination is evidenced by a special vividness of the memory images, which under certain circumstances acquire the strength of sensory impressions. This occurs particularly in the different delirious states, where there is almost always present a pronounced disturbance of apprehension. Another example is found in some of the anxious states of melancholia, manic-depressive insanity, and of the psychopathic states, in which the patients detail their fears with painstaking clearness and completeness.

In the excited stages of manic phases of manic-depressive insanity, of paresis and of catatonia, it is a question whether there really is an increase of the imaginative power. One might judge that there was no question as to this in the manic phases of manic-depressive insanity, but really the realm of ideas here is barely, if at all, enlarged, while it very often is even diminished. Some of these patients assert that they abound in ideas, and even in the circular depressive phases patients may make the same assertion, in spite of retardation. There is, however, good reason to believe that there really exists more of an increased distractibility and flightiness of the internal processes than an increased production of ideas.

A persistent increase in the activity of the imagination is found in a considerable group of psychopathic individuals, such as the morbid adventurer and inventor, who in the pursuit of their extravagant plans completely lose sight of the realities of life, keeping their gaze fixed only upon the results, while they never take into serious consideration the difficulties and insufficiencies of their methods. Then there is the dreamer, who gives himself up to reveries. Finally there are the morbid liar and swindler, who take the greatest satisfaction in the variegated pictures of their busy imagination.

Great activity of the imagination regularly accompanies an increased susceptibility of thought to external and internal causes. In normal individuals this trait is exhibited in children and women. Morbid suggestibility and susceptibility to autosuggestion are regular accompaniments of many psychopathic states, especially the hysterical conditions. They are manifest here not only in the accessibility of thought and feeling to striking impressions and persuasion, but also in the appearance of all kinds of physical symptoms which are released through the medium of emotional states.

Disturbances of Judgment and Reasoning. — Judgment and inference are the most complex products of the intellect. Since perception, memory, the formation of concepts, and the association of ideas are their necessary preconditions, they will be more or less affected by every imperfection of these processes. But this is not the only source of their derangement.

Human knowledge has two sources: experience, and the free action of the mind itself (imagination). Neither source is entirely independent of the other; empirical knowledge is never free from preconception and expectation, while even the wildest imagination employs material which originally came from experience. Nevertheless, we sharply differentiate empirical knowledge from pure belief, which arises from the recasting and interpretation of experience.

Primitive people do not draw this distinction. Their mythological interpretations and traditions are as credible to them as direct experience. Even in children invention and experience are sometimes only partially differentiated. Whenever invention can be easily tested by direct experience the line between the two becomes more and more sharply defined; but even here the natural incompleteness of our apprehension or our habits of thought may lead us into error. If the data furnished by experience is scanty or unreliable, imagination is free to fill the field with its own creations.

Empirical science has slowly supplanted many of the misconceptions of primitive thought, but superstition still survives among the uncultured; while even among the cultured there are beliefs which no experience or arguments can shake. The essential characteristic of these beliefs is their emotional significance for the individual. Dogmatic opinions, ideas firmly fixed by tradition, education, and habit, acquire an overwhelming emotional value, and not only persist in spite of experience, but even mould experience into conformity with themselves (cf. the force of prejudice). The emotional significance of such beliefs has its basis in their relation to vital interest. A feeling of helpless dependence and insecurity in the presence of the unknown and mysterious is the fertile soil of superstition in primitive races. Even in most highly cultured persons political and religious convictions, although more or less dependent on the rational elaboration of experience for their content, are characteristi-

cally inaccessible to opposition and argument.

These peculiarities of normal thought help us to understand the delusions of diseased consciousness. Deltisions are morbidly falsified beliefs which cannot be corrected either by argument or experience. They do not arise from experience or deliberation, but from belief. Although often associated with actual and falsified perceptions (hallucinations or illusions), they are always due to a morbid interpretation of the events arising in the patient's own imagination. The tendency so often encountered in health, to draw sweeping conclusions from insufficient data or to assume a causal relationship between purely accidental occurrences, becomes an important factor in morbid conditions; the most innocent events are construed as mystic symbols of secret occurrences, and simplest facts are full of mystery. The flight of a bird is an omen of good fortune; an accidental gesture reveals sudden danger.

Further proof of the subjective origin of delusions is found in the close relation which they maintain to the ego of the patient. Just as in health the self forms the point of reference for our thoughts and feelings, so in disease the mysterious creations of the imagination are most intimately connected with the patient's own welfare. The delusions are, consequently, never indifferent to the patient except in cases of advanced deterioration. They are not only referred to the self, but they exercise a marked influence over the patient's emotional attitude toward his environment.

Delusions are inaccessible to argument, because they do not originate in experience. Experience, therefore, is unable to correct them as long as they remain delusions. Only in convalescence, when they become a mere memory of delusions, can they be recognized as false. At the height of the disease they are as firmly established as reason herself. So long as the morbid conditions which give rise to them persist, the delusions are unchanged. If they are relinquished or modified, the change is not due to argument, but to a change in the morbid condition. Our argument may drive the patient to admit non-essential points, but the delusion serenely reasserts itself, notwithstanding the most evident self-contradiction. Even when the external object of reference or support is destroyed, a new one is quickly found. The delusion needs no other support than the absolute conviction of the deluded.

Vivid emotional states, such as fear, sorrow, anger, joy, and enthusiasm are important factors in the origin of delusions. Even in health, anxiety and enthusiasm create for us, in the consideration of any subject, fears and hopes which really have nothing to do with the subject matter. In morbid conditions, sorrow and fear exert the strongest influence on the falsifications of ideas. *Clouding of consciousness* is sometimes a factor in the development of delusions, especially in delirious states. Delirium tremens and fever delirium, for instance, present a host of fantastic delusions with but very little emotional disturbance. Moreover, delusions which are firmly believed one day may be recognized as false the next, clearly indicating a morbid condition of consciousness, which rendered their correction impossible. We have an example of this in dreams, where we are unable to detect or correct those contradictions which are perfectly clear to us on awakening. Without doubt, therefore, we must regard the clouding of consciousness as an essential preliminary condition for the development of delusions.

In paresis, senile dementia, and dementia praecox, delusions appear in which neither emotions nor disturbances of consciousness play a prominent role. The *psychic weakness,* which is a prominent symptom in these diseases, seems to favor the development of delusions. But congenital mental weakness shows only a slight tendency to the development of delusions, and likewise many cases of senile, paralytic, and precocious dementia run their course without delusions. The real cause for the delusions cannot, therefore, lie in the psychic weakness of itself, but only in the accompanying conditions of excita-

tion, which permit all sorts of delusional fancies to spring up in the patient's mind. It can be easily demonstrated that delusions originate most freely during heightened or depressed moods.

Another source of delusions may perhaps be found in those peculiar ideas which in health are accustomed to occasionally "pop" into our heads, and whose origin we are unable to account for. While they have no power over us, for the patient, on the other hand, they bear the stamp of absolute certainty, even though soon changed for others. They often intrench themselves firmly in his thoughts and dominate experience, feeling, and conduct.

After this preliminary consideration of all the facts relative to the origin of delusions, we are led to the assumption that *the essential factor is an inadequate functioning of judgment and reason.* In health we are accustomed to judge all our fancies according to the standard of our own past experience, and to regard as invention that which does not conform to our knowledge. The patient either does not perceive the contradictions between his fancies and his former experience, or he disregards it and hides it under assumptions which are even more fanciful. Clearly the patient has lost, not only the impulse, but the power, to oppose, correct, or suppress his delusions. The cause of this disability was formerly sought in the peculiar attributes of the individual ideas. The doctrine of "monomania," which held that the "fixed idea" was only a circumscribed disturbance of an otherwise healthy psychic life, was based upon this assumption.

The development of delusions is thus seen to be based on the general disturbance of the entire psychic life. They are probably incited by emotional fluctuations which transform slumbering hopes and fears into imaginary ideas. *But the fact that these ideas become delusions and acquire a power which even the senses cannot destroy, can only be explained by an inadequate functioning of judgment, dependent on impassioned emotional excitement, clouding of consciousness, and weakness of the*

reasoning power.

The character and duration of delusions differ according to their mode of origin. Those which originate in *emotional disturbances* change with the patient's mood, and usually disappear with the emotional disturbanceDelusions of delirium, which are determined both by *clouding of consciousness and emotional disturbances,* are variegated fantastic pictures recurring in manifold forms, with little or no mental elaboration or coherence. They likewise disappear with the clearing of consciousness and the subsidence of the emotional disturbance. Delusions depending both upon *mental deterioration and upon emotional disturbances* do not vanish with the fading of the emotional states. They are gradually forgotten, but are never corrected by reason. Such delusions occur in paresis, dementia praecox, and senile dementia. In these psychoses the forgotten delusions may reappear for short periods during emotional exacerbations. With continued moderate emotional excitement delusions may be firmly held and even elaborated, as in the paranoid forms of dementia praecox.

Persistent delusions are of two types, the *systematized* and the *unsystematized.* If systematized, the individual delusions form a part of a system; *i.e.* they all center about some one or more definite objects, and whenever new delusions develop they are absorbed into this system. Such delusions are usually expressed in a logical manner. The unsystematized delusions may ultimately disappear, as in dementia praecox, end stages of chronic alcoholism, paresis, and senile psychoses, or they may become permanent through frequent repetitions, without systematization, as in the paranoid form of dementia praecox. The progressive and uniform systematization of the delusions without marked mental deterioration constitutes *paranoia* in the strict sense of the word. In this form the delusions become the basis of a thoroughly elaborated, but falsified, apprehension of self and the environment; but even here a decided weakness of judgment is probably always demonstrable. The somewhat similar system of coherent delusions, sometimes found in paresis and dementia praecox, are always of shorter duration.

Practically all delusions center in the *self,* either as *self-depreciation* (depressive delusions) or as *self-aggrandize?nent* (expansive delusions). Among depressive delusions, those of *self-accusation* stand closest to the normal life. Many normal persons torment themselves with the belief that they are unlucky. In states of morbid depression the idea of guilt may be associated with the patient's every action. He believes that he is constantly injuring and deceiving others; his past appears to him as a series of abominable deeds and terrible crimes. He is an irredeemable, unfeeling creature, repudiated by God and damned, and is consequently about to suffer a fitting punishment, arrest, the scaffold, the stake, or whatever else his ingenuity can invent.

Related to these delusions are the general *fears of poverty, loss of work,* or *some other misfortune about to befall themselves or relatives.* In progressing mental weakness this form of delusions may become *nihilistic,* when everything, the patient included, is non-existent or less than nothing. A large group of depressive delusions are those of *persecution.* They originate during periods of indisposition, discomfort, or anxiety. Mistrust and suspicion are excited by peculiar coincidences and misinterpreted remarks. Newspaper articles and popular songs contain references and even indirect insults. All assertions of love and friendship are disbelieved. At this time, also, there usually appear hallucinations, especially auditory. The patient sees himself involved in a network of secret hostilities and imminent dangers which he cannot escape. All are joined against him and gloat over his misery. Men call after him, whisper to each other, shun him, spit in front of him, etc. Food and drink have a peculiar taste, as if poisoned, etc.

Delusions of *jealousy* also play a prominent r6le. The patient notices a coolness in marital relations, detects fond glances and secret signs, finds in letters arrangements for secret meetings. The wife is embarrassed by his unexpected return home, tries to conceal something, coughs in a significant manner, the room is darkened. Outside some one pounds on the door, a form scurries by the window, the last child does not resemble its father, etc. Indeed, these delusions as cited by the patient are sometimes presented with such good foundation that it is difficult to distinguish them from ideas of infidelity that are actually justified. Delusions of infidelity occur principally in chronic alcoholism and cocainism, but also in senile mental disorder.

In advanced mental weakness the persecutory ideas often assume a very *fantastic form.* Absurd somatic delusions of transformation and witchery, such as telepathy, magical, electrical, or hypnotic influences, are common forms. Sexual delusions are especially common, varying from mysterious sexual excitation to imagined childbirth during stupor. All these evils may be attributed to any individual or group of individuals from the neighbor or husband, to fraternal or political societies.

In *hypochondriacal delusions* the object is some alleged incurable disease. Harmless physical symptoms are regarded as signs of syphilis, sexual excess, paresis, etc. With the onset of deterioration the delusions become absurd and fantastic.

Expansive ideas may also be referred to a somatic basis. Thus, feeble paretics extol their beautiful voice, their gymnastic dexterity, although they cannot produce a single musical tone or even stand on their feet. Closely connected with the hypochondriacal ideas are such expansive ideas as that the excretions are gold, Rhine wine, etc. Sometimes delusions with a depressive content acquire the significance of expansive ideas. Patients state that they will die at once in order to be translated to heaven; they send invitations to their own execution, which is to be conducted with great pomp.

The delusion of *mental soundness,* in spite of deep-seated mental disease, constitutes an *absence of insight* into the disease. This absence of insight is almost universal in morbid states; many patients not only consider themselves perfectly sane, but remarkably intelligent, as in paresis and paranoia. The external relations of the patients, the social position and property, are similarly transformed by expansive delusions. Noble descent, close relation to the temporal and spiritual authorities, even association with supernatural powers, are among the most frequent forms. With further development the patient becomes the President, the Pope, Christ, or God. On the other hand, patients boast of their untold wealth and vast estates, including whole continents or the world itself, while vague plans of gigantic undertakings fill their minds.

Depressive and expansive delusions are by no means mutually exclusive. They may co-exist or follow one another very closely. The victim of persecutory delusions discovers an adequate cause of this persecution in exceptional ability, natural right to great possession or high positions. His detention is the result of jealousy or intrigues. These relations are not the result of logical elaboration, but rather spontaneous and independent consequences of the internal condition of the patient. In dementia pracox the appearance of expansive ideas following delusions of persecution indicates a decided progress of mental weakness.

Disturbances of the Rapidity of Thought. — The normal rapidity of the association of ideas and concepts varies so greatly in different individuals, and sometimes even in the same individual, that it has been impossible to establish a standard by which morbid deviations can be accurately estimated. We are, however, able to recognize two disturbances; namely, retardation and acceleration of the train of thought.

Retardation occurs even in healthy individuals as the result of physical and mental fatigue. Some unpleasant emotional states produce the same result. It also occurs during the intoxication produced by alcohol, ether, chloroform, chloral, and to a moderate degree after the use of tobacco. This disturbance is characteristic of the depressive and mixed forms of manic-depressive insanity, is found in the end stages of dementia praecox and paresis, and in congenital imbecility. Moderate retardation appears also in melancholia. *Acceleration* is less frequent than retardation. In normal life it is produced only by some forms of emotional excitement, and by such drugs as morphine, caffeine, and ethereal oil of tea. In morbid states genuine acceleration is probably never found. In flight of ideas the thought may appear accelerated, but even here real delay can usually be demonstrated.

Disturbances of Capacity for Mental Work. — The capacity for mental work is independent of the rapidity of thought. It is scarcely to be measured by direct experimentation, although it forms a most important symptom of mental disease. In normal life the capacity for mental work is determined by the residua of past efforts. These residua condition the increase of capacity, which we call *practice*. In morbid states the effects of practice are usually lessened and rapidly disappear, particularly in congenital imbecility.

The capacity for mental work stands in inverse ratio to susceptibility to fatigue. *Increased susceptibility to fatigue* is very general in most forms of insanity. We find it in exhaustion psychoses, dementia precox, congenital imbecility, and paresis, where it is often the first striking symptom of the disease. In neurasthenia it is often masked by increased nervous irritability.

Recovery from fatigue is effected by relaxation and especially by sleep. Melancholiacs and neurastheniacs recover very slowly from the effects of mental, emotional, and physical activity. This is the result, in part of diseased mental tone, in part also it results from disturbances of sleep, not only in amount but depth. It has been shown that in conditions of simple overwork the sleep is light, attains its greatest depth very slowly, and shows an incomplete abatement of its profoundness in the morning.

Finally the capacity for work is markedly decreased by *distractibUity*. It can arise from insufficient intensity of the goal ideas, from unusual vividness of individual presentations, or finally from an increased susceptibility to distracting influences. Inadequacy of the goal ideas is probably the cause of distractibUity in paresis and dementia praecox. The vividness of individual presentations is seen in the distractibility of acute exhaustion psychoses, and especially in manic-depressive insanity, and probably also in excited periods of dementia praecox and paresis. The increased susceptibility to distracting influences is a regular symptom of neurasthenia, where quite insignificant forms of irritation may become altogether intolerable.

Disturbances of Self-consciousness. — The sum total of all those presentations which form the complex idea of our physical and mental personality constitutes selfconsciousness. This is the permanent background of our mental life, and exercises a characteristic influence on the course of all our mental processes. In content as well as scope, self-consciousness is determined by the experiences of each individual. It is a familiar phenomenon in dreams that one may carry on a complete dialogue; indeed, one may be completely taken back by some particularly striking expression of his interlocutor. Apparently in such cases the unity of self-consciousness is lost, which in the waking state permits us to oversee all our thoughts and inner impulses at once. Such a *dual personality* or *splitting* of self-consciousness often occurs in mental disease. Possibly the first indications of this are found in those cases in which sense deceptions appear to the patients as strange phenomena of external origin. Whenever a patient suffering from delirium tremens overhears some derisive dialogue about himself, or plans of a threatening nature being devised against him, there is no doubt in his mind that these are of external origin and not the hallucinatory expressions of his own thoughts and fears. Unbeknown to himself he plays the r6le of two different persons. Splitting of self-consciousness is often observed in dementia praecox, where the patients refer to foreign influences and enemies residing within their bodies, the thoughts and actions of which they differentiate very clearly from their own. Some hysterical symptoms may be similarly explained.

The temporal connections of one's personality with the past may be disordered in such a way that the memory of certain periods of life of longer or shorter duration are completely lost. If during any such period of life there has been no development, self-consciousness remains on the same plane that it was at the beginning of the period; in this case the interval is bridged over by means of falsifications of memory or inferences. The patient depends upon inferences in the interruptions in self-consciousness occurring in clouding of consciousness, sleep, fainting, befogged states, and delirious conditions, and on fabrications in Korssakow's psychosis where loss of memory is produced by disorder of the attention. The so-called condition of *"double consciousness"* represents another form of disturbed self-consciousness where there is a more or less regular alternation of different states in each of which there is memory only for the experiences of similar previous states. Thus two different personalities are dovetailed, each of which has at its disposal only a part of the total experience of the individual. As a rule, one of these personalities belongs to an earlier stage of development than the other, and consequently does not possess all the skill and knowledge that the other commands. Sometimes there takes place a reversion to a particular period of the individual's past life, which has been conspicuous because of certain experiences. This condition, called *ekmnesia* by the French, may be induced experimentally by hypnosis, and is characteristic more especially of hysterical insanity.

Self-consciousness is no fixed mental construct, but it changes continuously with experience. So disease processes are able to falsify it, though not in like manner. The cause of this is not clear. The alteration of self-consciousness in the depressive stages of manic-depressive insanity is often very striking, while in melancholia it may be insignificant in spite of the extensive delusional conception of the environment. Also in delirium tremens the patients have the most fantastic experiences without suffering any alteration of self-consciousness. Since the most extensive alterations of self-consciousness occur in paresis, dementia praecox, and in manic-depressive insanity, the hypothesis is plausible that this disease symptom is related to disturbances of will. On the other hand, we are accustomed to ascribe disturbances of the will in large measure to the character of the psychic personality.

The particular form of the falsification of self-consciousness is determined by the morbid disposition. Thus in manic patients the peculiar condition of self-consciousness leads to the development of expansive ideas, which in reality are nothing more than a playful expression of the emotional elation. In the depressive and stuporous phases of manicdepressive insanity the patients become not only depressed and abject, but they even feel physically altered — turned to stone, dead, and transformed into other individuals, such as the devil and animals. Similarly the paretic in accord with his expansive and pessimistic ideas comes to believe that his body is variously altered. In dementia praecox this condition, although present, is less pronounced, and in contrast to paresis and manic depressive insanity is not infrequently associated with ideas of some sort of external influence which produces the alteration. In paranoia, the disturbance of self-consciousness is very slight and confined to the delusional overestimation of the patient's abilities.

In advanced deterioration, self-consciousness ultimately disappears. In dementia praecox and paresis this is the usual terminus of the mental life. It is to be especially emphasized, however, that this is not the result of deterioration, but a special symptom of these diseases. In some cases, on the other hand, even when the store of ideas is much impoverished, the patient still retains his self-consciousness and can give an account of his own condition. This is particularly common in epileptics. Even in presbyophrenia, where, on account of the marked disturbance of attention, experiences disappear entirely from memory and are replaced by the freest invention, self-consciousness is retained.

C. DISTURBANCES OF THE EMOTIONS

Every sensory impression which sustains any intimate relation to man's welfare is accentuated in consciousness by a concurrent feeling of pleasure or pain, depending on its apparent tendency to advance or retard the general aims of life. Therefore, the feelings are a direct indication of the attitude of the ego to the perceptions of the external world. According to Wundt, one can distinguish three opposite states of feeling, which rarely exist alone, but almost always accompany mental processes in various combinations; namely, pleasure and displeasure, excitement and calmness, perhaps preferably retardation, and finally tension and relaxation. Disturbances of the emotional life often form the first striking symptom of disease. But the recognition and estimation of these disturbances is difficult, because we lack an adequate normal standard. Even in health the emotions show marked personal peculiarities, closely allied to the abnormal.

Diminution and Increase of Emotional Irritability. — The *diminution of the intensity of the emotions* is their simplest and most frequent disturbance. In normal life one's interest in the environment is reflected in more or less intense fluctuations of his emotions. Diminution of these emotional accentuations indicate indifference toward the impressions of the external world. This is characteristic of most forms of mental deterioration, of which it is one of the first and most striking symptoms. Emotional indifference may be marked even when external impressions are well apprehended and elaborated. This striking disproportion between disturbances of the intellect and the emotions is most pronounced in dementia praecox. In paresis, on the other hand, mental elaboration is disturbed to a much greater degree than the emotions.

All phases of the emotional life seldom suffer equally. Naturally the patient loses most easily those feelings which are not directly connected with the changes of his own ego, but are related to the more remote, external world, and further those feelings which have lost their sensory properties and are aroused only through the higher mental processes as concomitants of general ideas and moral principles. The active interest of the patient becomes exclusively selfish. He loses all pleasure in mental work, and all feeling for the higher claims of propriety, morality, and religion. Consideration for his environment, his family, relatives, and finally for mankind in general, has no influence on his conduct. He loses the sense of shame and lacks all comprehension of the conventions of social intercourse. *Emotional deterioration* is very often the first striking symptom of dementia praecox, and advances with the progress of the disease. It regularly occurs in senile dementia, and sometimes is an early symptom of paresis. In its simplest form it appears, also, in simple senility. Emotional deterioration is also prominent in many forms of congenital imbecility, especially the so-called "moral imbecility," in which the patients show a certain shrewdness in the attainment of selfish advantages which often conceals the real severity of the disease.

Lower or sensuous feelings possess a greater momentary intensity, but are at the same time more transitory than the higher moral aesthetic sentiments, which accompany and determine our thoughts and actions throughout our entire life, and act as checks on sudden emotional impulses of the lower order.

The absence of these checks in imbecility gives rise to sudden, but transitory, outbursts of passion. Without a firm foundation for the emotional life a mere trifle, a word, the tone of the voice, suffices to plunge the patient from the most blissful self-complacency into the most profound despair. This is an especially prominent symptom in paresis. The emotional indifference characteristic of the end stages of dementia praecox is regularly accompanied by such emotional ebullitions. A permanent characteristic of emotional indifference is lack of insight. The retardation of depressed manic-depressive patients sometimes presents a superficial similarity to the emotional indifference of the deteriorated, but the former realize their condition, and often complain that they are forsaken and desolate. An especial *vivacity* of the emotions is characteristic of women and children. The emotional states are highly unstable and are readily influenced by momentary conditions. The great ease with which vivid feelings appear and disappear is characteristic of some of the psychopathic states. This condition underlies the syndrome of hysteria. In this disease ideas have such an intense emotional tone that a powerful influence is exerted not only over the will but also over such physical processes as are, in general, not under voluntary control; as, breathing, circulation, pulse, muscles of the bladder, rectum, and hair, secretions of the glands, as well as the accuracy of movements and the clearness and intensity of sensations.

A temporary increase of the emotional irritability is seen in some of the excited stages of paresis, catatonia, and in manic phases of manic-depressive insanity. Since the vividness of the temporary emotional state forces the restraining influence of the higher feeling completely into the background, this condition is accompanied by the important phenomenon — *change of mood.* A similar condition is observed in the intoxicated individual, in whom the exuberance of feeling is so often accompanied by abrupt change of mood. In this condition it is possible for one to influence markedly the tone of feeling of the patient except in catatonic excitement, where negativism prevails.

Morbid Temperaments. — The same experience may arouse wholly different mental attitudes in different individuals, according to the constitutional tendency to certain tones of feeling, the temperament of the individual. Because of the infinite variety of the combinations of feelings it is almost impossible to describe all the different types of temperament. In the morbid field this difficulty

is even greater; hence we must content ourselves with a brief sketch of only some of the forms.

Since displeasure exerts in general a stronger influence over our mental life than pleasure, we would expect to find it playing the more prominent r6le in morbid states. This *increased susceptibility to the unpleasant* leads to a tendency to discover in all of life's experiences only that which is unpleasant. The past is crowded with sad experiences and the future a source of anxiety. The individual's own wellbeing is the centre of his thought, and every insignificant ailment is regarded as a sign of threatening disease. The dejection which in normal life accompanies sad experiences gradually wanes, but in disease even a cheerful environment fails to mitigate sadness, indeed, it may even intensify it.

Whenever morbid sadness is accompanied by an inner tension, the emotional state becomes one of *apprehensiveness.* The patient feels a lack of security and freedom, together with a lack of confidence in his own ability. He awaits with apprehension the outcome of every act, and doubts its justification and fitness. In this state his own physical condition is a very fruitful source for the development of all sorts of doubts. There develops a self-torture and an exaggerated feeling of liability. This type of feeling furnishes the basis for the morbid fears to be described later, and also is often seen in the incipient stages of melancholia.

When this increased susceptibility to the unpleasant is associated with excitement, there exists what is known as *an irritable disposition.* This is characterized not only by a general tone of displeasure toward everything, but by an emotional excitement which demands expression and is held in check only by a constant struggle. This lack of control means a persistent variation of the emotional equilibrium and a condition of instability with occasional violent outbursts of feeling, which sometimes take the form of despair and sometimes of anger. Despair is encountered chiefly in congenital neurasthenia, while anger is found especially in the epileptic and

hysterical constitutions (Irabundia Morbosa).

Morbid sensitiveness to the outer world does not always lead to passionate outbreaks, but sometimes produces that type of temperament termed *sedusiveness.* Seclusiveness is not accompanied by that passionate feeling of anger that goes with the defiance of a normal individual, but it indicates a sort of shrinking from the impressions of life with a more or less clear consciousness of one's own insufficiency. Conversation with strangers, entering a new environment, unusual demands, and difficulties appear to a patient as unsurmountable obstacles. This condition underlies the conduct of many of the merely " peculiar " individuals. A history of such peculiarities often antedates the outset of dementia praecox.

The pronounced feelings of pleasure are found in those happy *sunny dispositions* that are always in good humor, see things on the best side, and are most enthusiastic. Associated with this state there is often a pressure of activity, which incites the individual to various changing unsuccessful pursuits; a combination which also exists in manic-depressive insanity.

Another modification of the emotional life is *fanaticism.* Here also there develops prominently types of feeling, especially of a religious and sexual nature, which control thought and action. These individuals may exhibit the most extraordinary feeling of happiness that rises above all external sadness and adversity. The hysterical constitution arises from this sort of a basis. Closely related to these fanatics are the *morbid swindlers* with their great love for adventure, and for the exciting and the unusual. The exaggerated joy in their own inventiveness forces all deliberation into the background. Hysterical symptoms also exist here.

A closely allied disposition is *morbid frivolity,* characterized by superficiality of the emotions. Here there is an increased susceptibility to superficial distractions while serious things are not taken seriously. Life in general is regarded as a joke. Associated with this morbid frivolity, which is an essential element in some forms of imbecility and weakmindedness, there is regularly a defective development of the higher feelings, a selfishness and instability of the will.

A common characteristic of this condition of frivolity is an exaggerated self-consciousness. The patients' own abilities and work appear to them in an especially favorable light. These patients not only grossly overestimate themselves, but have a corresponding lack of sympathy for others. This selfish onesidedness of the tone of feeling exists in many born criminals, also in the pseudo-querulants, where it is combined with great irritability. It is probably also a favorable soil for the development of genuine querulants and perhaps the allied forms of paranoia.

Morbid Emotions. — Morbid emotions are distinguished from healthy emotions chiefly through the lack of a sufficient cause, as well as by their intensity and persistence; furthermore the tone of feeling usually corresponds to some of the well-known mixed feelings. Even in normal life moods come and go in an unaccountable way, but we are always able to control and dispel them, while morbid moods defy all attempts at control. Again, morbid emotions sometimes attach themselves to some certain external occasions, but they do not vanish with the cause like normal feelings, and they acquire a certain independence.

By far the commonest form of the unpleasant morbid emotions is *fear,* which may perhaps be regarded as a combination of a feeling of displeasure with an inner tension. It influences the whole physical and mental condition more profoundly than any of the other emotions. The inner tension is exhibited physically by the facial expression, bodily attitude, convulsive action of the muscles, in a moan or an outcry, in an act of defence or escape, in attacks on the surroundings or the patient's own life. Besides this there is apt to be precordial oppression, palpitation, pallor, increased respiration, tremor, and sometimes perspiration and an increased de-

sire to urinate and defecate. In morbid conditions fear is usually without an object at first. The patients feel afraid without knowing why, and indeed are often well aware that their fears are groundless. In the constitutional psychopathic states the indefinite fear often assumes peculiar forms, as the feeling of homesickness and the like. In acute mental disturbances the indefinite anxious forebodings become fixed into more or less definite fears. Extreme fear, like all extreme emotions, is always accompanied by a clouding of consciousness.

Fear is not maintained at the same intensity for any considerable length of time, but shows remissions, and aggravations, the latter especially at night. Fear is most pathognomonic of melancholia of involution, where it is seldom absent. It occurs frequently in depressive forms of manic-depressive insanity, but may be absent. It occurs also in the befogged states of epilepsy, in delirium tremens, and in the beginning of catatonic excitement. Paresis sometimes presents fear in its most extreme form.

A large group of disturbances characterized by fear is found in the so-called *compulsive fears, phobias.* These fears are sometimes associated with some personal experience or idea which has given rise at some time to fear. In the lightest forms such fears are encountered in normal individuals, but here they lack the persistency and obtrusiveness which characterize the phobias.

The compulsive fears are characteristic of some forms of the psychopathic states, but may appear transitorily in manic-depressive insanity. These compulsive fears include the fear at the sight of or contact with certain objects, as spiders, knives, needles, etc.; also the fear of being alone on deserted streets, the fear of crowded rooms, of open or closed doors, etc. (see pp. 499-503). These patients are tormented by the idea that their clothes do not fit properly, that they themselves are soiled or poisoned by contact with others, that they might have swallowed needles or fragments of glass, that in tearing up any scrap of pa-

per they might have destroyed valuable papers, etc. Other closely allied disturbances are the feelings of discomfort which arise whenever individuals are compelled to come into any sort of relations with others, as in erythrophobia, morbid blushing.

While fear has been designated as sadness with inner tension, simple *dejection* is defined as sadness with inhibition; in other words, anguish with a feeling of insufficiency. The basis for this emotional state is found in the sorrow arising in the person himself, which impresses itself upon all of the experiences of life. As the result of this, the entire past seems but a series of misfortunes and failures; the present is troubled and dark, and the future dubious; all sorts of sad thoughts and forebodings arise, which may lead to delusional ideas of self-reproach and persecution, but the most painful is the feeling of desolation. Patients feel neither pleasure nor sorrow; indeed, they do not respond emotionally to any of the impressions of the outer world. One patient expressed himself by saying that he felt " like a cinematograph. To be sure I see things well enough, but I don't feel them." The normal pleasure in mere existence gives place to a feeling of weariness of life.

The alteration of the tone of feeling which is characteristic of some of the circular depressive phases of manic-depressive insanity as a rule is accompanied by a retardation of thought and action. The patients regard their condition as the most agonizing; they feel as if they were inwardly dead, had become heartless and morally desolate. They frequently entertain ideas of physical alteration. In reality these patients are not without feeling, as may be judged from their occasional attempts at suicide. The retardation may suddenly give place to excitement.

Sadness with excitement is occasionally observed in manicdepressive insanity, occurring either as an independent phase or as a transitional stage between different phases of the disease. In this case the mood is sometimes sad, sometimes anxious or passionate, the patients expressing themselves in wailing and moaning, in states of anxiety, or in outbreaks of irritability. The latter form is particularly common. The patients are fretful, discontented, at variance with themselves and their environment, and annoyed by trifles. They grumble and growl in the most intolerable manner and show outbursts of passion on the slightest provocation. An emotional state of this sort combined with exaggerated conceit and an attempt to be sarcastic is sometimes encountered in syphilitic insanity. Many of the emotional states of the hysterical patient exhibit a mixture of sadness and excitement with passionate irritability.

The epileptic presents a special type of emotional disturbance; namely, *a simple dejection with a feeling of weariness of life*. Occasionally it is associated with a feeling of inhibition, but usually there is a sort of homesick feeling with an indefinite yearning and inner restlessness, which leads to suicidal attempts, indulgence in alcohol, or aimless wandering. Yet irritability with sudden violent outbursts of great intensity is quite common. In the epileptic befogged states a tense anxious feeling predominates, sometimes combined with great irritability. Furthermore in all of these emotional states there may be a mixture of a sexual or ecstatic feeling of pleasure.

The *morbid feelings of pleasure* are less frequent than those of displeasure. They occur especially in alcoholic intoxications and alcoholic psychoses, manic-depressive insanity, paresis, dementia praecox, morphin and cocain intoxication. The feeling of increased strength, enthusiasm, and enterprise which results from alcohol probably originates in the facilitation of the release of motor impulses in the brain, while further action of the drug causes irritability, restlessness, and aimless activity. In the manic forms of manicdepressive insanity in which there is a similar combination of pleasurable feelings, irritability, and pressure of activity, the emotional disturbance is believed to have a similar origin. This belief is substantiated by physiological experimentation. In both conditions there is no insight into the disorder. The emotional attitude in both bears the stamp of a *wanton happiness,* and self-confidence is greatly increased.

The high spirits so characteristic of the chronic alcoholic represent another type of morbid feeling of pleasure, and are designated *drunkard's humor.* The same state may exist in delirium tremens where, however, it is mingled with a sort of concealed fear. Its origin is unknown, but may however, arise from the drunkard's insusceptibility to humiliation and his moral apathy to vice. In paresis the pleasurable feelings are apt to be marked, especially the *feeling of well-being.* In this disease, however, these feelings often exist unaccompanied by motor excitement, and in spite of the expansive ideas, there is absent the lack of restraint and fresh energy that is so characteristic of the manic exhilaration. In the later stages of paresis the feeling of well-being subsides to a silly thoughtless happiness without a trace of the irritability which is found in the later stages of the alcoholic. In dementia praecox, during the excited stages, pleasurable feelings take on the form of a silly, purposeless hilarity and exuberance with outbursts of silly laughter, which, in contrast to the hilarity of the manic forms of manic-depressive insanity, seem to bear no relation to the patient's ideas and environment.

Cocain, morphin, tobacco, and the bromides also produce characteristic feelings of well-being. In tobacco smoking the feeling of agreeable contemplation is due purely to a soporific effect; the bromides produce a feeling of wellbeing by relieving a state of inner tension. The feeling of *ecstasy,* which occurs especially in epilepsy, and sometimes in hysteria, seems to be very similar to the dreamy state which follows opium smoking. The origin of morbid feelings of pleasure is very difficult to determine, both because they may arise from a great many different disturbances, sometimes somatic and vasomotor, sometimes primarily emotional, and sometimes intellectual. Different types of feeling may exist at the same time or may succeed each other rapidly, as seen in the mixture of fear and humor in the alcoholic and of ecstasy and anger in the dreamy states of the epileptic.

Disturbances of General Feelings. — General feelings are those emotional states which stand in close and inviolable relation to self-preservation, such as feelings of fatigue and hunger. They are to be regarded as admonitions, which gradually develop out of the experience of countless generations into involuntary and instinctive impulses. In ordinary life these feelings inform us of our bodily needs, and they imperiously exact actions adapted to the circumstances. The performances of these actions can usually be inhibited by conscious volition, although often only by means of great self-denial; the feelings themselves are, on the contrary, only thoroughly silenced when the indicated need is relieved in some way or other. In normal life a general feeling may disappear when we pay no heed to it. We are able to overcome weariness when work demands our strength; hunger abates when we are unable for a long time to satisfy it. When at last we have the opportunity to attend to our needs for rest and food, we miss at first the painful weariness and hunger which makes the restoration of our strength so easy. Only when we have rested for some time do we again experience a feeling of weariness, while hunger gradually returns as soon as we begin to eat.

In normal life the performance of mental and physical work is accompanied by a feeling of pleasure. The basis for this experience lies in the fact that the formation and maintenance of personality depends upon activity. If this feeling of pleasure is absent, one regularly develops a form of *ennui.* This is the form of ennui that develops from idleness and soon forces one to some sort of endeavor. To a normal man enforced idleness is most irritating. Among the insane this form of ennui is usually absent because the patients, even although unemployed, are completely absorbed in their own morbid mental processes. The appearance of this ennui in a patient may, therefore, be regarded as a favorable sign; yet one must be cautious not to confuse it either with the feeling of discontent that is often referred to by the dejected patients as ennui, or with the pressure of activity of the manic patients. The complete absence of ennui in dementia praecox is a very important symptom. Here there is a complete loss of volitional impulse from which the desire for activity takes its origin. The patients can in spite of clear consciousness lie abed weeks and months without in any way becoming uneasy at the lack of activity. Their lack of ennui always indicates a profound disorder of the mental life, and especially accompanies progressive deterioration.

A wholly different significance attaches to that unpleasant feeling often designated as weariness which accompanies excessive exercise as a sign of warning. This form of weariness generally indicates in a normal individual an actual need for rest; in other words, *fatigue.* Patients sometimes fail to show their fatigue, although there is real need for rest. In many excited states, especially in manic forms of manic-depressive insanity, there is often a complete absence of fatigue in spite of the fact that the patients are exhausted by continual restlessness.

The feeling of *hunger* is similarly disturbed in these same psychoses. In paretic and catatonic patients there is often a senseless voracity, although the well-nourished patients have no need of such an amount of nourishment. In the constitutional psychopathic states and in hysteria, without any perceptible relation to the state of bodily nutrition, there may be a prolonged absence of the feeling of hunger, which is suddenly replaced by gluttony.

Severe disturbances of the feeling of *nausea* are almost always signs of a far-advanced deterioration. Such patients consume the most disgusting things, even their own dejections. Not infrequently they swallow nails, stones, pieces of glass, or animals, not only with suicidal intent, but constantly overpowering their nausea from pure greediness. These patients also lose those feelings which cause us aversion at the mere contact with filth or dirt and impel one to keep clean, not only the body, but the whole environment. They recklessly soil themselves, even intentionally, with their own food, their own saliva, urine, and even feces.

The feelings of physical *pain* are often abolished. In conditions of excitement, especially with intense fear, even severe injuries produce no sensation at all, although consciousness may be perfectly clear. Such patients pluck out their tongues or eyes, cut open the abdomen, etc., deeds which would be utterly impossible for a man with a normal sense of pain. This insensibility to physical pain is often found in demented patients, especially in paretics, in whom, to be sure, the destruction of the nervous conducting paths is an essential antecedent. The absence of the sensibility to pain encountered in the hysterical and epileptic patients is essentially different; in these conditions the threshold of pain only appears to be raised.

There is finally a group of feelings which pertain to the maintenance of the race rather than to self-preservation; namely, the *sexual feelings.* Among bewildered and excited patients the *feeling of shame* may pass wholly into the background; yet one sometimes observes distinct evidences of the feeling of shame in the great excitement of manicdepressive cases when it is not overpowered by increased sexual feelings. The rapid disappearance of the feeling of shame even without sexual excitement is a striking symptom of dementia praecox. Such patients denude themselves recklessly, speak shamelessly about sexual matters, and masturbate persistently and openly. These patients also tend to employ obscene language (copralalia) and gestures.

Sexual feelings in mental disease are either increased, abolished, or perverted. *Sexual indifference* occurs in many forms of the constitutional psychopathic states, and particularly in hysteria, also in morphinism. An *increase of sexual excitability,* which is more frequent, is found in some idiots, but in a more pronounced degree in dementia praecox, and also in the excited stages of paresis, the manic forms of manic-depressive insanity, and in senile dementia. *Perverted sexual feelings* are those in which sexual feelings occur exclusively in connection with persons of the same sex, associations with certain objects, or accompanied by brutality (see p. 92).

D. DISTURBANCE OF VOLITION AND ACTION

All disturbances of the psychic life find their final expression in volition and action. The idea of a definite aim (some change either in ourselves or our environment) forms the starting-point of a volitional act. This idea is accompanied by feelings which are converted into impulses for the attainment of that aim. The direction of any action is determined, therefore, by an idea, while its performance is. determined by the intensity and the duration of the accompanying feelings.

Morbid disturbances of volition manifest themselves in the most varied ways: the energy of the volitional impulse can be diminished or increased; its release facilitated or impeded; or the direction can be modified by external or internal influences; morbid impulses can forcibly suppress the normal will; or natural impulses can assume morbid forms; finally, the conduct of the insane is naturally influenced by all those disturbances which occur in other spheres of their mental life, although the volitional process itself presents no disturbance.

Diminution of Volitional Impulses. — The complete suspension of volitional activity is termed *paralysis of the wM.* It is produced by extreme fatigue, profound alcoholic intoxication, and in the narcoses of chloroform, chloral, and morphin. It is characterized by an absence of energy. Ordinary impulses find no issue in action, while even the most powerful incentives of personal well-being and moral claims fail to influence the patient. A more or less complete paralysis of the will occurs in the end stages of progressive mental deterioration: senile dementia, dementia praecox, and paresis. This is characterized by a marked diminution of personal initiative, except in gratification of the lower, selfish, and vegetative impulses, such as greed, gluttony, and sexual desire. If left to themselves, the patients are content to sit around, inactive, displaying very little animation and staring vacantly into space. In dementia praecox it can often be shown that the patients have not lost the voluntary control of their actions, but normal incentives fail to influence them. In the end stages of deterioration the only movements are involuntary and reflex. Similarly, defective volition appears in congenital imbecility as the result of defective development.

Increase of Volitional Impulse. — The universal indication of the increase of volitional impulse is *motor excitement.* But we are really justified in speaking of an increase of volitional impulse only when there is a marked disproportion between the intensity of the excitation and the importance of the motives. In alcoholic delirium, for example, we find marked unrest which cannot be explained by the patient's delusions, hallucinations, or emotions, but must be referred to a morbid motor excitation. Patients will not remain in bed, show a pronounced restlessness, and constantly busy themselves as if employed in some occupation. In alcoholic intoxication, increase of volitional impulses begins with simple loquacity, and increases to brawling, screaming, and aimless activity. In chronic cocain intoxication (see p. 210) there develops a peculiar motor excitability which seems to form a transition to the morbid *pressure of activity* which is a characteristic symptom of manic-depressive insanity (see p. 387), and is sometimes found in exhaustion psychoses and paresis.

In the lighter hypomaniacal disturbances this pressure of activity takes the form of general instability and *busyness,* great talkativeness, and a tendency to animated gesticulation. Such patients collect all sorts of useless things, begin countless undertakings which they never finish, and, when unrestrained, travel aimlessly about. In more marked excitement the goal ideas become more and more inconstant, and one can hardly detect any purpose at all in their ever changing, incoherent activity. Patients scream, laugh, sing, dance, disrobe, tear their clothing, smear themselves, wash in their own urine, destroy everything they can reach, and pound incessantly with their hands and feet.

Catatonic excitement furnishes a picture essentially different from that of the manic pressure of activity. In the manic excitement, all impulses lead to more or less purposeful actions, though they might at first appear purposeless and senseless. In catatonia, on the contrary, we have to do with movements which at most have no definite aim. Although the characteristic excitement in catatonics is often more moderate, the movements are entirely purposeless. Such patients make grimaces, contort the body, run about, clap their hands, and utter a succession of senseless noises. These movements are not pure volitional acts, as there is no antecedent idea of their purpose. Patients themselves often assure us that they do not know why they perform such absurd antics.

Impeded Release of the Volitional Impulse. — The strength and rapidity with which a volitional impulse is converted into action is dependent, not only on its own intensity, but also on the resistance which it has to overcome. Thus, fright and fear may present obstacles to the realization of our intention, which can be overcome only by the most strenuous exertion of the will.

The *psychomotor retardation,* which is the most important disturbance in the depressed states of manic-depressive insanity, is probably due to a similar increase of resistance. Such patients require special exertion of the will for almost every movement. All the actions are characteristically slow and weak, except when a powerful emotional shock breaks through the resistance. The retardation may become less pronounced under the influence of continued effort. In severe cases independent volitional action is almost impossible. In spite of every apparent exertion, the patients cannot utter a word or at best answer only in monosyllables, and are unable to eat, stand up, or dress. As a rule they clearly recognize the enormous pressure lying upon them, which they are unable to overcome. The name "*stupor*" is usually applied to these disturbances, but they are only superficially related to the stupor of catatonia.

In *catatonic stupor* the release of movements in itself is not rendered difficult, as action is occasionally both rapid and powerful. But every impulse is almost immediately followed by the release of an opposing impulse which prevents the consummation of the act. Thus, we often see the desired movement begin all right, but it is immediately interrupted and extinguished by the opposing impulse. Here the impulse is not hindered by internal resistance, but is simply quenched by a counter impulse. In contrast to the retardation, in which there is a continuous hindrance, one might refer to this as a *blocking.* As soon as the blockade is raised, the counter order disappears, and the action proceeds without the slightest difficulty.

As a result of this *blocking of the will* many reactions which normally occur without special act of volition are suppressed at their inception. The patients will not look up when accosted, or shake hands when the hand is proffered. If one threatens them with a knife, or pricks the eyelid, they may perchance shrink away, but they never make any welldirected effort to protect themselves; they continue to he in the most uncomfortable positions, and will sit for hours in the sun, when by taking a couple of steps they could reach the shade. Possibly the persistent holding open of the eyelids, the regular swallowing of saliva, and the retention of urine and feces may be explained in this way. The whole attitude of the patient becomes strained and unnatural.

In blocking of the will there is no lack of impulses, but rather a balance of counter impulses. Hence we do not find the lassitude characteristic of retardation but a *rigid tension*, which discloses the play of opposing influences. Movements take place with an excess of tension which extends almost equally over all associated groups of muscles: the resulting action depends on relatively slight preponderance of one group of muscles over the opposite group. Hence both station and movement appear tense and stiff. Occasionally the relative strength of impulse and counterimpulse varies, sometimes one and sometimes the other gaining the upper hand. A movement suddenly stops and then just as suddenly begins again. It proceeds by jerks and is awkward and clumsy. Possibly it is the consciousness of all this opposition that leads to the innervation of more remote muscle groups. The entire limb is apt to come into play for the simplest movements, which thereby become ponderous and indefinite.

Facilitated Release of Volitional Impulses. — Both the impressions of the outer world and our inner experience develop in us continually more or less tension of the will, which tends to relieve itself in the most varied expressions. Part of these operations are independent of voluntary control. The greater part of them, however, are subject to inhibition through voluntary effort. The ease with which impulse is converted into action depends upon the development of the inhibitions which we control. Our mental development means in general an increase of inhibitions. The child reacts immediately, while growing self-control enables the man to suppress numberless impulses, before they develop into action. The female sex with its heightened emotional irritability tends to remain on the plain of the child.

The restraining power of the inhibitions naturally depends on the strength of the impulses and the intensity of the emotional state, from which they originate. On the other hand, there are well-recognized influences that facilitate the release of impulses and thereby lessen the resistance to the conversion of an impulse into action. This operates to a greater or less degree in all forms of psychomotor activity. Whenever movements are continued there arises a certain degree of excitement which means a diminution of inhibition. Indeed, it has already been pointed out that morbid inhibition is gradually reduced by activity. Still more evident is the increase of

excitement in manic and catatonic patients when their restlessness is not restrained. An unrestrained discharge of impulses always makes it more difficult for the patients to control themselves.

A most significant diminution of inhibition is produced by alcohol. Ether and cocain have a similar effect both in the acute and chronic intoxications.

The facilitated release of volitional impulse is a constant symptom in some forms of morbid constitution, especially in hysteria. In this disease the intensity of the emotions leaves little room for the reasoned action, hence these patients sometimes suddenly find themselves performing strange and incomprehensible acts, as thieving, cheating, and self-mutilation, apparently at variance with their intention.

Heightened Susceptibility of the Will. — The motives of action have two sources: external stimuli; and those relatively constant principles of action which arise from within rather than from without, and render the individual's conduct more or less independent of his surroundings. The control of actions by these general principles is lacking only in children and unstable individuals. In diseases this control is lost in weakness of the will, increased psychomotor excitability, and in conflict with overwhelming morbid impulses.

Weakness of will is found in all forms of imbecility, where the fixed principles of action are lacking. There is no internal unity or consistency in conduct. The chief characteristic is a hypersuggestibility, through which the patients become the prey to every accidental influence. This condition is found in its purest form in paresis. Similar phenomena are induced through suspension of these fixed principles of action by means of hypnotism.

Transient hypersuggestibility is found in catalepsy, where often the limbs of the patient will remain in any position in which they are placed until, as the result of extreme muscular exhaustion, they tremblingly obey the laws of gravity. In this condition there is often found a moderate, but constant, muscular resistance called cerea flexibilitas, in which

it is possible to mould the limbs into any desired position. Less often patients are found who will repeat for some time any simple movement, once started, or who will laboriously imitate everything done in their presence — echopraxia. In echolalia the patient involuntarily repeats every word he hears, although at the same time giving evidence of considerable elaboration of impressions by his ability to solve simple problems. Indications of these symptoms, especially cerea flexibilitas, are occasionally observed in the most varied diseases, such as hysteria, epilepsy, manic forms of manic-depressive insanity, paresis, and alcoholism; but the whole group of symptoms is most pronounced in dementia praecox, especially the catatonic form.

Distractibility of the will is a morbidly easy translation of ideas into action. It usually accompanies heightened susceptibility of the will, but is differentiated from it by a reaction to internal as well as to external stimuli. It is to conduct what the distractibility of the attention is to intellection, and effectually prevents all permanent volitional control of action. Sudden resolutions are half carried out only to yield to new ones. The patients are wholly under the influence of the environment, whether good or bad. Distractibility of the will is found in certain conditions of manic and delirious excitement. It accompanies hysteria and some forms of imbecility as a permanent personal characteristic.

Interference and Stereotypy. — The carrying out of any simple act is in general determined by the goal idea. Since our movements are usually governed by the principle of economy, we seek to reach the goal with minimum expenditure of strength and time. In case this principle is clearly transgressed, or if the act is clearly inappropriate, we have a disturbance of conduct which is provisionally called interference, in which the correspondence between intention and accomplishment is interfered with by the interpolation of incongruous impulses. Here, apparently, incidental impulses break into the natural flow of conduct. A similar condition obtains in the blocking of the will. One may regard the blocking of the will as a special case in which the incidental impulses are directly opposed to the original impulses; then interference would be regarded as a crossing of the original impulses by the incidental impulses in various directions. The blocking of the will would then be only a special form of the general disturbance which may be described as a *crossing of the voluntary impulses.* Both symptoms belong to catatonia.

The incidental impulses may influence action in many different ways. The simplest form is probably seen in the reiterated repetition of chance impulses. Normally every impulse, as soon as the aim is realized, is forced into the background by other impulses. But where the pursuit of any definite aim is disturbed and there still remains a general pressure of activity, any impulse once released has a good chance to be repeated as long as the active residua of the impulse are not obliterated by new aims. Such an impulse becomes, so to speak, an incidental impulse which breaks through the more or less aimless operations of the will and becomes more insistent with each repetition. This disturbance is called *stereotypy* (Kahlbaum).

Whenever stereotypy is marked (a) by a blocking of the will we find a continuous tension of definite muscle groups; whenever it is marked *(b)* by crossing of voluntary impulses we find a reiterated repetition of the same movement. (a) In *muscular tension* the patients remain in the same place and attitude for an almost incredible length of time in spite of the greatest discomfort. They stand in the same corner, kneel in a definite place, lie in bed with legs curled up and head extended, so rigid that they can be lifted like a log. Others grip a piece of bedspread with their teeth, or convulsively grasp a piece of bread or torn-off button. The expression of the countenance is also rigid, mask-like, the forehead drawn up as if in surprise, the eyebrows elevated and the eyes often wide open. The eyeballs are often turned sidewise and the lips are protruded like a snout.

(6) *Stereotyped movements* have an unlimited variety. The patients turn somersaults, rap rhythmically, walk about in peculiar places, hop, jump up and down, roll and creep on the ground, pick at the clothing or hair, and grit the teeth. These movements can be repeated innumerable times, for weeks or even months. In all these movements the patients are absolutely reckless of themselves and their environment. *Mannerisms* are a kind of stereotyped movement, consisting of ordinary movements peculiarly modified. The patients walk with a peculiar gait, drag one foot, go in straight lines or in circles, hold their spoons at the very end, eat in a definite rhythm, and shake hands with stiffly extended fingers. Mannerisms are especially common in speech. Grunts, lisping, peculiar words, phrases, and inflection, and numerous repetitions of the same words are among the most frequent forms. Stereotypy is a characteristic of the catatonic forms of dementia praecox, but also occurs in exhaustion psychoses and in paresis, where it is only a transient symptom.

In the end stages of catatonia there is occasionally observed a form of stereotypy which is scarcely the same as that just described. It consists of peculiar rhythmical movements, especially rocking the body while sitting and standing, nodding or shaking the head, clapping of the hands, etc. This symptom always indicates a complete deterioration of the will. It is likewise observed in the most profound idiocy. It is a fair hypothesis that these movements are the expression of certain primitive arrangements of our nervous system, which in the absence of the higher processes determine the activities.

In stereotypy voluntary activity never proceeds to a goal. Even when the patients are active their activities move in a circle. On the other hand, there is a type of crossing of impulses in which the incidental impulses produce only a *superfluous embellishment* of the intended act. The act is finally accomplished, but only after all sorts of additions and deviations. The patients skitter along, go backward, walk on their knees, bend away backward, or drag one foot: they extend their hands in wide circles, or with sudden swoops or stiff jerks. In shaking hands they touch one's hand only with the little finger, or with the back of the hand. In eating they grasp the spoon by the tip, arrange the food in little piles, or count seven between each mouthful; the water is drunk in little sips or after long pauses. The bed clothing and their garments are arranged in a peculiar way. The catatonic grimacing may also be regarded as belonging here.

From this embellishment of conduct there are regular transitions to those disturbances which have been termed by Schiiles *derailment of the will,* where acts are completed very differently from the way in which they are begun. For instance, in grasping the spoon to eat the patients may twirl it about in a circle, then lay it down again, or in carrying a glass of water to the mouth upset it on the table, suddenly turn it upside down, and return it to the table.

Also in their speech it is often observed that the patients will suddenly stop and begin anew with another thought, which in turn is just as abruptly left for another, so that the goal idea is finally lost sight of. It is in this way that desultoriness arises (see p. 40). In this crossing of impulses many of the acts stand in no definite relation to any goal idea. The patient suddenly beats his companion, perches himself like a bird on the foot of the bed, grips his finger in the anus, stands on his head, or filths on his dinner plate. Occasionally, aggressive and violent attacks originate in this way.

In this derailment of impulses one gets the impression that the original purpose in the act is forced into the background; for instance, the patient will exert the greatest effort of the will when started in a certain direction when he could easily succeed by making a little detour. He will push persistently against a locked door toward which he has started when he could easily leave the room by an open door close at hand.

Diminished Susceptibility of the Will. — In the description of the blocking of the will it was shown how, under certain circumstances, every impulse of the will can be rendered ineffective by counter impulses. The blocking of the will is but a partial symptom of a very general disturbance; namely, the impulsive resistance to every outer influence of the will, which by Kahlbaum has been designated *negativism*. In negativism there is a blocking of all external impressions, an inaccessibility to social intercourse, and an opposition to every request; and it may even extend to the regular performance of contrary actions (the negativism of command), and finally to the suppression of nature's demands, as in micturition.

In this way conduct in every respect becomes just the opposite of that which is striven for and that which would be expected normally. Patients do just the opposite of that which they are requested to do: press their teeth together when asked to show their tongue, close the eyes when an attempt is made to examine their pupils, and refuse to answer questions — *mutism,* although they sometimes speak spontaneously. They offer the most powerful, but almost always passive, resistance to every external encroachment: will not allow any one to dress or undress them, will not bathe or take care of themselves, and offer strenuous resistance to compulsory feeding, but when unmolested eat greedily. The feces are often retained with the greatest exertion, especially if the patients are taken to the closet. As soon as they are returned to bed, the evacuation immediately takes place. They persist in leaving their own bed and crawling into others, likewise they will smear and spoil their own food, although it may be even better, and steal or fight for that of their companions. The impulsive character of its origin is most clearly demonstrated in the occasional cases of negativism to requests. Such patients continue lying on their back if requested to arise, or they turn around if asked to go forward, and remain silent if told to speak.

Negativism is not due to voluntary opposition. Patients sometimes admit after the attack that they do not know why they acted as they did. Negativism, stereotypy, and loss of will probably all have the same basis. They often occur in the same patient, and may be easily made to pass into one another. These various disturbances of the will are most frequent in catatonia, and are sometimes found in a less pronounced form in paresis, senile dementia, and idiocy.

Catatonic negativism must not be confused with the conscious resistance of terrified patients. In catatonia there is no conscious reason for resistance, and no persuasion can overcome it. It is not influenced by pain, and the manner of resistance is always constrained and often absurdly inappropriate. The *stubbornness* of imbecility, epilepsy, hysteria, paresis, and senile dementia is closely allied to negativism, but in contrast to negativism it always starts with an idea, and is more or less influenced by persuasion, new ideas, and emotional changes. Moreover, in stubbornness the general emotional attitude is fretful, irritable, and unruly. The patient shows fight, and is often dominated by confused, malevolent delusions, whereas the negativistic patient shows great equanimity, seldom defends himself, and almost never attacks, but merely resists.

Compulsive Acts. — *Compulsive acts are those which do not arise from normal antecedent consciousness of motive and desire, but seem to the patient to be forced upon him by a will which is not his own.* As a rule, the patients struggle against the morbid impulses; often caution those about them at their approach, and adopt measures to prevent harm to others. The accomplishment of the act is accompanied by a feeling of relief, and is usually followed by clear insight into the nature of the act, accompanied by chagrin and remorse.

Compulsory acts are generally accompanied by great emotional excitement, and stand in close relation to compulsory ideas and fears already described (see p. 69). These disturbances all originate on a basis of congenital morbid endowment, and are all a part of the symptoms of the constitutional psychopathic states.

Impulsive Acts. — *Impulsive acts are distinguished from compulsive acts, in that they do not seem to the patient to be influenced from without, but are the direct expression of a sudden overwhelming impulse, which gives no chance for reflection or resistance.*

They are found in the most varied morbid conditions. Probably the pressure of activity in manic forms of manicdepressive insanity is of this type. Here belong also the wanderings and assaults of the epileptic (see p. 446), the excesses of the dipsomaniac, as well as the morbid impulses of hysteria, self-inflicted injury, theft, and fraud, Their origin does not lie in definite feelings of pleasure or dislike, but in marked motor excitement. The outbursts of the catatonic are thoroughly representative of impulsive acts, although the basis lies not in a pleasurable or unpleasurable feeling but in a powerful pressure of movement. The patient is controlled by the consciousness that he must do this or that, without a definite reason and without forethought, although he sometimes appreciates the foolishness of his act. Occasionally there is an idea that his limbs are controlled by an invisible power, as God, the devil, or some electrical influence. The patient's consciousness is dominated by one blind impulse without clear motive or realization of the outcome. There is no opportunity to resist the impulse. The execution is rapid and reckless, and the patients are correspondingly dangerous. This is clearly seen in the impulsive acts of the catatonic, such as the shouting, sudden attacks, denuding, the senseless attempts to strangle themselves, to cut out the tongue, and to gouge out the eyes.

Morbid Impulses. — A disturbance of the natural impulses is a symptom of all general morbid changes of volitional action. In paralysis and inhibition of psychic processes all the appetites are diminished; in excitement, on the other hand, appetites are increased, especially sexual desires. The latter seldom lead to actual assault, but manifest themselves in ambiguous phrases, abusive language, and by more or less reckless masturbation: in women, by shameless exposures, extreme uncleanliness, or incessant washing with water, saliva, or urine, combing and unloosing the hair; in lighter forms, by adornment and flirtation, by an alternation between seductive, shamefaced, and sentimental manners, by hand pressing, letter writing, significant glances, and the like. Less frequently in manic excitement there is found an increased desire for food, although restlessness usually hinders the patients from taking sufficient nourishment. On the other hand, excessive greediness is not infrequently found in idiots, paretics, and especially in catatonics. Incredible quantities of the most unpalatable and disgusting things, sand, stones, seaweed, feces, etc. , are sometimes devoured by such patients. In these last cases there is not a simple increase of healthy impulses, but probably a simultaneous perversion of the appetite both in nature and direction. The same is true of the well-known excessive desire for eating suddenly manifested by pregnant women. Much more numerous, however, are the morbid sexual impulses, which in recent years have been most thoroughly investigated. The most pronounced of these are the *contrary sexual instincts,* in which the sexual feelings and desires are exclusively directed toward members of the patients' own sex.

Sadism consists in the attempt to increase or induce sexual excitement by brutality. In the final stage of its development actual sexual congress is a matter of indifference. In *masochism,* on the other hand, the endurance of pain increases sexual excitation or may be substituted for it. The satisfaction of sadism appears to arise from the feeling of absolute power over the victim, while that of masochism arises from the most complete subjection to the will of another. In *fetichism* particular articles of clothing or parts of the body become either the necessary adjuncts for satisfactory coitus, or the simple observation or contact with the fetich may satisfy

the sexual impulse. The most common fetiches are boots, shoes, handkerchiefs, underclothing, and finally velvet and furs.

Besides the perversion of normal impulses as seen in the above, there is a group of morbid impulses which seem to bear no relation to normal life. Such are *kleptomania,* the irresistible impulse to steal all manner of worthless and useless things; *pyromania,* the impulse to burn. Both these usually arise on the basis of an epileptic or hysterical endowment.

The whole series of abnormal impulses are partial symptoms of a general morbid endowment, and indicate congenital degeneracy. It is possible that kleptomania and pyromania should be regarded as compulsive acts. The impulse appears as an obtrusive compulsion which is resisted as long as possible, while the performance of the act is accompanied by a feeling of relief.

Disturbances of Expression. — The movements by which patients express their ideas, feelings, and impulses are among the most important clews to morbid psychic impulses. A full delineation of the symptoms of the various disease types occurs in the clinical portion of this work. In this place we confine ourselves to a few characteristic indications.

Dementia praecox is indicated by lack of interest, notwithstanding accurate apprehension, by listlessness, strained attitudes, senseless grinning or laughter, with sudden impetuous movements. In dementia praecox the change that occurs in the character of movements is very striking, particularly the loss of grace. The catatonic movements are either stiff and wooden on account of the superfluous tension; or careless and listless as a result of an insufficient expenditure of energy; and again they are gross and awkward because associated groups of muscles are involved in the movements. The naturalness of the movements is destroyed by the tendency to ornamentation, which gives them the appearance of being affected, and finally there is a lack of uniformity in the movements of expression.

Paretics may often be recognized by their awkward friendliness and production of silly expansive ideas. Depressed patients sit around collapsed and flaccid, with troubled expression. Their movements are slow and laborious. The apprehensive patients are restless, bite their nails, and wring their hands. In extreme retardation, they lie motionless in bed with fixed expression and whisper their answers with great exertion. The manic-depressive, on the contrary, moves rapidly about, talks, cries, sings, plays tricks on his fellows, and busies himself with all sorts of things. The hysterical patients arrange their clothing and hair to make an impression. The paranoiac endures his hospital confinement with dignity, carrying with him the documents which prove all his pretensions.

Alterations of speech and writing are of the greatest diagnostic value. Delusions are usually betrayed by the content of the communications. In manic patients there is incessant babbling, with a tendency to puns and rhymes. This is also found in excited paretics with more or less disturbance of articulation. In both diseases speech may be reduced to an incomprehensible gibberish, though from different causes.

In retarded patients speech is low and difficult. Melancholiacs express their thoughts laconically, and often keep up a monotonous lamentation. Catatonics are often mute for weeks at a time, and then suddenly begin to speak fluently or sing, although more or less confusion of speech is always present. Their stereotypy is manifested by constant repetition of the same words, phrases, or even senseless syllables, while they frequently make up entirely new words.

Disturbances of writing correspond both in content and form with those of speech. The manic-depressive patient fills sheet after sheet of paper with large, showy, and hastily written characters, which are often illegible even to the writer. The paretic's writing shows omission, misplacement of words and syllables, blots, untidy corrections, and uncertainty. Hysterical patients use innumerable marks for emphasis. In melancholiacs the individual characters are incomplete, small, and crowded. The same is true in retardation. Catatonic patients cover the paper with unintelligible scrawls, endlessly repeated — *written verbigeration.*

In psychoses associated with brain lesions there are apt to be present disturbances of speech and writing such as aphasia, paraphasia, agraphia, paragraphia, perseveration, inability to read and to combine letters into words and syllables, indistinct enunciation, scanning or monotonous speech, also ataxia in writing.

Conduct arising from a Morbid Basis. — Since conduct is the expression of the entire psychic life, we readily understand why it is more or less seriously disturbed by morbid changes in any part of the psychic individual, while, on the other hand, no isolated act can be taken as an infallible index of the exact morbid condition. Delusions of sinfulness impel patients to penance, self-mutilation, or suicide. Delusions of persecution lead to mysterious precautions, to misanthropic isolation, to restless wandering, or even to outbursts of rage and murderous attacks against supposed enemies. Hypochrondriacal delusions may lead to revolting smearing, self-mutilation, or injurious and absurd curative attempts, often with the evident purpose of attracting attention and sympathy.

Mental excitement very soon leads to conflicts with the environment, to breaches of the public order, and quite often to resistance to civic authority. Patients behave in a reckless and striking manner. They are ungovernable, irritable, and violent under contradiction and restraint. At first they act as if intoxicated, and later become still more restless and even dangerous. There is usually also a tendency to sexual excesses, in which they indulge without regard to decency or morality. Such excited states are regularly accompanied by all sorts of mad pranks, destruction of property, adventurous journeys, brawls, and public scandals. When associated with expansive ideas, the patients purchase large amounts of useless stuff, prepare for mythical undertakings, and spend

large sums of money. The idea that everything in their neighborhood belongs to them induces the patients to innocently appropriate whatever they happen on, to embezzlement, or to fraud.

Paranoiacs systematically prepare their claims, address letters to prominent officials, and publish pamphlets. In their attempts to compel notice they appear on the street in unusual costumes, attack prominent persons, and create public scandals. Love-letters, proposals, etc., are directed at the supposed secret lover. The religious paranoiac founds a church and seeks a martyr's crown.

METHODS OF EXAMINATION

In mental disease it is of the utmost importance that the student employ a definite routine method of examination of the patient. Any method to be satisfactory must include the (a) anamnesis of the family, and (6) personal history previous to the disease, (c) the anamnesis of the disease, (d) and finally the status praesens.

(a) The importance of heredity as an etiological factor necessitates a careful consideration of the *family history,* not only as regards the presence of mental and neurological diseases, but also evidences of defective physical constitution. This can never be elicited by simply asking the general question if there is a history of insanity or nervous diseases in the family, but it requires a detailed inquiry into the habits, traits, and physical illnesses of all the members of the direct branches of the family, laying particular stress upon mental peculiarities, alcoholic and other addictions, and criminal tendencies. *(b)* The *personal history* should begin with an inquiry into the conditions attending gestation and birth, such as, exhausting diseases, deprivation, severe emotional shocks, mental anguish, and birth trauma. In infancy there is the presence of infectious diseases and their sequelae, convulsions, head injury, paralyses and the tardy appearance of walking and talking, and in childhood, the progress in school and conditions accompanying puberty and menstruation, also the existence of masturbation, sexual impuls-

es, peculiar emotional manifestations, timidity, morbid temperaments, religious experiences, etc. If married, the conditions attending child-bearing should be known, as well as severe illnesses, such as, typhoid fever, injuries, mental shocks, and deprivation; and if employed, the character of the work, the materials handled, the sanitation and undue physical and mental strain, excessive indulgence in eating, drinking, and amusement, and also drug habituation. Personal idiosyncrasies, exaggerated egotism, one-sided intellectual development, with attainments in one field and lack of development in another, should be included in your list of inquiries. In eliciting such facts it should be borne in mind that general questions are wholly inadequate. It requires close and detailed questioning, and even then important facts are very apt to be overlooked.

In determining the cause of the disease one should guard against mistaking for causes the actual early symptoms of disease; such as the excesses of the paretic, the self-condemnation of the melancholiac, and the masturbation of the hebephrenic.

(c) In eliciting the *anamnesis of the disease* particular attention should be paid to the character of the onset and the symptoms to date. In securing this information it is usually most satisfactory to follow out the outline prescribed for making a mental status; *i.e.* elicit information concerning the presence of hallucinations or illusions at various periods, of disorder of orientation, attention, memory, train of thought, judgment, and in the emotional and volitional fields.

It is often difficult to determine the actual date of onset of the disease because the initial change in disposition is sometimes so insidious that the true significance of certain peculiarities is not appreciated until emphasized later by the occurrence of the more striking symptoms. In case there have been one or more previous attacks of mental disease there should be the same careful inquiry not only into the character of the symptoms presented at these periods and their duration, but also particularly as to whether the patient fully recovered or suffered residual defects in some field of the mental life.

(d) *Status prcesens.* This examination should include observations of both the physical and mental conditions of the patient. In view of the fact that many persons are particularly sensitive about undergoing a mental examination it is desirable to begin with the physical examination. During it there is always opportunity to frame questions in such a way that the answers will give valuable information as to the mental state; as, for instance, the memory can be determined by questions as to the date of appearance of certain physical signs, or the orientation may be ascertained by questions as to those who are caring for them, by whom their food is prepared, etc. Indeed, the great variety of physical symptoms to be inquired into offers sufficient chance to cover all fields of the mental status; even hallucinations and illusions of hearing and sight may be disclosed by the examination of the senses of hearing and sight.

The general survey of the body should include the state of nutrition, the present body weight compared with earlier weights, the presence of anaemia or cachexia, signs of premature senility, or delayed pubescence, also evidences of socalled physical stigmata, as harelip, malformation of the palate, of the ears, or sexual organs, albinism, congenital strabismus, malposition of the teeth and eyes, etc. Trauma, scars, and residuals of previous diseases should not be overlooked, and particularly those of syphilis. The physical examination should be careful enough to eliminate such chronic diseases as chronic nephritis, uraemia, diabetes, pernicious anaemia, Graves' disease, tuberculosis, syphilis, lead poisoning, and chronic gastritis. The condition of sleep and of the gastro-intestinal tract needs special attention because of the frequency with which disturbances exist in these fields.

In the examination of the nervous system, the measurements of the cranium will give some indication as to the development of the cortex, but it is of more importance to observe the disproportion between the cranium and the rest of the body. The circumference of the skull taken along the line just above the external occipital protuberance and the glabella should measure in an adult between 48 and 56 centimeters, while the distance between the extreme lateral points as taken by craniometer should be between 14 and 15 centimeters. The examination of the eye grounds should not be omitted, as it often reveals vascular sclerosis, which might otherwise escape notice. Likewise, a careful examination of the ears sometimes discloses a sufficient cause for peripheral hallucinations.

Then the *muscular system* should be examined. First determine the condition of muscular tonicity by employing passive movements and examining the tendon reflexes. Both of these may be difficult on account of lack of cooperation and inability to secure complete relaxation of the limbs; hence it is important to have the patients in a comfortable and restful attitude, such as in a recumbent position, with their attention distracted by engaging them in conversation, giving them figures to add or something to read aloud. In eliciting the knee jerks, if the patient is lying on his back, place left hand beneath the knee and gently lift it, allowing the foot to rest on the bed. If you find the leg relaxed, strike the tendon at any time. Frequently the patient will not relax until you have raised the knee high enough so that it will support itself in that position. If the patient is sitting, he should recline backward in an easy posture, with both feet squarely on the floor and brought as far forward as possible without causing the toes to leave the floor.

The ankle clonus is best elicited now by slipping the right hand under the toes and sole of the foot and quickly jerking the foot upward for a few inches, so that the weight of the elevated leg and thigh rests on your hand. The Achilles jerk is determined by asking the patient to stand leaning forward and supporting his weight by placing his hands on the top of a table or back of a chair. The ankle is then lifted in the rear and allowed to rest on your knee, when the tendon is struck. The wrist and jaw reflexes should also be determined.

The muscles should be examined further by palpation and by the exercise of active movements which will determine the presence of paralysis (flaccid, spastic, or accompanied by contractures), as well as disturbances of coordination. Such movements are the voluntary raising of the legs while the patient is recumbent, attempts to touch the knee, to touch the end of the nose with the forefinger with or without closed eyes, standing erect with eyes closed and feet close together, closing the eyes, opening the mouth, and protruding the tongue upon command, and then reversing the order. These tests should also include voluntary writing, and speech, as well as the enunciation of different words, such as "electricity," "Massachusetts artillery brigade," "around the rugged rock the ragged rascal ran." The movements employed above will also demonstrate tremors (fine, coarse, fibrillary, and retractile of the tongue), which should be noted.

The mechanical irritability of the muscles and the nerves is then determined by percussion of the muscles, and the mechanical stimulation of the peripheral nerves. The nature of spasms should also be investigated (epileptic, hysterical, choreic, and athetoid). Finally, the irritability of the muscles and nerves to electricity, wherever there are indications for its use, should be determined, since disturbances in it as well as in all of these other fields may have distinct bearing upon the general brain condition.

Following this the sensibility should be tested, including the sensations of pain, touch, and temperature, for areas of hyperaesthesia, analgesia, and paraesthesia. For this purpose the simplest implements are the best; namely, a camel's hair brush, a needle, and small bottles of hot and cold water. It may also be necessary to examine the stereognostic sense.

Vasomotor, secretory, and trophic disorders should be recognized and recorded, particularly cyanosis of the extremities, dermography, glossy skin, canities, alopecia, onychogryphosis, naevi, herpes, scleroderma, and hyperidrosis; the various trophic disorders of the bones and joints, including spontaneous fractures and haemotama auris.

In the examination of the pulse there is nothing to be found peculiarly characteristic of any special form of mental disease. The blood pressure in fearful and depressive states is usually elevated, and depressed in manic states, corresponding with the vasomotor symptoms ordinarily accompanying these states. The fall in blood pressure observed in the end stages of paresis is in accord with the progressive terminal cardiac weakness. The examination of the blood has been thus far unproductive of characteristic disorders. In any given psychosis the blood states may vary considerably in the different stages. In the psychoses studied by us—dementia praecox, manic-depressive insanity, and dementia paralytica — the only apparently characteristic blood states were those found in dementia paralytica, where there was a progressive anaemia and a progressive increase of polymorphonuclear leucocytes accompanying the advancing course of the disease and the presence of a leucocytosis accompanying paralytic attacks. The chemical investigations of the urine, gastric contents, and of body metabolism, while still fruitful fields for study, do not warrant routine examinations except in the matter of urine and gastric contents to obtain indications for treatment.

"Blood Changes in Dementia Paralytica," American Journal of Med. Soc, Vol. 126, p. 1074.

"A Contribution to the Study of Blood in Manic Depressive Insanity," American Journal of Insanity, LIX, No. 4, 1903.

A careful physical examination should include in doubtful cases the examination of the cerebrospinal fluid for the purpose of differentiating between functional or organic diseases. As much depends upon the technique, the method is briefly stated. With the strictest aseptic precautions the needle is inserted between the fourth and fifth lumbar vertebrae, and three or four centimeters of fluid withdrawn. This is immediately centrifugalized 10 minutes — if the speed is 3000 revolutions, or 30 minutes — if only 2500 revolutions can be obtained. The supernatant fluid is poured out of the glass and then a pipette is carefully introduced into the bottom of the tube and the sediment all withdrawn. This is thoroughly mixed by blowing it out into the tube and sucking it up again, when three drops of equal size are dropped on three slides, which are allowed to dry in the air. The slides are fixed by a half-hour immersion in equal parts of absolute alcohol and ether, stained with a few drops of Unna's polychrome methylene blue, washed in water, then in alcohol, cleared in xylol, and mounted in balsam. With a magnification of 300 to 400 times the presence of three or four lymphocytes in a single field may be regarded as normal. At least three lumbar punctures are necessary for a final decision. The bacteriological examination of the cerebrospinal fluid as well as of the blood has thus far yielded such varying results in the hands of different observers that a routine examination cannot be recommended for diagnostic purposes.

The most difficult part of the examination is securing the mental status. In this matter much depends upon the acuteness of the observer, as the patient often enough cannot be depended upon for cooperation. Unfortunately, we have no scientific standards for determining the mental symptoms, but must depend upon the simplest psychological tests; namely, the asking of questions.

For convenience and thoroughness of examination it is most important to always have before one an outline of the method of examination. If for purposes of record or otherwise, and particularly in medico-legal cases, it is necessary to write down the observations, it is always best to write in full the question and the answer verbatim as given by the patient. Upon subsequent examinations the same questions should be asked, and the answers compared. The general arrangement of this outline should follow closely the presentation of the general symptomatology; *i.e. disturbances of perception, clouding of consciousness, disturbances of apprehension, of attention, of memory, of orientation, of the train of thought, of judgment, of the emotions, and of the volitions.* 1. Disturbances of Perception *(hallucinations and illusions).*— Hallucinations can oftentimes be most readily elicited by asking the patient directly if he hears *voices* or sees *pictures* or *visions,* or, if this question is not understood, if he hears noises or voices when no one is about him. Frequently the patient does not consider the hallucinations as a peculiar sensory experience and will answer your questions negatively. Then he should be questioned closely as to how he sleeps nights, and whether or not he is disturbed. Again, he may be questioned as to whether or not intimate associates, shopmates, employers, or business associates, whom you know to be absent, converse with him. Such questions often elicit the desired evidence of hallucinations. Sometimes sense deceptions are elicited only when one seeks for the basis of certain delusions held by the patient, when, for instance, he will admit that he believes he is persecuted because of remarks that he hears. Patients observed assuming listening attitudes and addressing remarks to unseen persons, or gesticulating earnestly in a definite direction, or persistently spitting out or casting aside good food without adequate reason, may be regarded as suffering from sense deceptions, although these are denied by them when questioned directly. In the matter of religious hallucinations, such as the voice of God, one should be particularly careful not to mistake the " *voice of conscience"* or the *"voice of the heart"* as genuine hallucinations, a distinction which some patients are loath to admit. Again, sometimes what in many appear to be true hallucinations are not such, but are really genuine perceptions. In this matter one cannot exercise too great care. What has been indicated in reference to hallucinations and illusions of sight and hearing refers equally well to the hallucinations and illusions of the other senses.

2. Clouding of Consciousness and Disturbances of Apprehension. — The determination of *unconsciousness,* of *befogged states,* and of *diminished sensibility* depends mostly in clinical practice upon the patient's reaction to definite stimuli, such as one uses in any neurological examination; namely, the test of pain and touch sense by the use of the needle, of hearing by the use of speech, of sight by writing tests or the perception of colors. Further, the comprehension of simple or confused pictures (medleys) placed before the patients gives an insight into these defects. Many elaborate tests, such as Hipp's chronoscope and the apparatus of Ranschburg, have been devised for the accurate determination of the process of perception, which are not wholly suitable for general application or for bedside use. 3. The Disturbances of Attention *(blunting, blocking, retardation, passivity,* and *distractibility)* can usually be determined in a satisfactory manner by the use of the progressive adding and subtracting test, such as, subtracting 7 successively from 100 down to 0. The variations in the rapidity and the occasional blocking afford good demonstrations of the stability of the attention. The introduction of distracting influences during the test, such as dropping a cent upon the floor, will bring out distractibility of attention. In the application of such a test one must always take into account the social grade of the individual as well as the degree of his education. 4. Memory *(defects in the impressibility, retentiveness, accuracy, and fabrications of memory).* — The retentiveness of memory is usually determined by a series of questions directed toward the retention of certain school knowledge, such as the multiplication table; or the uninterrupted adding or subtracting of 3, 7, or 12, the time required being measured by a stop-watch. The retentiveness in patients sensitive to being subjected to such tests can be estimated only by asking questions concerning the past personal experiences or facts in history.

The impressibility of memory can be most readily determined by asking the patient to repeat numbers of more than one figure which are dictated to him; also unfamiliar combinations of syllables. This may be done both orally and by writing. Again, he may be asked to recognize in a group of pictures a certain picture which has previously been shown to him. Questions directed to ascertaining recent occurrences in their daily lives, such as what he had for dinner yesterday, what the nurse or doctor is doing for him, may be asked. In the determination of both the retentiveness and impressibility one must never demand from an uneducated person more than he ever acquired. The accuracy of memory and the fabrications will already have been elicited by the questions asked in reference to remote and recent personal experiences.

5. Orientation *(apathetic, amnesic,* and *delusional disorientation* and *perplexity).*—The orientation as to time, place, and persons is determined by such questions as: "What is the date of the month, the day of the week, and the season and year?" "Where are you now?" "What is the name of the place, of the building and its character, and of the city?" "Who are these persons about you, their duty here, and what is your mission here?" In case the patient is not disposed to or is unable to respond, his orientation as well as his power of apprehension can be determined by watching carefully his conduct in his environment; for instance, noting the names with which he addresses his associates, his religious observances, his ability to find his way about in familiar environment, etc. 6. Train of Thought *(paralysis of thought, retardation of thought, compulsive ideas, simple persistent ideas, perseveration, circumstantiality, flight of ideas, desultoriness).* — If the patient is at all communicative and has answered the foregoing questions, you already have had some opportunity to judge of the wealth of his store of ideas, or the degree of its impoverishment, if present; also to some extent of all of the other disturbances of the train of thought, and particularly the retardation of thought. If the patient is productive and volun-

teers much speech, there is usually little difficulty in determining the presence of simple persistent ideas, *circumstantiality,* flight of ideas, and desultoriness. In case the patient is not productive, the disturbances in the content of thought can be elicited by requesting him to recite connectedly the incidents of some recent personal experience; such as the detailed account of the nurse's method of caring for him or the account of the journey to the hospital. It may be necessary in order to keep the patient talking to continually urge him by interjecting " Yes, yes," or, " Is that so?" In this way circumstantiality, flight of ideas, and desultoriness is usually detected. Another method is to peruse the voluntary writings of the patient, particularly home letters.

There are many more accurate tests for determining the associations of ideas. Of these, the one most easily carried out at the bedside is to give the patient any sort of a word, such as "horse," and then ask him to speak aloud the ideas first arising in his mind, which you may write down, or you may ask the patient himself to write down all ideas occurring to him in a definite period of time after being given the initial word. In this way one can obtain some conception of the relationship between the inner and external associations, of the prominence and frequency of fixed associations, senseless and sound associations, of uniformity and the desultoriness of the train of thought, as well as the wealth of the store of ideas, the tendencies to sudden cessations, or the tenacious holding of a single idea.

7. Judgment *(delusions).* — Usually by the time one has reached this stage of the examination real delusions have been actually expressed or some hints have been accidentally dropped which will serve as a basis for further questioning. In determining delusions, direct questions are less pernicious than in eliciting some of the other mental symptoms. One may ask the patient if he is troubled in any way, if the affairs at home are moving smoothly, if his business is successful, and if he is at all apprehensive of his welfare, etc. Should

your patient show considerable reserve and refuse to speak of personal matters, as often happens immediately after his liberty is restrained or he is placed in a new environment, one must be tactful in approaching the matter of delusions. Sometimes the simple direct question as to why he has been deprived of his liberty or submitted to the care of the physician may be sufficient. Again, it may be necessary to introduce a subject of much interest to him, such as his employment, literature, or travelling, or he may be asked to express his judgment as to cost of manufacture of the material with which he works, the contentions of trade unions, the utility of trusts, or his opinion of the countries in which he may have travelled. A free discussion of a matter of general interest, but at the same time bearing upon the individual's livelihood, usually uncovers some of his delusions, if any be present. In the case of women, domestic difficulties, church or social relations, and especially neighborhood differences, are usually fruitful sources for discussion and inquiry. The various somatic delusions are most often brought out by questions as to the health of all the various organs of the body. The evidence of systematization of delusions can often be best determined by asking directly, "What is the object of all this? " or, "Do these various ideas bear any relation to each other?"

Defective judgment in other matters than delusions will usually be established by such general discussions as those advised above or by such questions as, " What do you think of the restriction of your liberty?" "How much does it cost you to live?" "Are you receiving sufficient wages, and do you live within your income?" "Figure up your cost of living." "Who aids in the support of your family, and do they do as much as they should?" etc.

8. Emotional Field *(emotional deterioration, increase of emotional irritability, sad disposition, irritable disposition, seclusiveness, sunny disposition, fanaticism, morbid frivolity, fear, phobias, dejection, sadness, feelings of pleasure, feeling of well-being, disturbances of hunger, nausea, pain, and of the sexual feelings.)* — In this field one has to depend rather more upon observation than upon interrogation of the patient, as there is large opportunity for simulation and falsehood. Most patients if asked if they loved their parents would say " Yes " even though they might be totally barren of all affection and exhibiting profound emotional deterioration. One rather has to rely upon the observations of others as to relations which the patient maintains with his family, in his work, and in his social environment, which would exhibit increased and diminished emotional irritability and persistent sadness or elation. Likewise one cannot depend upon the patient for accurate observations as to whether or not he is of a sad, sunny, seclusive, or irritable disposition, or given to fanaticism or morbid frivolity. The persistent feelings of fear, of sadness, and of well-being usually become apparent to one during a prolonged examination and do not need special inquiry. Yet in this matter one sometimes must ask the patient directly how he feels, or whether or not he is fearful or dejected. The disturbances of the general feelings of pain, of hunger, nausea, and of the sexual life are more readily determined by observation of the conduct than by questioning.

In questioning those most intimately associated with the patient one may ask such questions as these: whether or not there has been a change of disposition; previous to illness was the individual of a sociable, cheery, or melancholy disposition; was he fond of solitude, was he silent, timid, courageous, irascible, suspicious, or proud and egotistical; is he now fond of his family or apathetic, is he fulfilling his family and business obligations, or is he negligent, disrespectful, or insensible to the feelings and interests of others; is he fulfilling his religious obligations, or does his general conduct show unnatural fear, sadness, or exaltation.

We have at best no very accurate means of measuring the emotional side of the life of the patient. Feelings of displeasure, of pain, fear, and anger can be created experimentally in various ways and by hypnosis, and the latter method has been employed by Lehmann to determine the influence of emotional states upon respiration, pulse rate, and blood pressure. Furthermore, the writing scale and the ergograph, which are used to measure the finer expressions of the will, are serviceable in measuring the outward expressions of emotional excitement.

9. Volitional Field *(paralysis of the will, pressure of activity, psychomotor retardation, stupor, blocking of the will, muscular tension, hypersuggestibility of the will, catalepsy, cerea flexibilitas, exhopraxia, distractibility of the will, interference, stereotypy, mannerisms, negativism).* — Here also one must depend to a large degree upon observation of the conduct, both spontaneous and in obedience to command or suggestion. Thus paralysis of the will can be determined by watching the patient's voluntary movements, also the reaction in response to the call to dinner or when requested to attend some simple duty. Pressure of activity, retardation, stupor, and blocking of the will, as well as muscular tension, are usually evinced before one has reached this stage of the examination. The methods of physical examination are sure to bring out these defects as well as cerea flexibilitas and catalepsy. If not, one has simply to grasp the arm and place it in an awkward and uncomfortable position or to command the patient to perform certain movements, as walking, shaking hands, or writing. If negativism is present, it also will be elicited by these methods. Distractibility of the will, interference, stereotypy, and mannerisms are elicited by similar commands.

The observation of the conduct by nurses and others should be inquired into, as in this way the varying periods of mutism, negativism, muscular tension, and tendency to eat the food of others and to get into others' beds, to stand in awkward and statuesque positions, can be elicited, which may not be present at the time of your examination.

In the finer analysis of disturbances of volition, particularly psychomotor excitement, retardation, and tension, Kraepelin suggests the writing scale, by which one can determine the path of the writing, the rapidity, and the pressure. Also the ergograph, invented by Mosso, can be employed to measure the strength of the movement, the effect of retardation, fatigue, and muscular tension, as well as the rapidity with which the contraction and relaxation of the muscles follow under the influence of the impulses of the will. Both of these instruments, however, have their drawbacks which render their routine application unsatisfactory. The more severe disturbances in the release of the volitional impulses can be measured by the use of the watch, such as in counting as rapidly as possible from 1 to 30, rapidly repeating the alphabet, or in simply raising the arm.

FORMS OF MENTAL DISEASES CLASSIFICATION OF MENTAL DISEASES CONSIDERATION OF THE FACTORS ENTERING INTO A PROVISIONAL CLASSIFICATION

The principle requisite in the knowledge of mental diseases is an accurate definition of the separate disease processes. In the solution of this problem one must have, on the one hand, knowledge of the physical changes in the cerebral cortex, and on the other of the mental symptoms associated with them. Until this is known we cannot hope to understand the relationship between mental symptoms of disease and the morbid physical processes underlying them, or indeed the causes of the entire disease process. There are still other difficulties to be encountered in obtaining that fundamental knowledge necessary for a scientific classification of mental diseases. In the first place, it is almost impossible to establish a fundamental distinction between the normal and the morbid mental state, as was frequently indicated in our discussion of the general symptomatology. It is equally difficult sometimes to distinguish between the transition states existing between different forms of recognized types of mental disease. Again, the symptoms of the disease are apt to be greatly influenced and exaggerated by the morbid hereditary basis which underlies so many forms of mental disease. Finally, as the functions of dif-

ferent parts of the brain differ, hence the character, intensity, and location of the morbid process influence greatly the gradations in the form of the mental disease.

Clearly, then, there is at present no sure foundation upon which to construct a final standard classification. Nevertheless, there is always a demand for some grouping of our knowledge as a basis for practical work, particularly in teaching. Judging from experience in internal medicine, the safest foundation for a classification of this kind is that offered by pathological anatomy. Unfortunately, however, mental diseases thus far present but very few lesions that have positively distinctive characteristics, and furthermore there is the extreme difficulty of correlating physical and mental morbid processes.

Likewise it has been impossible thus far to establish a classification upon an etiological basis. Although there are some agents that produce very definite symptoms, such as alcoholic intoxication, certain acute infectious diseases, head injury, and particularly the more profound types of hereditary degeneracy, yet very many individual cases of insanity are wholly without any distinctive etiological factors. And furthermore, one often has to admit that any single pathogenic factor may make itself known by a great variety of symptoms. Again, the causes of mental disease often work in conjunction with each other, rendering it extremely difficult to ascertain the relationship between the causes and the symptoms.

The most popular method of classifying mental diseases has been the so-called clinical classification. The grave defect here arises from the fact that there is apt to be an overvaluation of some symptoms resulting in the accumulation in one group of all cases having in common some one striking symptom. In this way all sad and anxious emotional states came to be regarded as melancholia, all excited states as mania, and delusional states accompanied by hallucinations as paranoia. The difficulty becomes apparent when a single case thus classified presents during its course

the characteristics of several groups. It is, therefore, essential, as was pointed out by Kahlbaum, to distinguish between transitory mental states and the disease form itself. The scientific conception of the disease demands knowledge not only of the present state, but also of the entire course of the disease.

Judging from our experience in internal medicine it is a fair assumption that similar disease processes will produce identical symptom pictures, identical pathological anatomy, and an identical etiology. If, therefore, we possessed a comprehensive knowledge of any one of these three fields, — pathological anatomy, symptomatology, or etiology, — we would at once have a uniform and standard classification of mental diseases. A similar comprehensive knowledge of either of the other two fields would give not only just as uniform and standard classifications, but all of these classifications would exactly coincide. Cases of mental disease originating in the same causes must also present the same symptoms, and the same pathological findings. In accordance with this principle, it follows that a clinical grouping of psychoses must be founded equally upon all three of these factors, to which should be added the experience derived from the observation of the course, outcome, and treatment of the disease.

In the classification presented here there are treated first of all those forms of insanity that are produced by external causes; namely, those psychoses that arise in connection with infectious diseases, those that follow upon severe exhaustion, and finally those produced by intoxicating agencies. Next are considered the psychoses presumed to bear some relation to the products of faulty metabolism and autointoxication. Our knowledge of these is definite only in reference to thyrogenous insanity; but there are certain points of similarity which would indicate that dementia praecox and dementia paralytica should also be classed here.

The forms of insanity arising from diseases of the brain, the organic dementias, comprise the next group. Here external causes also play some role, as, for instance, the syphilitic lesions, head injury, and cerebral embolism. Next come the insanities associated with the involutional period: melancholia of involution, senile dementia, and the presenile state with delusions of prejudice.

The next group comprises manic-depressive insanity in which a morbid constitutional basis occupies a prominent position. The same condition obtains to a still more marked degree in that gradual morbid transformation of the entire psychical personality designated paranoia, which is described next.

In epileptic insanity, which comes next, besides the prominent morbid constitutional basis, there often exist other morbid conditions as head injury, arteriosclerosis, and infectious diseases. The epileptic attacks sometimes date from some particular revolution in the physical organization. These facts give to epilepsy an intermediate position between auto-intoxication, organic brain disease, and hereditary mental diseases. We do not, however, believe that the disease group recognized to-day as epilepsy presents a clinical unity. Further knowledge probably will disclose in it several different disease processes. In hysteria, while the faulty constitutional basis is prevalent, the various forms of mental disorder seem to be released wholly through the action of the emotions.

Closely associated with hysteria are the insanities of degeneracy. The morbid constitutional basis encountered here varies greatly and it is often impossible to differentiate the several different forms of psychosis. Yet one may formulate two large groups; namely, the constitutional psychopathic states and the psychopathic personalities. The former comprise those morbid constitutional states which are recognized by being more circumscribed, as developing gradually at first, or as appearing only at times; the latter include the characteristic morbid developmental forms of the entire psychic personality, which are justly regarded as an expression of degeneracy. In some instances this division is inadequate.

Finally there are described those forms which indicate a restriction of mental development — an incomplete development of the psychical personality. Sometimes the basis for this lies in a faulty development of the body, but more often there exist in the undeveloped brain disease processes, which produce a partial destruction of the tissue, thereby rendering mental development impossible. Strictly speaking, these latter cases should be regarded as organic brain diseases. We are not yet in a position to distinguish accurately between restricted development and diseases of the brain, and furthermore, the mark of congenital weakness predominates to such a marked degree in the clinical pictures that any distinction between both of these groups which are so intimately related from an etiological standpoint hardly commends itself. Indeed, we might go even a step farther and consider these forms of defective development as states of mental weakness which were produced by profound mental disease in the earliest stages of development. Also in these cases the development of psychical personality was destroyed at the outset.

In concluding the subject it should be emphasized that many of the disease pictures differentiated in the following pages are but attempts to present a part of our observations in a form suitable for teaching purposes. It must be admitted that even to-day it is impossible, in spite of honest efforts, to create a "system" of psychiatry that will include all cases. Attempts of this sort that have been made only bring confusion. While this assertion may prove somewhat disquieting to the student, to the investigator it means a frank acknowledgment of real conditions and an honest effort to establish accurate and fundamental knowledge from our clinical experience.

I. INFECTION PSYCHOSES

The mental disturbances here described are supposed to develop primarily from toxins of infectious diseases.

They are *fever delirium, infection deliria,* and *post-febrile psychoses.*

Fever delirium follows rather closely the clinical course of the fever, and in a measure depends upon it. The infection delirium corresponds to the initial deliria of other authors, appearing at, or near, the onset of infectious diseases, independently of fever. The remaining group includes the various forms of mental disturbance which follow the infectious disease, developing during or following the fever, and which are apt to lead to permanent mental enfeeblement. Other writers describe these under the various diseases which they accompany; as, typhoid delirium, pneumonic delirium, influenza insanity, and insanities following exanthemata. The mental symptoms arising from the toxins of the different infectious diseases cannot as yet be sufficiently differentiated to permit of their being considered as characteristic of the corresponding disease. The only distinguishing features are the physical symptoms characteristic of the different diseases. It is still a question whether the changes in the cortical neurones are due directly to the toxins produced by the micro-organism, or to an autotoxin developing within the body as a result of the infectious disease.

A. Fever Delirium
The clinical picture of fever delirium presents four different grades corresponding to the intensity of the toxic action upon the cortical neurones, varying from moderate irritation to paralysis and finally to complete destruction.

Etiology. — The form of febrile disease has very little influence on the type of delirium, which apparently is modified only by the rapidity of the development of the fever, its intensity, and duration. There seems to be little ground for the claim that the mental disturbance occurring during typhoid is more or less characteristic. Besides the toxin produced in the febrile disease, the rise in temperature, acceleration of metabolism, and disturbance of circulation should be regarded as causative factors. In addition there should be included alcohol, which plays such an important rôle in pneumonia, giving rise to symptoms characteristic of delirium tremens, such as illusions and hallucinations of many moving objects of great sensory vividness, the occupation delirium, tremor, and a mixed emotional state showing both elation and anxiety. Furthermore, the individual's power of resistance is of importance. It is well known that children, women, and nervous men show a tendency to develop delirium with any severe form of fever.

The pathological anatomy exhibits mostly a disappearance of the cortical cells very similar to that which can be produced experimentally by the application of superheated air to test animals as well as many other deleterious agents.

Symptomatology. — In the lightest grade of fever delirium there is irritability, some restlessness, general hyperesthesia, insomnia with anxious dreams, a feeling of numbness in the head, and a desire to be left alone.

In the next grade there is a marked clouding of consciousness; illusions and hallucinations largely dominate ideation, producing a dreamy confusion of thought. The designs on the carpet and ceiling appear as moving forms or grinning faces, the bedpost assumes the form of an angel. Frightful outcries or beautiful music are heard, patients have airy floating sensations, and are led about through gorgeously decorated rooms. These dreamy experiences are interrupted momentarily by a return to normal consciousness. The emotional attitude becomes either much exalted or depressed, and motor activity increases greatly.

In the third grade the disturbance of consciousness becomes very pronounced. The patients prattle constantly, the content of thought showing even greater dreamy confusion. There are many varied emotional outbreaks and frequent wild impulsive movements, which soon become irregular and uncertain, indicating the onset of paralysis. The intense restlessness is interrupted by short periods of sleep.

In the fourth grade the movements become absolutely purposeless. At this time carphologia appears with subsultus tendinum. The utterances become indistinct, and consist in mumbling over incoherent words and sentences. From this the patient may enter into a state of coma vigil, when, in spite of open eyes, he is oblivious to all his surroundings and unable to indicate his desires. The urine and faeces are passed involuntarily.

The intensity of the motor activity varies in different individuals, sometimes reaching an extreme degree and at other being confined to spasmodic twitching or choreiform movements of the extremities, or merely of the face and tongue, the latter producing peculiar enunciation.

Course.—The duration of the psychosis in three-fourths of the cases does not extend beyond one week, and usually the delirium subsides with the temperature. Some of the delusional ideas held during the disease may be retained for a long time.

The prognosis is naturally poor because of the severity of the initial disease. If the delirium advances to the third or fourth grade, at least one-third of the cases die. Where there is hyperpyrexia the prognosis is extremely doubtful. A few cases emerge from the fever delirium into an exhaustion psychosis, or may end in dementia. Finally, the delirium may be the starting-point of other psychoses, as manic-depressive insanity, dementia praecox, or dementia paralytica.

Besides the treatment of the initial disease, the ice cap should be applied to relieve cerebral hyperaemia. Cold baths or cold packs with friction are most serviceable. In case of cardiac weakness one must be cautious in the use of the bath, and if necessary administer a cardiac stimulant. For this purpose strong coffee is valuable. Antipyretics are not only useless, but often aid in producing and intensifying the delirium. One of the most important indications is constant attendance, both to prevent harm to others and injury of the patient by escaping out of doors or jumping out of windows. If the excitement becomes excessive, one should resort to the prolonged warm bath (see p. 140). This measure rarely fails to bring quiet. In addition, however, a clever, reassuring nurse is most essential. The method of applying strait jackets and restraint sheets so much in vogue in private homes and general hospitals should be decried. If impulsive movements are a prominent feature, it may be necessary to improvise padded beds with high sides, or to resort to padded rooms. The use of hypnotics and narcotics is harmful and distinctly contraindicated. Furthermore, the proper use of hydrotherapy usually renders their administration unnecessary.

B. Infection Deliria

This group comprises psychoses which appear to stand in intimate relationship to the specific toxaemia of certain infectious diseases, including the *initial deliria* of typhoid and smallpox and the deliria accompanying malaria, acute chorea, and influenza. There are also grouped here deliria that develop in some septic states, as well as those occurring in toxic states of a less specific nature and presenting the course of the so-called " Acute Delirium."

Initial Deliria. — Of the infection deliria, the initial delirium of typhoid is best known. Nissl has reported on the pathological anatomy in one case in which there was distention of the vessels of the cortex, with increase of white blood corpuscles and pronounced degenerative changes in the nerve cells. The cell bodies were swollen, the chromophiles were dissolved, and the processes diffusely stained for some distance. Karyokinesis was observed in nuclei of the glia cells. These changes, which are similar to those produced by experimental intoxication, tend to prove that we have to do with a psychosis depending upon intoxication.

Aschaffenburg 1 distinguishes two forms of initial delirium of typhoid. In the first the delirium is not accompanied by psychomotor activity, but there are numerous and pronounced hallucinations and delusions, mostly of a threatening and persecutory nature; such as, cursing voices, visions of frightful and threatening forms, and ideas of poisoning and personal injury. The emotional attitude is usually one of intense anxiety and sadness. The patients are often productive and relate adventurous experiences.

The other form, which, indeed, may develop directly from

'Aschaffenburg, Allgem. Zeitschr. f. Psychiatrie LII, 75.

the first, is characterized by great psychomotor activity. The delirium usually develops rapidly with marked hallucinations, incoherent delusions, delirious confusion of thought, sometimes flight of ideas, also an intensely anxious emotional state, together with senseless impulsive movements. During the initial delirium the sleep is greatly disturbed, and there is little appetite; on the other hand, there is usually but slight rise in temperature, and the pulse is not accelerated. The recognition of the type of delirium at the onset may be rendered difficult by the absence of the characteristic typhoid symptoms, which may not appear until the delirium is well established. Farrar 1 lays stress upon impaired associative activity, fallacious sense deception, with developing delusions, disorientation, psychomotor excitement, and anxious affective states. He also calls attention to certain prodromal symptoms, which may exist from a few hours to many days, as, nervousness, insomnia, and nocturnal restlessness, and believes that cases with a sudden onset are more uniformly fatal and occur particularly in individuals with a faulty heredity. *The initial delirium of smallpox* usually develops between the third and fifth days, and is characterized by a short violent course. The symptoms are similar to those observed in the initial delirium of typhoid, but are characterized by an even greater clouding of consciousness, and violent conduct with a tendency to commit suicide, in which respect one is reminded of the epileptic befogged states. Tremor and convulsions sometimes develop. The symptoms subside with the appearance of the eruption, but occasionally extend over into the pustular stage. It rarely happens that the psychosis passes over into a condition of dementia. The recognition of the smallpox delirium depends wholly upon the fever, the physical symptoms, and circumstances pointing to this

infectious disease. Farrar, "On Typhoid Psychoses," Medical Reports of the Shepard and Enoch Pratt Hospital, 1903. Vol. 1, No. 1, p. 42.

Another type of mental disturbance characteristic of smallpox may develop between the eruption and pus fever, in which the patients present only vivid hallucinations of sight and hearing, while in other respects they remain well oriented, clear in thought, and orderly in conduct. The varied visions and voices simply annoy them without causing much effect.

The course in these initial deliria is frequently characterized by partial remissions during the daytime, in which the patients continue somewhat clouded and do not wholly regain insight into their condition. The duration of the symptoms rarely extends beyond one week, and usually is much shorter. The delirium usually clears with the onset of the fever, but it may pass over into the characteristic fever delirium.

The *outcome* is distinctly unfavorable, as forty to fifty per cent. of the patients die.

The infection delirium accompanying *malaria* is distinctly intermittent, either accompanying or replacing the fever. It occurs most frequently in the tertian and quotidian forms, and rarely in the quartan. The delirium may appear only in the early stages of the disease, during this time replacing the fever for a few days. The symptoms develop suddenly, and consist of states of marked anxious excitement with profound clouding of consciousness and a tendency to reckless violence. All of these symptoms suddenly disappear after a few hours' duration, and are followed by profound sleep, from which the patient awakes with little or no memory of the attack. The delirium always responds readily to the use of quinine.

The delirium that accompanies *acute chorea,* particularly when associated with acute polyarthritis and endocarditis, seems to belong to the group of infection psychoses. It is characterized by a clouding of consciousness with a peculiar dreamy confusion of thought, some hallucinations and delusions and

emotional irritability. These patients apprehend single impressions fairly well, but continue disoriented and are inattentive and distractible. Their speech is characterized by monotonous disjointed sentences, in which they occasionally weave incidental observations. While they may hear voices calling, see strange visions, and express persecutory or fearful delusions, these ideas are not clear and are never elaborated further. The emotional attitude varies, as at times they are anxious, at others elated, and occasionally show outbursts of passion.

This mental picture is accompanied by a condition of almost constant choreic excitation, in which the characteristic choreic movements continue in an exaggerated form both day and night, preventing sleep and also interfering greatly with nutrition. The duration of the psychosis is from a few days to a few weeks, and not infrequently terminates fatally.

Other infectious diseases that may give rise to a delirious state which apparently depends upon a toxaemia, are *influenza, hydrophobia,* and certain *septic states.* In the first there is apt to be clouding of consciousness, delirious hallucinations, confusion of speech, and anxious excitement. Sometimes there is also present paralysis of speech and deglutition, as well as polyneuritic symptoms. The psychosis accompanying *hydrophobia* is a delirium in which hallucinations predominate. In the septic states the patients may develop a delirium in which there are many hallucinations, clouding of consciousness with disorientation, low and indistinct mumbling, and attempts to grasp at invisible objects. At times the condition is one of pronounced delirious excitement. M6bius, Neural. Beitrage, II, 123,1894; Zinn, Archiv f. Psy. XXVTII, 411, 1896; Krafft-Ebing, Wiener Klin. Rundschau, 1900, 30. 'Hogyes, Lyssa, Nothnagel's Handbuch der Pathologic u. Therapie, V, 5, 88, 1897.

Finally, there is a group of cases which seem more properly classified here than elsewhere. It includes those *delirious states thai sometimes accompany fu-*

runcvJosis or follow a slight physical illness, angina, intestinal catarrh, obstinate constipation, etc., or may occur in the course of any other type of psychosis, which suddenly takes a turn for the worse. Some would include this particular type of delirium with certain other states of marked excitement, and denominate them all "Acute Delirium." The delirium seems to arise from a recent active infectious involvement of the cortex, as shown in the pathological anatomy, by an acute destruction of the nerve cells, sometimes including the fibres, in addition to an increase of the glia, and vascular changes with diapedesis of leucocytes and occasionally an escape of the blood corpuscles.

The patients become sleepless, bewildered, and distractible. Numerous hallucinations of sight and hearing appear, and incoherent expansive and persecutory delusions are expressed. They prattle away, sometimes pray, and finally speech may be resolved into a repetition of a few senseless words and syllables. Emotionally, they may be anxious, elated, or irritable. The activity is greatly increased and accompanied by impulsiveness, with pounding, dancing, yelling, etc. Food is usually refused and the patients fail rapidly. Temperature develops; and there appear ecchymoses or fat embolism, furunculosis, gangrene of the lung, severe catarrh of the nose, gangrene of the mouth, sometimes parotitis and retention of urine and feces. In the vast majority of cases the delirium runs a fatal course in from one to two weeks.

An accurate differentiation of this form of psychosis based alone upon the symptoms is at present almost impossible. The delirious states which sometimes develop in *paresis* and *catatonia* are recognized only by the previous history of symptoms characteristic of these diseases antedating the delirium. *Collapse delirium,* which may arise from an identical toxic state, can be distinguished only by the relative observations that in it the clouding is less profound, the activity less turbulent, while the hallucinations and delusions are more vivid, and in the speech both dis-

tractibility and flight of ideas prevail.

The *treatment* of these different infection deliria depends in some measure upon the treatment of the underlying physical disease. In view of the toxic origin of the disease a thorough flushing of the body combined with infusion of normal salt solution is excellent practice. One may employ the prolonged warm bath (see p. 140) for relieving the motor excitement. Sufficient liquid nourishment is always indicated, which may have to be administered by stomach or nasal tube. The bowels must be kept open, for which purpose high rectal injection of normal saline solution may be used twice daily. Furthermore, the mouth should be cleaned by frequent swabbing. In case medicinal sedatives seem advisable, alcohol and paraldehyde are well recommended, but powerful narcotics and sedatives should be sedulously avoided. Failing heart action should be supported by the use of caffein, camphor, or ether.

0. Post Infection Psychoses

These psychoses are in general characterized by a more or less pronounced degree of intellectual and emotional weakness, together with, in most instances, pronounced delusion formation and a prevailing sad or anxious emotional attitude. The postfebrile psychoses described here by no means include all of the psychoses appearing after the febrile period in infectious diseases. The exhaustion psychoses as well as most any other form of mental disease may develop during this period. The first symptoms often, but not always, appear before the fever wholly subsides.

The mildest form of postfebrile infection psychosis is represented by those cases in which after the subsidence of the fever in a severe attack of infectious disease, the patients fail to show their former physical and mental energy. They are dull and sluggish, and are very susceptible to fatigue. They cannot collect their thoughts, and find it difficult to read and write, are indifferent, idly lie abed, and let things go as they will. Orientation is undisturbed and there usually are no hallucinations, although tran-

sient hallucinations may appear after closing the eyes, when for a few moments they hear unintelligible sounds, see faint visions, or experience peculiar bodily sensations which are interpreted by them as grave symptoms. In emotional attitude they are sad and troubled, sometimes irritable, and occasionally at night they suddenly develop a state of great anxiety. They may at times exhibit a distrust of their surroundings, transitory fear of poisoning, hypochondriacal ideas, and even delusions of persecution, which may give rise to aggressive attacks and attempts at suicide. In actions they are inclined to be reserved, sort of stupid, and reticent about their delusions. Physically, sleep and appetite are poor and body weight much reduced.

This mild form follows particularly influenza and polyarthritis, and whooping cough in children. It is occasionally seen in tuberculous and choreic cases. After a *duration* of a few weeks to a few months, *improvement* gradually sets in, provided the underlying physical disease has cleared up. This syndrome, although suggestive of *chronic nervous exhaustion,* may be differentiated from it by the fact that the symptoms are more severe and stubborn, and do not improve under rest and relaxation. Furthermore, there is not the same clear insight that exists in chronic nervous exhaustion.

A second group of postfebrile infection psychoses is characterized by more pronounced symptoms; namely, prominent hallucinations, fantastic delusions, and active excitement with anxiety. When the symptoms first appear, which is always during the febrile period, there is complete disorientation with marked confusion of thought, and very many hallucinations which may involve all of the senses. After the temperature subsides and the symptoms of the initial disease disappear, the patients gradually become somewhat oriented and more composed, but the hallucinations and delusions persist. They still hear threatening voices, see grinning faces looking in at the window, and must get out of the bed and at them. Some one pulls the bedding, the food is not genuine, they are poisoned, no one is willing to do the right thing for them, etc. Emotionally, they are dejected, anxious, and ill-humored. Sometimes, in outbursts of passion, they attempt suicide and become violent. They are apt to be obstinate, quarrelsome, constrained, and resistive. Physically, there is faulty nutrition and insomnia. As the appetite and sleep improve, the hallucinations and delusions disappear. The patients gain insight into their condition, begin to busy themselves, and resume their accustomed conduct, but for some time they continue to show an unusual susceptibility to fatigue, and an absence of the wonted mental and physical energy, together with weakness of memory. A few cases never completely recover. A fatal termination is rare, and always due to exhaustion or some complication. The *duration* varies from several months to a year. This form follows especially typhoid, smallpox, articular rheumatism, and sometimes develops during tuberculosis.

In adults, there may be some difficulty in differentiating this condition from *melancholia of involution* developing during an attack of some infectious disease. It, however, may be distinguished by the greater prominence of hallucinations, the predominance of delusions of persecution over self-accusations, and the great irritability in contrast to the anxiety of the melancholiac. It may be differentiated from *dementia pracox* by the greater affect and disturbance of apprehension and orientation at the onset of the disease, and by the absence of negativism and stereotypy, from the depressive phase of *manic-depressive* insanity by the absence of psychomotor retardation.

The *third and* severest form of postfebrile infection psychosis is characterized by a severe delirium which soon passes over into a condition of stupor. In spite of improvement in the physical condition the patients continue dull, and incapable of perceiving and elaborating external impressions, and have poor memory and judgment. Emotionally, they are indifferent, sometimes peevish.

They may be quiet or childishly restless. They lie abed unable to take their food or care for themselves, and have to be petted and handled like small children. Physically, they fail markedly in nutrition, and occasionally give evidence of severe cerebral disorder, as hemiplegia, disturbance of speech, and epileptiform attacks. The *prognosis* is dubious, as after an extended course of many months only one-half of the cases recover. The other cases improve gradually but present as residuals, weakness of will-power, poor judgment, forgetfulness, poverty of thought, and apathy. This form follows chiefly typhoid fever, and sometimes malaria. It may be distinguished from the stupor of the *catatonic state* by the absence of negativism, and from the stupor of the *manic-depressive* by the absence of retardation and the presence of faulty memory.

The *treatment* of all these three types of postfebrile infection psychosis is mostly symptomatic, with very careful nursing, rest in bed, nutritious diet, and cautious watching.

Still another group of postfebrile infection psychoses is the "Cerebropathia psycbica toxamica," which was first described by Korssakow' (Korssakow's "Psychosis," "Polyneuritis Psychosis," "Neurocerebrite Toxique"). It is characterized by a pronounced disturbance of that element of memory which we call impressibility, also by disorientation and the physical signs of polyneuritis, associated sometimes with a delirious excitement or stupidity. The symptoms of this form of polyneuritic psychosis are very similar to the alcoholic polyneuritic psychosis (see p. 184), and can be distinguished only by their more prolonged course and the history of the underlying physical state. The *duration* of the psychosis extends over many months, in case death does not occur, and the *outcome* is rather more favorable than in the alcoholic cases. The *treatment* is practically the same as that outlined in the other forms, with the exception that some attention must be paid to the muscular atrophies, which demand the use of electricity and massage after the subsidence of the acute neuritic

symptoms.

Korssakow, Gazette russe hebdomadaire clinique, 1889, No. 57; Meyer in Raecke, Archiv f. Psych., 1903, Bd. 37, H. I; Turner, Jour, of Ment. Sci., October, 1903; Miller, Am. Jour. f. Ins., LX, No. 4, 1904; Frie auder, Monatschr. f. Psych., VI, 4491; Raimann, *idem.*, XII, 329.

There is still another form of postfebrile infection psychosis, different from any of the preceding forms, which is characterized by the sudden appearance of active excitement with clouding of consciousness, flight of ideas, and fantastic expansive delusions, simulating the symptoms of the expansive paretic. Following a few indefinite prodromal symptoms there appears first, usually during the febrile period, considerable restlessness, then disorientation, distractibility, and hallucinations of sight and hearing, and finally the most elaborate grandiose delusions. The patients also fabricate extensively. Emotionally, they are sometimes irritable, sometimes elated, but always changing rapidly from one state to another. There is absolutely no insight. In addition, the patients are productive and show a flight of ideas with a tendency to rhyming. The restlessness is so great that they cannot remain in bed. Little food is taken, sleep is scanty, and nutrition suffers greatly. This form follows typhoid. In part of the cases the *course* is rapid and the *outcome* favorable. After some months the excitement and the delusions gradually disappear. The patients, however, continue to be irritable, susceptible to fatigue, and upon slight mental application easily develop again flight of ideas and delusional fabrications, and may show a characteristic silly elation even when convalescence is well established. In a considerable number of cases dementia ensues. This form may be distinguished from *paresis* by the absence of physical signs. The treatment consists mostly of continued rest in bed, prolonged warm baths to alleviate the excitement, a nutritious diet, and very careful nursing.

II. EXHAUSTION PSYCHOSES

The exhaustion psychoses, collapse

delirium, amentia, and chronic nervous exhaustion, include those forms of mental disease that seem to arise from excessive exhaustion or insufficient restoration of the nervous elements in the cerebral cortex. The term "exhaustion " is most applicable to those psychoses that immediately follow a severe and radical change of the physical organism, such as that produced by acute diseases, excessive loss of blood, and childbirth. But even here one cannot always exclude the possibility of a toxaemia arising from an infectious organism or from the destruction of tissue. A more accurate knowledge may result in these forms being grouped elsewhere and ascribed to other etiological factors. This occurred in the case of "acute dementia," which is now classed in the group of post infection psychoses, except when it represents a phase in catatonia or manic-depressive insanity.

Collapse delirium and *amentia,* though they run a slightly different course, have many symptoms in common; namely, a profound disturbance of apprehension and of the coherence of thought, as well as hallucinations, flight of ideas, and psychomotor excitement. Exhaustion arising from more prolonged mental and emotional stress, or extended physical illness, produces the less acute but more chronic psychosis, *chronic nervous exhaustion* (acquired neurasthenia). *A.* Collapse Delirium

This psychosis is characterized by an acute onset with *profound clouding of consciousness, great incoherence of thought, dreamy hallucinations, a changeable emotional attitude, and great psychomotor activity, a rapid course, and a fairly favorable prognosis.*

Etiology. — Collapse delirium is a rare form of insanity. Among the exhausting conditions giving rise to it, childbirth is the most prominent; others are loss of blood, excessive mental strain, emotional shock, and deprivation with anxiety. The acute diseases which may lead to this condition are pneumonia and erysipelas. Oftentimes a fright occurring while the patient is in a weak condition acts as the exciting cause.

Pathological Anatomy. — Unfortunately but few cases have been examined pathologically. Alzheimer, in a case which seems to belong to this group, found throughout the cerebral cortex a fine granular disintegration of the chromatic substance, and without much involvement of the nucleus or increase of glia.

Symptomatology. — Following a few days of insomnia and restlessness, the patients rapidly become disoriented and everything about them seems changed and unnatural. Numerous dreamy *illusions* and *hallucinations* appear; the designs on the carpet assume the form of threatening figures, gas light appears like the sun, neighbors pass to and fro, beautiful music is heard, and patients pass through all sorts of dreamy experiences.

They become very talkative, the content of speech showing great incoherence with a *flight of ideas,* many alliterations, rhymes, and repetitions, which may be sung as well as spoken. Numerous *delusions* are expressed which are incoherent, changeable, and both exalted and depressive. In *emotional attitude* patients are much exalted and sometimes erotic; depression with anxiety, however, may predominate the emotional tone. Occasionally there is irritability with exhibitions of passion. Wandervereammlung d. suedwest Neurolog. u. Irrenraetze an Baden-Baden, 1897.

The *motor excitement* is very pronounced; patients remove their clothing, race about the room, overturn furniture, and pound the door. They are both destructive and untidy, and often exhibit the most reckless and impulsive movements. They prattle away incessantly, sometimes in a whisper, now at the top of their voice, and again gesticulating and clapping their hands. The *attention* cannot be attracted and questions are rarely answered. They will not obey requests, but almost always exhibit a purposeless resistance to everything, even to bathing and dressing.

Physically. — There is great insomnia. If the patients sleep at all, it is only for short intervals. Likewise they take

but little nourishment, and in many cases require mechanical feeding. The condition of nutrition is wretched, and there is a marked loss of flesh and physical weakness. The skin is pale and clammy, the temperature usually subnormal, and the pulse weak and irregular. The reflexes are usually exaggerated. Tremor is sometimes present and there is a tendency to acute decubitus.

Course. — The duration of the disease is brief, sometimes of only a few hours or days, and rarely lasting over one to two weeks. The return to consciousness is usually sudden, often following a sound sleep. When the patients awaken, the hallucinations and illusions have disappeared; they are conscious of their surroundings and ask for nourishment. They may continue talkative, perhaps showing a flight of ideas, some exaltation, grumbling, and fretful manners for several hours and even days. Brief relapses sometimes occur. As soon as nourishment is freely taken, the weight increases rapidly.

Diagnosis. — The differentiation from infection delirium has already been considered (see p. 130). The *epileptic befogged states* are distinguished by the greater clouding of consciousness, a more uniform emotional tone which is mostly anxious or ecstatic, and the fact that the activity does not conform to the thought or the emotional expressions. The *catatonic excitement* is recognized by the clearer orientation, and the characteristic catatonic movements. The delirious excitement of *dementia paralytica* can be differentiated only by the history of preceding mental deterioration and the presence of characteristic physical signs. The delirious mania of *manic-depressive* insanity, in the absence of a history of previous attacks, can be recognized only by a greater disturbance of apprehension and the very vivid hallucinosis. *Amentia* is differentiated by the longer course and distractibility of the attention.

Prognosis. — Recovery from the mental disorder is usual if the patients do not die from collapse.

Treatment. — The important indications are first to *maintain nutrition* and next to alleviate the excitement. The patients must, therefore, receive a sufficient quantity of liquid nourishment, in the accomplishment of which it is often necessary to resort to forced feeding by stomach or nasal tube. A little alcohol (one to two ounces) added to the milk and egg is extremely valuable. Broths and peptonized meats may be given in small quantities. Where mechanical feeding is contraindicated, because of vomiting or abrasion and hemorrhage of the mucous membrane, nutrient enemata can be substituted. Failing in this one can always resort to the hypodermoclysis of normal saline solution, one to two pints, with the expectation of securing excellent results, especially if there is impending collapse. The infusion should be given under low pressure in the back, rump, or breast.

In the alleviation of the *excitement,* by far the most efficient remedy is the prolonged warm bath, into which the patient should be placed at once and kept there until the excitement subsides. The bath should be maintained at ninety-five to ninety-eight degrees F. all the time. The patients may remain in the bath without fear of harm for hours and even days at a time, but usually they become quiet in less than an hour, when they should be returned to bed. As soon as the excitement reappears, they should again be placed in the bath. If the patients exhibit fear in entering the bath and require holding, the bath can do but little good. In such cases, one may give a hypodermic injection of hyoscine hydrobromate, - to *jfe* grain, or trional, 15 grains, shortly before the bath for the first few times. As soon as the patients become accustomed to the bath they usually like it, and some even fall asleep in it. If the bath is not available and one must resort to hypnotic and sedative drugs, hyoscine hydrobromate to grain and paraldehyde forty-five minims to one drachm may be relied upon for the best results. One should not be persuaded to overload the system with sedatives in an effort wholly to subdue the excitement in the hope of securing quiet for others. Excitement, of itself, is by no means the most serious symptom. It

is sufficient if you succeed in procuring even a few hours' sleep and prevent the patients from wholly exhausting themselves. Prolonged warm baths properly applied usually render unnecessary the use of sedatives. If the patients collapse, hot coffee by mouth or rectum, strychnia, dignitatis, or hypodermic injections of camphorated oil are indicated.

It is best that the patients be isolated in a quiet place, with sufficient attendance to control them at all times. Constant attendance must be enforced in order to prevent injuries, and this must be observed until convalescence is well established. Mechanical restraint should not be employed; a padded bed or room is preferable. During convalescence the same indications obtain here as in convalescence from any acute disease: careful feeding, graduated exercise, and freedom from all forms of excitement. Finally, one must be assured of complete recovery before the patients are permitted to resume their usual occupation or responsibilities. A good index of this is found in the weight, which should always return to normal.

B. Acute Confusional Insanity (amentia)

This form of exhaustion psychosis is characterized by the *rapid appearance of numerous illusions and hallucinations, clouding of consciousness, and motor excitement, with a duration of two to three months.*

Etiology. — The conditions of exhaustion giving rise to amentia are chiefly childbirth, also acute illnesses, excessive loss of blood, excessive mental strain, and night watching. An emotional shock may be the final exciting factor. Women are more frequently affected than men. Cases of amentia represent about one-half to one per cent. of the admissions to hospitals.

Symptomatology. — At first the patients are anxious, restless, and forgetful, sometimes complaining of numbness and confusion in the head, and inability to gather their thoughts or concentrate their attention. In the course of a few days disorientation appears; the surroundings seem changed, and they do not recognize relatives. *Hallucina-*

tions of the different senses appear. They see strange faces and hear strange voices, birds are flying about, lions are roaring, poisonous powder is thrown at them, and they are threatened and cursed by strangers. The numerous hallucinations form the basis for many depressive *delusions,* which are dreamy, incoherent, contradictory, and often repeated. Their children are dead, the home is lost, they are to be hung, are under the influence of some magnetic power which draws them about, and in the end will consume them. In a few cases the delusions are expansive; they then believe themselves exalted to some high position, possessed of great wealth, or they have journeyed around the world. They will convene Congress, and send an army to Cuba. They sometimes fabricate extensively.

The *attention* is attracted by the surroundings and the patients endeavor to grasp what transpires. It is usually possible, also, to direct the train of thought by objects held before them, by movements and gestures; but they understand readily only the simplest occurrences. Some patients claim that everything is changed, things are not genuine, the chairs and windows are not the same to-day as yesterday, the thermometer is not correct, the clock is not right, and the papers are incorrectly dated. Often the patients appreciate this inability to understand things, and complain that they cannot "think right " or that some one "has made them crazy."

There is marked *disturbance of the train of thought.* The patients are unable to complete one idea before others interrupt, producing a flight of ideas. Words and sounds caught up from the surroundings find a place in their expression, though not necessarily influencing or directing the train of thought. The speech is sometimes made up of single, incoherent, and disjointed words and phrases. Occasionally sound associations and rhymes are heard. In spite of distractibility and flight of ideas, one occasionally finds the patients holding to single indefinite ideas, usually of persecution. The *consciousness* is much clouded. The persistence of clouded consciousness, with difficulty in arranging the impressions and ideas, is a characteristic and striking feature during the intervals when the patients are quiet and present a normal emotional attitude.

The *emotional attitude* varies considerably, sometimes with prevailing happiness, but more often with depression. Alternations of the attitude are characteristic; for short periods the patients may be elated, and hilarious, with perhaps some sexual excitement, when they suddenly become excited and irritable, or they may even be dull and stupid.

In the *psychomotor* field there is a marked pressure of activity. They move about restlessly, crawl in and out of bed, destroy clothing, pound and beat, but the movements are not very quick, are performed without display of much energy, and are planless. The motor excitement is distinctly intermittent, there being intervals of complete quiet.

Physically. — The sleep is much disturbed, the appetite is poor, and sometimes there is complete refusal of food. The body weight falls, but the condition of nutrition is better than in collapse delirium. The deep reflexes are increased, the pulse slow, and the temperature subnormal.

Course. — The height of the disease is usually reached within two weeks, during which time there may have been remissions of a few hours or even a day with clear consciousness, insight, and disappearance of hallucinations. From this tune the symptoms present characteristic fluctuations. The more active symptoms may disappear, and the patients become more coherent in speech, when again they develop excitement. Genuine improvement develops gradually. Even after they have become clear, long conversations or letter-writing tend to create confusion. In the lighter cases, which are the more numerous, even after the patients have become quite clear, the emotional attitude may show a slightly elated or depressed condition, as seen in hyperactivity and garrulity, or distrust, anxiety, and irritability. The entire course is from three to four months. In the severer cases, lasting some months, even when the patients have become clear, a few hallucinations may persist for a short time, and occasionally indefinite and transitory expansive or depressive delusions are expressed. The patients may appear unnatural and irritable and show outbursts of passion. Even after all the symptoms of the disease have disappeared, the patients are very apt to show increased susceptibility to fatigue, while for many months emotional shocks or injuries are prone to create relapses. The weight rises rapidly during convalescence.

Diagnosis. — The manic form of *manic-depressive* insanity is distinguished from amentia by the fact that there is less disturbance of apprehension than of the psychomotor sphere; in the manic state, in spite of great motor excitement, the patients usually give evidence of at least a partial comprehension of the environment. Again in amentia the movements are slower, more planless, and less precipitous, and, in quiet intervals, when there is no activity, the patients are still hazy and confused. The condition of *catatonic excitement* is distinguished by the fact that the catatonic patients in the midst of the greatest excitement are usually able to comprehend their surroundings, to reckon time correctly, to recognize persons, and to record some passing events. The amentia patients even during quiet are somewhat disoriented and fail to recall passing events. Furthermore, the characteristic catatonic features are absent. To be sure, catalepsy and automatism may be present, but genuine negativism, verbigeration, stereotypy, mutism, and mannerism are absent.

Prognosis. — Death rarely occurs except as the result of suicide, of collapse during the intense excitement at the onset, or precarious physical conditions; as, heart failure, sepsis, and phthisis. The patients almost always fully recover their mental health.

Treatment. — The indications for treatment are identical with those in collapse delirium; namely, maintenance of nutrition and the alleviation of the excitement (see p. 140). On account of the great tendency to relapse, one should be extremely careful about allowing the patients to enter an environment in which they might be subjected to an emotional shock. For this same reason, one cannot resist too long the entreaties of the patients and their relatives that they be allowed to enter their accustomed life, before they have regained their normal weight, the menses have reappeared, and the emotional attitude has become wholly stable.

0. ACQUIRED NEURASTHENIA
Chronic Nervous Exhaustion
Acquired neurasthenia is characterized by a *diminished power of attention, distractibility, defective mental application, difficulty of thinking, an increased susceptibility to fatigue, increased emotional irritability, and a great variety of physical symptoms, mostly subjective, including hypochondriasis.*

Acquired neurasthenia must be clearly distinguished from the psychopathic states or congenital neurasthenia (see p. 155). No doubt there are many transitional states between the two diseases, and especially where both defective heredity and exhaustion are prominent factors. The difference in the symptoms, their course and outcome, in individuals free from hereditary taints, it seems, is sufficiently distinctive to justify the restricted use of the term acquired neurasthenia.

Etiology. — The real nature of the disease has been most logically pointed out by Mobius, who claims that there is a kind of chronic intoxication resulting from the effects of exhaustion upon nervous tissue, corresponding in a measure to the intoxication resulting from the prolonged excessive use of alcohol. This view, certainly, is helpful because it offers a clearer conception of the disease and aids in distinguishing between those cases which simply involve an accumulation of the effects of fatigue and those in which the morbid hereditary and inherently impaired powers of resistance play the essential r61e (congenital neurasthenia).

The rapid, irregular, and extravagant manner of living, with little relaxation and lack of sufficient and wholesome sleep in individuals actively engaged in business or taxed with the responsibilities of the household, is distinctively characteristic of the American people in the temperate regions, and accounts for the great prevalence of this disease in our nation. Besides excessive mental application, the worry attendant upon responsibility is an important factor. On the other hand, prolonged and excessive physical exertion is at times undoubtedly an important factor in producing neurasthenia, particularly excessive bodily exercise, as is occasionally seen in sports, such as golf, rowing, basket ball, etc. But of especial importance are our faulty methods of living, with insufficient relaxation and improper nourishment. Moreover, considerable depends upon the individual powers of resistance. This is particularly applicable to that considerable group of individuals, who always feel unequal to the demands made upon them and find themselves quickly and completely exhausted upon any strenuous effort.

Of the men, naturally those who are more talented, better educated, and more active, are the individuals who most often suffer from this disease. Indeed, it is a fact worthy of note that great capacity for work is frequently accompanied by greater susceptibility to fatigue. Women, because of their weaker powers of resistance and their greater emotional irritability, are more susceptible than men, particularly the overburdened mothers, teachers, and nurses. The disease may appear at all ages, but is most often met between the ages of twenty-five and forty-five, the period of life during which the greatest mental strain occurs. At an earlier age it is seen in ambitious students who apply themselves too closely to studies without relaxation. Occasionally symptoms, which differ in no respect from those described here, develop after emotional shocks and acute illnesses, especially influenza, childbirth, loss of blood, and operations. The "nervous weakness" which appears during convalescence from severe illness is only in part due to simple exhaustion. It is doubtful if the disease ever develops after a fright.

Symptomatology. — Prolonged work produces fatigue and with it difficulty of further application. Up to a certain degree, this fatigue, which may be considered as a safeguard against overwork, may be overcome by an increased exertion of will power, which in long and fatiguing work gives rise to a feeling of " increased effort." Associated with this there soon develops a characteristic feeling of disinclination and then a fagging of the will, and when this appears the danger of overexertion is relieved. While the increased exertion of the will can for a time balance the effects of fatigue through an increased expenditure of power, the effects of fatigue ultimately gain the upper hand and force one to cease work.

The first indications of exhaustion are when, under certain conditions, the increased exertion of will continues for some time in spite of the uncomfortable feeling of fatigue. This is what happens when work is performed under intense emotional excitement. The signs of fatigue, which call for relaxation, either do not appear or are overwhelmed, and work is prolonged beyond a permissible degree. This in time leads, on the one hand, to an exhaustion of the available supply of strength, which recuperates only very slowly, and is manifested by a sort of *prolonged weariness,* which persists after relaxation and is still present to some extent when work is again undertaken. It also involves an increased susceptibility to *fatigue* and a more rapid diminution of the capacity for work. On the other hand, under such circumstances, the increased exertion of the will also persists and brings with it an increased emotional irritability.

Unfortunately, there are as yet no experiments on the effect of prolonged overexertion on the mind. But we know from long experience, that, first of all, the *ability to continuously exert the attention fails.* The patient is easily distracted by little things and is inattentive. He is no longer able to think clearly and sharply, and requires much more time for his accustomed work. He is also apt to be forgetful of names and figures, so that the same work has to be done over

several times before he is sure of his results.

His susceptibility to fatigue is greatly increased, and his work is carried out only with constantly increasing difficulty, requiring greater exertion and more frequent rests. As the result of this difficulty of work, the patient also loses the wonted pleasure in his occupation. He finds that he is compelled to force himself to the work which he previously performed with ease and pleasure. He, furthermore, shrinks from new undertakings because of obstacles which appear unsurmountable.

Under the influence of these conditions, the *emotional attitude* also becomes changed. The patients become easily flustered, are ill-humored, unreasonable, peevish, faultfinding, irritable, and impetuous. Customary amusements fail to please, and they become discontented with their occupation. Trifling affairs, like the misconduct of a child, inconveniences at work, which normally would pass unnoticed, disturb them for hours and even days, and may lead to impulsive outbursts, which they later regret.

The patients have not only a keen insight into these defects, but also a tendency to exaggerate their symptoms. They assert that the memory is becoming profoundly affected, and that the judgment is failing. The physical symptoms are even more strongly exaggerated, which aids in increasing their misery. The excessive anxiety about their condition of health leads to a characteristic symptom, *hypochondriasis,* in which there is a tendency to pay undue attention to any trifling symptoms that may be present. They believe that they are suffering from some incurable disease, and especially the one most dreaded. There may be some genuine disorder, but the real symptoms are greatly enhanced by the attention habitually paid to them. Canker in the mouth is considered infallible evidence of syphilis, a cloudy urine indicates Bright's disease, and a cough means consumption. In the beginning these fears may not be considered in a very serious light, but when they interfere with the livelihood of the patients they may lead to such feelings of despair that the patients no longer hope for recovery, make their wills, and not infrequently attempt suicide.

The appreciation of their incapacity creates a feeling of reserve, timidity, and a lack of self-confidence. They cannot trust themselves in public and fear fainting upon the slightest exertion. Associated with the loss of willpower, there should also be mentioned the tendency to compulsive thoughts and impulsive acts, which sometimes explain the suicidal attempts. Here are included the various phobias, which are fully described in the constitutional psychopathic states. In the strife to overcome impulsive ideas, the patients often reach an emotional crisis of short duration, with restlessness, wringing of the hands, crying and moaning, and even attempts at suicide. These states are more apt to follow continued excitations, such as prolonged visits or unusual noisiness.

Physical symptoms. — These form a very characteristic feature of the psychosis. Among the most important symptoms are headache, insomnia, general muscular weakness, paraesthesias, cardiac and gastro-intestinal disturbances. *Cephalalgia,* which appears early, may be expressed as a headache, a feeling of numbness or a pressure in the head, which interferes with work. This is usually situated over the eyes or in the occiput, and increases with exertion until it becomes unendurable. It is more prominent in the morning and passes off during the day. Sometimes there is a feeling of pressure, as if the head were held in a vice or by a constricting band. It may be associated with vertigo, dimness of vision, roaring in the ears, or painful pressure points in the scalp.

Insomnia is usually an aggravating symptom from the onset. The few hours of sleep, obtained either immediately upon retiring, or in the early morning, after hours of restless tossing, are unrefreshing and disturbed by dreams. In some cases, there is an unnatural drowsiness which causes the patients to fall to sleep at all times and particularly after some exertion. General muscular weakness is always in evidence; patients are always languid, and tire easily upon walking or from slight muscular effort.

Both the superficial and deep reflexes may be increased. Rhythmic twitchings are occasionally noticed, particularly twitching of individual muscles and especially those of the eye. Moderate stuttering is sometimes complained of. There is slight tremor of the eyelids and hands, but usually a marked fibrillary tremor of the tongue. Subjective sensations, variously located, are prominent, such as paraesthesias or feelings of formication in the trunk and limbs, also darting pains and burning sensations.

The patients are usually alarmed by various cardiac sensations; such as a gnawing or burning sensation, palpitation and precordial pain and pulsations in different parts of the body. The pulse rate varies considerably and is easily influenced by work or emotional excitement. Associated with the cardiac disturbances or occurring independently, there may be vasomotor disorders; as cold extremities, localized sweating, and blushing or abnormal dryness of the skin.

The appetite is variable and anorexia is frequent, but the *nervous dyspepsia,* gastric and intestinal, is by far the most prominent digestive disorder. When the stomach is empty, there is usually present a gnawing sensation which is quickly relieved by eating. Gastric fermentation, probably due in part to deficiency of the digestive fluids, especially hydrochloric acid, causes distention of the stomach, accompanied with discomfort and pain. Extending into the intestines, the fermentation gives rise to borborygmus and colicky pains, the latter of which may be severe enough to simulate genuine colic. The digestion is usually not impaired sufficiently to create disturbances of nutrition, but in severe cases it may even cause cachexia and anaemia. The bowels are usually constipated and the tongue coated. Diarrhoeas are apt to appear for short periods, and may be persistent for a considerable time.

In the sexual life there is more often a loss of sexual desire, but in a few cases there is a tendency to excessive indulgence, although at the same time patients may complain of impotence.

In those cases in which there is frequent recurrence, the patients tend to become chronic invalids of a most distressing type. They go the round of physicians, pass from one sanitarium to another, taking all kinds of drugs. Mentally, they pass into a state of lethargy in which all thought centers about their own misery. All attempts at business are abandoned, and the cares of the household are renounced. They betake themselves to the seclusion of a charitable institution with its freedom from annoyances, or if they remain at home, demand the utmost consideration for every whim. They have no thought for the maintenance of the family or appreciation of the burden which they create. The increasing demand for sympathy leads to prevarications and to various assumed contortions, in order to assure the physicians or friends that they are in a critical condition. The daily greeting from one patient was, " My God, doctor, I am dying! Just feel of my abdomen. Have you no compassion for a dying man?" A female patient remained in bed for years, and when received at the hospital from the hands of a tender-hearted mother, had not had her hair combed in two years, and one of her toe nails had grown to the length of five inches. It is this class of patients who eventually become habitues of morphin, cocain, chloral, antipyrin, and other drugs.

Course. — The onset of the disease is gradual. It may, however, develop rapidly, following an acute illness, especially influenza and also childbirth. There is a great variation in the prominence of the symptoms. A daily improvement toward evening is characteristic. Under stress of circumstances, the patients are usually able to pull themselves together for a special occasion, but the following day witnesses an exacerbation of the symptoms. The course is often protracted and the convalescence gradual.

Diagnosis. — The differentiation of neurasthenia from other forms of mental disease is of the greatest importance because of its bearing upon the prognosis and treatment. In the first place it is necessary to exclude organic disease of the internal organs. The diagnosis of neurasthenia should rather be reached by a process of exclusion, after a most thorough physical examination.

The psychoses most apt to be confounded with neurasthenia are dementia paralytica, dementia praecox, and melancholia of involution. The difficulties in *dementia paralytica* arise only in the first stages of the disease. Signs of nervousness without definite cause in a man of healthy constitution, appearing for the first time in middle life, should at least arouse suspicion of dementia paralytica. In neurasthenia the alleged memory defect varies from day to day, is easily corrected upon effort, and does not show the defective time element which is so characteristic of the defective memory in the paretic. Neurastheniacs complain of mental impairment, but are able to amend errors in writing and speech, while the real mental defect in the paretic is unrecognized, or, if recognized, its extent is not appreciated. The defect, therefore, in the work of a neurastheniac is quantitative, while that in the paretic is qualitative. The symptoms of the neurastheniac ameliorate as the day advances, so that the evening finds him at his best; on the other hand, the paretic usually awakens refreshed, and more capable, but fatigues more during the day. Again, the neurastheniac has a keen insight into his condition, and tends to exaggerate his symptoms, but the paretic has little or no insight, or, if present, he rather minimizes than exaggerates his symptoms. The sensory disturbances of the neurastheniac are mostly subjective, while those of the paretic are objective. The presence of the characteristic physical signs of paresis should leave no doubt; such as, Argyl Robertson pupil, increased myotatic irritability, ataxia in speech and gait, tremor of the facial muscles and of the tongue, epileptiform or apoplectiform attacks, etc.

The depressive phases of the other psychoses, especially *dementia prœcox* and *melancholia,* are distinguished with difficulty, particularly where these psychoses follow some acute disease, or appear in neuropathic individuals who have succumbed in the struggle with more favorably endowed associates. While the neurastheniac is ill-humored and irritable because he appreciates that his mental ability is impaired, his emotional attitude becomes happier just as soon as some external excitement or a jolly company allows him to forget his troubles, or as soon as he is relieved of the responsibilities of his occupation, and can secure the benefit of rest and relaxation. In the despondency of other psychoses there develops a feeling of anxiety and sadness without any good reason, which, under the influence of distraction, is not only not alleviated but may even be intensified. The diminution in the power of comprehension and the ill-humor at the onset of dementia praecox is recognized especially by the dulness of the patient, his indifference to the future, and sometimes also by the senselessness of his hypochondriacal complaints.

Where the external causes of exhaustion are comparatively insignificant one naturally suspects that there is at the bottom a constitutional nervous weakness, which demands not rest and relaxation but exercise and occupation. While very sharp distinctions cannot be drawn between these states, yet there are some symptoms in *congenital neurasthenia* which are rarely, or to only an insignificant degree, found in simple neurasthenia; namely, the great susceptibility of the individual symptoms to mental suggestion, especially the abrupt fluctuations of the emotional attitude, the anxious states, and the lack of strength.

Prognosis. — The prognosis in simple nervous exhaustion is regarded as favorable, but it depends upon the extent to which the exciting causes can be removed, as well as upon the individual's powers of resistance. Under proper treatment most patients greatly improve, but the probability of a return of the disease sooner or later becomes much greater, if the patient must enter his old environment and undertake the same responsibilities that lead to the first breakdown. The more frequent the recurrence of the disease, the less liable is the patient ever to regain his former health.

Treatment. — Where possible, it is the duty of the family physician to bear in mind prophylaxis. Individuals who are handicapped by a defective heritage must be well guarded during their development, with due attention to moral and physical hygiene. Later, when it becomes necessary to enter actively into the severer duties of life, the limitation of mental application and physical exertion, together with the avoidance of worriment and anxiety, must be constantly kept in mind.

In the treatment of the disease after its development, the individuality of the physician is of prime importance; he must recognize and utilize his power of influence over the patient in addition to various therapeutical agencies. It requires confidence in order to inspire the patient and to lift him from his morbid anxiety and depression. *Isolation* with a changed routine of life demands immediate attention. In the lighter cases a trip to the mountains or a sea voyage to relieve the asthenic condition, or where this is impracticable, removal from the customary surroundings into a quiet, restful, but attractive place, will accomplish the same result.

Next, *insomnia* must be combated. Enforced rest in bed with change of environment, removal of cares and relaxation, and the establishment of a fixed routine usually relieve the sleeplessness. At any rate, one should not have to employ sedatives until the patient has had a chance to react to the new method of life. Before resorting to the use of drugs, the simple hypnotic measures should be exhausted; such as, warm liquid nourishment upon retiring, a hot bath, gentle massage, etc. If it seems necessary to resort to drugs, then employ the triple bromides in five-grain doses repeated every half hour for five doses if necessary, administered on alternate nights with trional, veronal, or somnos.

Hydriatics are of great service in this disease, the most serviceable methods being the cold ablutions, the spray, the simple douche, and the dripping sheet. In the last method, which may be carried out at home, after a cold ablution, eighty-five to seventy-five degrees, the patient standing in warm water, or on a dry surface, with a cold towel about the head, a linen sheet dipped into water seventy-five to fiftyfive degrees, is wound dripping about the patient, the nurse at the same time applying friction until a thorough reaction takes place. The douche, as carried out at bath institutions, is of great value.

In the more severe cases, the secret of successful treatment lies in a well-regulated routine suited somewhat to the tastes of the individuals, but requiring of all a definite amount of sleep, nourishment, mental and physical exercise, alternated with rest and relaxation, together with baths and outof-door life. All of this may be carried out under the supervision of a physician who is willing to spend time and thought in attending to the details. The relative amount of exercise and forced rest must vary in individual cases. The anaemic and debilitated who have been exhausted by long suffering or the prolonged care of invalids, together with anxiety and worriment, require forced rest for a few weeks with a full nutritious diet, massage, and passive movements. Others, from the beginning, need graduated daily exercise, which must be purposeful and suited somewhat to the tastes. The diet, also, must depend upon the condition of the nutrition. Where indigestion or constipation exists, the usual means should be used to counteract these conditions, always giving preference to physical agencies. Electricity and massage are of value, but only secondary to the above methods. Sometimes local treatment is called for in correcting uterine troubles, errors of optical refraction, or in removing nasal obstructions.

Finally, the patient should not be considered suitable for discharge until you have placed her beyond the danger of relapse. This involves on her part a thorough understanding of the conditions leading to her breakdown, and requires an inculcation of the correct principles of living and working and an appreciation of her own limitations. Such training should be established early, and throughout the period of treatment no opportunity should be lost in impressing these ideas upon her mind.

III. INTOXICATION PSYCHOSES

The term intoxication psychoses is here used in a narrow sense to include all psychoses arising from toxic substances taken into the body.

They are divided into *acute* and *chronic intoxications,* according to the length of the time during which the toxic substances have been ingested.

1. ACUTE INTOXICATIONS.

The acute intoxications are characterized in common by a delirious state of short duration, with pronounced psychosensory disturbance, dreamy fantastic delusions, pleasurable emotional attitude, often with conditions of ecstasy, and without much motor excitement.

The number of toxic substances, including ptomaines, which might be mentioned here is large. The transitory character and the infrequency of the toxic deliria make them of little importance to the clinician. They are, however, of great scientific value to investigators, who are able to study pathologically and psychologically the effects of the different toxic substances. Some of them which are characterized by peculiar mental symptoms will be mentioned here. The mental state produced by *chloroform* is characterized by hallucinations of sight only. In *santonin* poisoning there are hallucinations of sight in which everything appears yellow; *hasheesh* delirium is characterized by disturbance of the taste and muscle senses.

Hasheesh and opium smoking produce a complacent feeling of well-being, and of a dreamy, pleasurable existence. The *carbonic acid* narcosis is characterized by its short duration and the presence of pronounced sexual hallucinations. In the toxic condition produced by *atropin* there is a severe disturbance of apprehension, with isolated hallucinations, marked confusion of thought, elated emotional attitude, and active motor excitement. The course is either fatal or the psychosis clears very quickly with no recollection of the events.

The duration of all these conditions is short, from a few hours to a few days at the most. The prognosis depends entirely upon the severity of the intoxication. In diagnosis one must rely in great measure upon the knowledge of the circumstances and upon the physical signs. The treatment is limited to the employment of means to rid the body of the toxic substance, and the application of special antidotes.

The psychosis produced by lead poisoning, *encephalopathia saturninia,* is more frequent and differs from the above delirious states by its longer duration, characteristic nervous symptoms, and poorer prognosis. The physical symptoms usually precede the mental disturbance; that is, wrist drop, peroneal paralysis, tremor, pains in the limbs, and sometimes colic. The immediate prodromes are restlessness and headache. The onset of the delirium may be acute or subacute. There are many hallucinations of sight and hearing, great psychomotor disturbance, many delusions with great fear, and complete clouding of consciousness.

The speech is incoherent, and in the height of the delirium there are frequent reckless impulsive movements. There is complete insomnia, and very little nourishment is taken. The active excitement is followed by a condition of stupor or coma, sometimes antedated by stupor with excitement.

Epileptiform convulsions may also appear, and amblyopia is frequent. The convalescence is gradual, extending over several weeks. Some cases terminate fatally in coma. While most of the patients recover, there are many who, upon regaining clear consciousness, present a degree of mental enfeeblement in which simple apathy is a prominent feature. A few present progressive muscular atrophy, simulating dementia paralytica. The whole duration of the psychosis in favorable cases is from a few weeks to three months.

2. CHRONIC INTOXICATION

Of the many toxic substances whose continued use leads to disturbances of the mind, those best known and of most clinical value are alcohol, morphin, and cocain. Almost all nations, according to anthropological data, have had a drug whose habitual use has been a source of danger to its people. It is a striking fact that these substances have always been used first for medical purposes, and later continued for their exhilarating and alleged supportive effect.

A. Alcoholism

The acute intoxication of alcohol is described here rather than under the acute intoxications, because of its close association with chronic alcoholism.

Acute alcoholic intoxication produces at first a diminution of the power of apprehension and elaboration of external impressions, and an acceleration in the release of voluntary impulses. The perception of simple sensory impressions is difficult, sluggish, and uncertain. An attempt to solve a simple problem shows a distinct diminution in intellectual power.

In speech one can discern that the association of ideas most closely related to the motor elements of speech is prominent, such as the use of compound words and rhymes. The release of motor impulses is much accelerated so that those expressions find utterance most readily that are most familiar. The choice between two movements is precipitous, frequently incorrect, and sometimes already executed before the proper direction is determined upon. Later, or following larger doses, the psychomotor activity is displaced by paralysis, the rapidity and extent of the paralysis depending both upon the amount taken and the susceptibility of the individual. The muscular strength, at first slightly increased, is soon much diminished.

Even small doses influence the capacity for good mental work. Thoughts are not easily gathered, rendering the solution of complicated problems very difficult. This increases with the amount taken. A thoroughly intoxicated man is unable to comprehend what is said to him or what goes on about him, cannot maintain his attention or direct the train of thought. He has no conception of the significance or the bearing of his actions. The internal association of the train of thought is very much disturbed, as indicated by the tendency to the repetition of phrases and the use of commonplace remarks, also in the fondness for quoting obscene rhymes and in the use of jargon. Finally apprehension may be so far lost that he becomes insensible and unconscious. Memory of events of the intoxicated state is very meagre.

In the psychomotor field, at first, there is a light grade of overactivity, with the disappearance of the usual restraints which regulate the actions of our daily lives. He is active, gay, free and jolly, speaks and acts without restraint, and even becomes reckless. The ready release of motor impulses promotes the feeling of increased muscular strength. Later the motor excitation increases; the facial expression loses its character, each action is exaggerated; the voice is louder, and the smile broadens into laughter. He becomes profane, grumbles, and growls. He is hasty and passionate, and a single word or a trifling accident suffices to start a quarrel or to lead to an assault. Finally the excitation, as the disturbance of apprehension increases, is replaced by signs of paralysis, and there is a profound disturbance of speech, a staggering gait, and even complete motor paralysis.

The emotions at first give way to a feeling of well-being. There is a certain degree of exhilaration, and freedom from care. He becomes light-hearted and happy. Later irritability appears. Higher moral feelings are lost. He is shameless, and because of the increased sexual excitability is often led to filthy excesses.

The duration of the intoxication depends much upon the individual. It usually disappears quite rapidly, although ill effects may be observed for twenty-four to thirtysix hours later: headache, lassitude, nausea, and anorexia. Fatigue predisposes to rapid appearance of paralytic signs, even without the intervention of the period of excitation. Individuals who are rendered sluggish and sleepy are apt also to be quarrelsome, aggressive, mischievous, and even cruel.

As the result of experimental investigations of acute intoxication in test animals, Nissl has demonstrated a profound change in the cortical neurones, seen in the destruction of many cells, in the fading and the irregular amalgamation of the Nissl granules, the diminution in size and irregularity of the nucleus, whose membrane and nucleolus may finally disappear. Dehio has observed similar changes in Purkinje cells.

Chronic Alcoholism

Chronic alcoholic intoxication depends upon a chronic degenerative process in the central nervous system, and is characterized by a *gradually progressive dementia, with diminished capacity for work, faulty judgment, defective memory, moral deterioration, occasional delusions, infrequent hallucinations, and various nervous symptoms.*

Etiology. — Defective heredity is an important etiological factor, and is manifested by a diminished power of resistance in the individual. Some observers have reported as high as eighty per cent. of cases with defective heredity, in at least one-half of whom the father had been a chronic drinker. Head injury, according to Moli, in twentytwo per cent. of the cases, has been regarded as a factor in producing lessened resistance to alcohol. Male alcoholics greatly predominate. At Heidelberg only six per cent. were women. Hirschl, in Vienna, found among the male insane thirty per cent. alcoholics and among the women only four per cent. alcoholics. Alcoholism is more prevalent among those who come in contact with it, especially the bartenders, liquor dealers, brewers, and waiters. The extensive use of alcoholic drinks by many classes of society and the laxness of public sentiment in regard to it should also be regarded as etiological factors. Furthermore, the ignorance of most people as to its proven deleterious effects is in a measure an important element. There are thousands upon thousands who daily take a little beer, wine, or liquor because they are convinced that " it does them good," and strengthens them.

Pathological Anatomy.—In the brain, in advanced cases, there is regularly more or less chronic leptomeningitis and pachymeningitis with or without haematoma. The cerebrum is below normal in weight, its convolutions more or less shrunken, and its ventricles dilated, the ependyma of which in rare instances is granular. The larger vessels at the base and in the fissures present arteriosclerotic patches or atheroma, but the most characteristic lesion is the endarteritis, mostly localized, of the small terminal arteries of the cortex and other parts of the brain. The cortical neurones present a gradual sclerosis, called the "chronic change of Nissl." Nissl, in his experimental research with chronic alcoholism, in test animals, found a moderate thickening of the pia, especially at the base, destruction of many of the cortical neurones, with an increase of neuroglia, and besides these other extensive characteristic cortical changes, the meaning of which is still unknown. Alterations in the internal organs are equally prominent; namely, chronic gastritis, cirrhosis of the liver, chronic nephritis, fatty infiltration of the myocardium, and chronic endocarditis with greater or less degree of general arteriosclerosis.

Symptomatology. — There is a gradual and progressive enfeeblement of the intellectual faculties. The capacity for work is first to suffer. The power of mental application gradually fails, it becomes difficult to maintain the attention, and the susceptibility to fatigue increases. New and unaccustomed work requires unusual application and is accomplished only with difficulty. Patients prefer to continue in the same old ruts, and are indifferent in applying themselves to any mental work. Consequently intellectual development not only ceases, but retrogrades, showing an increasing lack in judgment and a poverty of ideas, enhanced by a gradual failure of memory. Finally there is in-

ability to acquire anything new, important facts are forgotten, and the past is recalled only as a somewhat confused and distorted picture. The defects of judgment and memory offer a fertile soil for the development of numerous more or less pronounced delusions. These delusions tend to show a striking lack of judgment, are peculiarly ideas of injury, which sometimes take their origin from isolated hallucinations, but more frequently from genuine perceptions which are falsely interpreted. In the more severe cases, a condition of advanced deterioration is reached.

Moral deterioration is a prominent and characteristic symptom. There is a profound change in moral character, and the patients soon lose sight of the higher ideals of life and the sense of honor. This is especially noticeable in their own estimation of their alcoholic habits. They disregard their depravity with nonchalance, and claim that the liquor, taken for their physical benefit, does them no harm. When reprimanded for continued inebriety, they accuse a friend of having given them the liquor, or claim that they are driven to drink by their wives. A faithful promise to abstain from further use of alcohol may be volunteered by an habitu6; but when encountered coming from a saloon an hour later, he fails to show any feeling of shame.

Some claim that their work necessitates stimulation; others take only as much as can be regarded as a food. It is of interest to note the variety of conflicting excuses offered by mechanics for the necessity of taking liquor: the cook, the fireman, and the iron moulder require it because of the great heat; while the night watchman, the truckman, and the iceman need it to keep off the cold. Many are driven to drink by unfortunate circumstances at home; the death of a relative, a sick child, and an ugly wife are frequent incentives.

The patients lose all affection for their families, become indifferent to the tears of their children, have little interest in their welfare, disregard the real infidelity of *their* wives, at the same time developing a certain exaggerated

feeling of self-importance, noticeable especially in conversation. They are unable to take matters seriously, and display an unnatural sense of humor, — *drunkard's humor.*

There is a corresponding increase of emotional irritability, which is more evident during intoxication. Patients are quarrelsome, engage in strife and abuse on small provocation, misuse their children, and are destructive of clothing and furniture. Their complete and abject submission when opposed by a superior force or when incarcerated is in marked contrast to their behavior at home. Their inoffensive behavior and attitude of humiliation before others often excites sympathy from the inexperienced.

They become entirely unstable, cannot remain at home, visit from saloon to saloon, tramp from one city to another, and engage in their usual occupation only for a few days or hours at a time, offering the excuse that they are physically unfit for continued labor. They leave the support of the family to the wife and children, whom they browbeat for enough money to keep them in liquor. Others degrade themselves by pawning clothing and furniture, and even steal in order to satisfy their appetite.

Physically. — The most prominent physical symptoms are: fine tremor, noticed first in the more delicate movements and later becoming general; muscular weakness with atrophy; uncertainty in gait; defective speech, sometimes thick, sometimes slurring, with occasional aphasic symptoms; peripheral neuritis; frequent headaches and sometimes vertigo. The tendon reflexes are often increased, rarely lost. In the sensory field there are frequently found areas of hyperaesthesia, anaesthesia, paraesthesia, as well as painful pressure points. Epileptoid attacks occur in about ten to thirty-five per cent. of the cases, usually during an attack of delirium tremens or at the conclusion of a spree, but also during the course of chronic alcoholism and even after more or less prolonged abstinence. They occur mostly in persons addicted to distilled liquors, and differ from genuine epileptic attacks in that they are infrequent, but unusually severe, while the absences, ill-temper, and befogged states peculiar to epilepsy are absent. Furthermore, the epileptic attacks usually, but not always, disappear with enforced abstinence.

In the sexual life there gradually develops, in spite of increased sexual irritability, impotency which often leads to jealousy and fornication. Furthermore, the progeny is rendered not only susceptible to alcoholism, but is particularly apt to exhibit evidences of defective physical and mental development, and also epilepsy. The rate of mortality of the children of alcoholic mothers is twice as great during the first two years of life as of non-alcoholic mothers. This rate also increases with successive childbearing, reaching as high as seventy-two per cent.

Prognosis. — The chances of recovery depend upon the extent of mental deterioration and the character of the treatment. If the patients already show moral deterioration, prolonged treatment is apt to be of little avail; each time they relapse into their former habits, becoming at last mental and physical wrecks. Cases when taken early and submitted to an extended treatment have a fair prospect of complete recovery. In many reputable inebriate institutions from one-fourth to one-third of their cases recover permanently.

Diagnosis. — The recognition of chronic alcoholism presents few difficulties in view of the history, the typical facies, and the physical symptoms, the latter being at times made more evident by the presence of neuritic symptoms.

Treatment. — The successful treatment of chronic alcoholism demands complete abstinence from alcohol in every form. A few patients are capable of carrying out this injunction successfully by themselves, but the vast majority, and especially those whose occupation brings them into bad associations, require the treatment afforded by a special institution for alcoholics. The success of this or any other plan of treatment in the chronic alcoholic is materially impeded by the general indifference of the environment and the attitude

of physicians. Very many physicians, wholly ignorant of the favorable results of treatment in reputable institutions, injudiciously advise the friends that it is of no use to waste money in a long sojourn at an institution. Even institution physicians are not beyond criticism in this respect, and will force the patient's discharge "as soon as the drink is out of him." If the patient himself does not appreciate the necessity of treatment or because of delusions resists any restriction of his liberty, then one must resort to a legal commitment to an institution, which is now possible in many states even for a period of two years.

As soon as the patient is committed to your care the alcohol can be suddenly withdrawn, except in a few cases where there is a disturbance of the heart. The abstinence symptoms, insomnia, anorexia, and occasional hallucinations, which arise in consequence of withdrawal, tend to quickly disappear, and should cause no alarm. Improvement begins in a few days, and progresses gradually. If the patient is received in a condition of drunkenness, ergot administered in fifteen-minim doses and repeated every two hours, or apomorphin given hypodermically, beginning with -£$ grain and repeated until vomiting sets in and the patient falls to sleep, are remedies well recommended to ward off delirium tremens and to restore the equilibrium of the patient. But for the benefit of the psychical effect, it is sometimes advantageous for the patients not to be relieved of all suffering. Severe cases require a hospital residence of nine to twelve months, or even longer. An index of the power of resistance may be found in the patients' insight into their own condition, and willingness to prolong hospital treatment.

In light cases it sometimes suffices to place the patient to live in a family and community where total abstinence prevails. Even here it is necessary that the patient be kept under close surveillance, especially during the first few months. A similar arrangement is sometimes an excellent plan to adopt for a time after discharge from an institution, particularly where the patient has to return to

an unfavorable environment. *Hypnotic suggestion* has been very successful in the hands of some physicians, both in establishing a disgust for liquor and in creating will power to combat the habit and withstand the enticements. Its employment, if successful, permits the patient to remain at work and with the family, rendering unnecessary a prolonged and expensive sanitarium residence. Much depends upon the personality of the physician in charge of the patient or the individual at the head of the family, who must inculcate the principles of temperance and rehabilitate the powers of resistance. A very important means for the assistance of the patient in his struggle against the alcoholic habit are the various temperance abstinence societies, the most powerful of which in this country are the Temperance Abstinence Society of the Catholic Church and the Good Templars.

Upon the basis of chronic alcoholism, there develops a series of characteristic psychoses: namely, *delirium tremens, Korssakow's psychosis, acute alcoholic hallucinosis, alcoholic hallucinatory dementia, alcoholic paranoia, alcoholic paresis,* and *alcoholic pseudopareses.*

Delirium Tremens

Delirium Tremens is characterized by the rather sudden development of numerous *fantastic hallucinations, mostly of sight and hearing, indefinite and changing delusions, principally of fear and often of a religious nature, with clouding of consciousness, restlessness, tremor, ataxic disturbances, with rapid course and good prognosis.*

Etiology. — The etiology of delirium tremens is by no means thoroughly understood. In the greater number of cases excessive alcoholism appears to be the important factor, though it is generally recognized that the disease may develop in connection with an acute febrile disease or some pronounced emotional excitement, as imprisonment and injury. Careful analyses of cases tend to show that bodily injury is really significant in not more than five to ten per cent. of cases, while the disease, pneumonia, occurs far more frequently (Bonhoeffer forty per cent.). It seems probable, therefore, that in chronic alcoholics, any disturbance which overtaxes the functional activity of the body or disturbs its equilibrium tends to produce delirium tremens; thus, severe chronic disturbances of the general nutrition are of great importance among the predisposing factors, such as that arising from gastritis, which occurs in most cases and prevents the taking of sufficient food for many weeks and even months. Furthermore, the symptoms of delirium tremens in no way resemble those of acute alcoholic intoxication, hence the delirium cannot be due to alcoholic intoxication alone. Again, the amount of alcohol ingested immediately before the attack seems to bear no definite relation to it, as, in some cases, the patients have had no alcohol for weeks; others develop the condition only upon its withdrawal, and in some it appears in spite of continued drinking. In the development of delirium tremens, other particular factors must be at work besides the excessive use of alcohol. Just what they are is not definitely known. It is believed that the numerous and severe organic changes accompanying chronic alcoholism play an important role and undoubtedly produce, as shown by the poverty of the blood and abundance of adipose tissue, profound disturbances of metabolism. Jacobson points to the presence of a decomposition material in the intestine; Hertz places delirium tremens on the same basis as uraemia; Elsholz finds blood changes indicative of a particular auto-intoxication; and Bonhoeffer suggests an intoxication arising out of the process of digestion, the product of which is normally secreted by the lungs, which intoxication is particularly apt to develop when the lungs become diseased, as so frequently happens in delirium tremens. But the findings in the blood and urine, which result directly from the action of the alcohol or indirectly through the fever, also the frequent occurrence of fever and finally the characteristic mental picture, point conclusively to the fact *that in delirium tremens we have to do not only with the simple increase of the chronic alcoholic intoxication, but with an es-sentially different sort of an intoxication to which the excessive alcoholism is only a predisposing factor.* The common occurrence of abortive attacks of delirium tremens, preceding for some time the genuine attack of delirium tremens, seems to distinctly favor this view, and to point to the additional fact that in delirium tremens there is only a sudden increase of disturbances which have been present some time, but in a milder degree.

Male patients greatly predominate in delirium tremens. According to Bonhoeffer seventy-four per cent, of cases occur between thirty to fifty years of age. The disease occurs more frequently in summer than in winter.

Pathological Anatomy. — Besides a pronounced degree of venous stasis and edema of the brain, which is usually present, Bonhoeffer 1 finds a marked degree of fibre atrophy in the radial fibres of the central convolution, in the fibretracts of the worm of the cerebellum, and especially in the columns of Goll in the cord, while there is little or no alteration in the parietal or Broca convolutions; these lesions are not found in simple alcoholism. In the large pyramidal cells and in the motor cells of the anterior central convolutions, the outline of the unstainable substance is more or less completely lost, and the processes are markedly stained for a considerable distance. Occasionally nuclear changes are observed. A number of cells appear to be destroyed. A similar condition prevails among the Purkinji cells. Nissl calls attention to a partial destruction of the cortical cells, and to a cell change, which is suggestive of other acute cell changes, in which there is staining of the achromatic substance, especially the axis cylinder processes, vacuolization in the cell substance and moderate swelling, besides chronic cell changes and an increase of glia. A part of these changes are due to chronic alcoholism, among which should be added miliary hemorrhages, which in places occur in great numbers, particularly about the nuclei of the eye muscles, as well as certain vascular changes. In the internal organs there are found fatty degeneration and fibroid myocarditis of the heart, cirrhosis of the liver, and acute and chronic alterations in the kidneys. Furthermore, Jacobson discovered in fortyfive of seventy-two autopsies an acute hyperplasia of the spleen, and in nine cases a hyperemia.

Symptomatology. — Among the first symptoms to appear are the *sense deceptions; illusions* and *hallucinations* of all the senses, but more especially of sight and hearing. These appear at first during the day and annoy the patients constantly. They are perceived with great clearness, and with the terrifying content produce a marked alteration in the emotions. The patients see all sorts of animals, large and small, moving about them; rats scamper about the floor, serpents crawl over the bedding, insects cover their food, and birds of prey hover about in the air. These forms almost always show more or less active movement, depending upon the restlessness of the body and the eye movements. Double sight is sometimes observed. This unsteadiness may in a measure account for the frequency with which the flitting and scurrying animals appear. Fantastic forms are seen, — mermaids, satyrs, and huge quadrupeds. Crowds press upon them, troops file by. The devil and his imps are omnipresent, peering in at the windows or crawling from under the bed.

Bonhoeffer, Monatsschr. f. Psychiatrie u. Neurologie, I, 229; Troemner, Archiv f. Psychiatrie, XXXI, 3.

The patients hear all sorts of noises,— the roaring of beasts, ringing of bells, firing of cannons, crying of distressed children. They are taunted by passing crowds, are threatened with death, are cursed, called traitors, thieves, and murderers. Paresthesias of the skin lead to the ideas that ants are crawling over them, that bullets have entered the body, and even the absence of wounds does not deter them from exposing limbs which have been shot full of missiles. Hot irons are being applied to their backs, and dust is thrown in their faces. They can detect the odor of gas, sulphur fumes are being forced through the keyhole. Real objects about the room assume life; the tufts on the bedding become creeping things, and the bedposts, demon guards. The content of the hallucinations is not always of a terrifying nature. Sometimes angels are seen; beautiful music is heard. God appears to them, announcing that they are Christs, and empowered to cast out devils; they are commanded to go to confession and to proclaim the gospel message; they are in beautiful surroundings, are richly dressed, in palatial quarters, attended by lovely maidens. Sometimes the scenes are of a lascivious character. Occasionally there is a mixture of the fearful and the beautiful, but more often, when there is a change of the emotions, the former is gradually replaced by the latter, as the course of the disease progresses. The hallucinations in a few cases, and especially after the height of the disease has been passed, are nothing more than a passing show for the patients; they then gaze at the hideous forms and listen to the various noises quite unconcerned.

The results of various experiments seem to indicate that the hallucinations and illusions originate in disturbances of the central processes. Hallucinations seen through a colored glass are not similarly colored. Also the hallucinations can be made to appear by directing the patient's attention to their sensory fields, and by asking them what they see and hear.

The various hallucinations may enter into the picture of an *occupation delirium,* when the patient is busy gathering up the gold lying about him, driving a flock of sheep, leading an orchestra, or addressing an audience. On the basis of these delirious experiences, the patients may develop a whole fabric of delusions concerning their environment and their experiences, but these delusions are never elaborated, do not influence the thought or action to any extent, and are quickly forgotten. There never develop delusional ideas in reference to the personality of the individual. The patients always know who and what they are.

The process of *perception* in itself, according to Bonhoeffer, does not present any very striking disturbances, the

pain, muscular and temperature sense of the skin, as well as the acuity of sight and hearing and the measuring of distances by the eye, being normal. The field of vision is sometimes restricted, the recognition of color is uncertain, and the tactile sensibility on the finger tips and the forehead is increased. The sense of equilibrium is sometimes very greatly disturbed, many patients being unable to sit up, to stand or walk, and very anxious to remain in bed. This, he believes, accounts for the disorientation of the body in space. Patients frequently complain that the floor is shrinking and that the walls are coming together, which may be due to disturbances of the eye muscles or of the labyrinthine sense.

Bonhoeffer, Der Geisteszustand der Alcoholdeliranten, 1897.

Disturbances of *apprehension* are prominent. There is defective interpretation of the impressions excited in the various sensory fields, with the result that the patients misinterpret noises, do not recognize pictures, and are unable to obtain any sharp and clear impressions. The disturbance becomes more apparent when the patients attempt to read. Instead of correct sentences, they read a senseless series of words and sound associations, noticeable especially when the type is small and indistinct. Sometimes there is no relation at all between the reading and the subject-matter. This same defect is sometimes due to aphasic disturbances.

The *attention* also shows marked disturbance. While it is possible.to hold the attention for a moment, — for instance, long enough to get a response to your reading test, — at the next the attention fails in spite of your efforts. The pronounced disturbance of attention makes the disturbance of apprehension appear even greater than what it is. Forcible language may hold the patients for a short time, but they usually relapse, and they note only those objects that especially attract them.

There is always a *moderate clouding of consciousness.* The surroundings are not correctly comprehended, and the ideas which are excited by occurrences

in their immediate surroundings are confused and contradictory. The greater degrees of insensibility are found only in severe cases and especially following epileptoid attacks. On the other hand, there is *profound disturbance of orientation,* except in the lightest cases. The surroundings are mistaken for the barroom, the church, or the prison, and strangers are greeted as old friends. Time orientation is also incorrect. Usually the duration of the illness seems to the patients much prolonged, even to months.

The *memory* for remote events is well retained. The patients recall correctly where they live and facts concerning their families and occupation, and the length of time they may have resided in different places. But the impressibility of the memory is greatly impaired, as may be determined by giving the patients a series of words or numbers to recall later. Memory for recent events is very defective, especially as regards the temporal arrangement. Fabrications of memory frequently appear.

The *train of thought* is mostly coherent, yet the patients show considerable distractibility. The goal ideas are flighty and not very well fixed. During a conversation trifling incidents or hallucinations may hinder the thought or lead it off into various directions. The patients experience difficulty in collecting their thoughts, are unable to recognize contradictions, and fail in trying to solve problems which require thought.

In *emotional attitude* the patients are anxious and fearful or happy and cheerful, depending upon the character of the hallucinations or illusions. They may change rapidly from intense fear to jolly laughter, and even indulge in witty remarks. Thus elation and the fear of death may rapidly follow each other, and in this way there may develop a mixture of concealed anxiety and humor, when it seems as though the patients, in spite of the dreadful pictures and fears, still recognize more or less clearly the humorous impossibilities and contradictions in their delirious experiences.

In *actions* the patients are more or

less restless and talkative. They are seldom able to engage in work, though occasionally a patient continues at his occupation until the disease is well established. Usually they take an active part in their numerous hallucinations. They plug the ears to keep out disagreeable noises, crawl under the bed to elude persecutors, escape from the window to get away from the sulphur vapors and the enemies waiting outside the door; they answer the imaginary voices, run to the station for protection, or amuse themselves with their beautiful surroundings and join in the happy company of imaginary revellers. Sometimes they are assertive and aggressive, demanding attention or carrying out divine commands. When in fear they sometimes commit assaults, but they rarely attempt suicide.

Many chronic alcoholics develop what in their own parlance is called a " touch of the horrors," which in reality is an *abortive form of delirium tremens.* Some of these cases come under the care of the family physician, but the majority of them go without medical attendance. The symptoms are those of the prodromal stage of delirium tremens. During a debauch or following abstinence or mental shock, there develops some paraesthesia, a vague feeling of fear, as if some one were constantly behind the patients, the slightest noise causing them to be startled. While in this state they have isolated hallucinations of sight and hearing. One patient saw for a moment a number of rats scampering across the floor, others were attracted by unnatural voices. It very frequently happens at night that some object appears at the window for a second and is gone. The patients are perfectly conscious, and appreciate their condition. Some of the physical signs of delirium tremens are usually present. The condition is of short duration, rarely lasting over a few hours or days. Berkley, Mental Diseases.

Physically. — Besides the various sensory disturbances, such as neuritic disturbances, paraesthesias, hyperaesthesias, and circumscribed areas of anaesthesias which may form the basis for illusions and hallucinations, there is sometimes a lack of insensibility which will permit the patients to sustain severe injuries without complaint. There is often present great muscular weakness. The muscular movements tend to be coarse and unsteady, and the gait uncertain and staggering. There is some ataxia and pronounced *tremor* of the tongue and fingers, and sometimes of the extremities and eyelids. Speech is often ataxic and paraphasic, with malposition of words and syllables, and in the severest cases may be slurring and unintelligible. Occasionally in the severe cases muscular spasms are noticed. Epileptiform seizures are frequent, occurring mostly before the attack, in ten per cent. of the cases one to two days before the outbreak, less often during the attack, and sometimes accompanied by transitory paralytic symptoms, such as hemiparesis. The tendon reflexes are exaggerated. Insomnia is marked from the first, and persists unless the patients become stuporous. The condition of nutrition suffers, because of the small amount of nourishment ingested, which is due in part to the delusions of poisoning and in part to the gastritis. There is apt to be a slight rise of temperature during the first few days, rarely reaching one hundred degrees. The pulse rate is low as well as the respiration, and occasionally there is profuse perspiration.

In a large percentage of cases the urine contains albumen and casts, which clears up with the psychosis. Elsholz finds in the blood a relative leucocytosis, with a diminution of the eosinophiles at the height of the psychosis.

Course. — The duration of the delirium varies from a few days to two weeks, rarely extending beyond three weeks. The improvement comes with sleep. The hallucinations usually fade away slowly, though sometimes they disappear within a night. With the improvement of sleep the physical symptoms disappear gradually. The memory of the events of the psychosis, in spite of great clouding of consciousness, is sometimes surprisingly clear, though it later tends to fade.

Not all cases show rapid clearing up of symptoms with the improvement of sleep. A few suffer a second attack after a few days or even a week of clear consciousness have intervened, and in spite of the fact that they have continued abstinent. Others show a complete alteration in the character of the psychosis after the hallucinations and illusions have disappeared, some developing the characteristic polyneuritis psychosis or the alcoholic hallucinatory dementia. A certain number of cases pass into alcoholic paranoia, to be described later.

In the more severe cases the physical signs become more prominent and there develop convulsions, muscular twitching, ataxia, and disturbances of the eye muscles. At the same time the insensibility and the incoherence increases, the movements become weaker and the pulse smaller, and finally death ensues, with sudden loss of consciousness or collapse.

Diagnosis. — The diagnosis of the disease is not difficult if previous history of alcoholism is known. *Fever delirium* and the *epileptic befogged states* may be confused with delirium tremens. In the former there is a more marked clouding of consciousness, and, especially in the epileptic condition, confused delusions of a religious character stand in contrast to the moderate restlessness without impulsiveness, the active hallucinations, and the muscular tremor of the alcoholic.

The *delirium of dementia paralytica* is differentiated from the alcoholic delirium by the previous history of change of character, evidences of failure of memory and judgment, paretic physical signs, and the more profound clouding of consciousness, with a change of personality.

Prognosis. — The outcome is usually favorable. In the unfavorable cases (three to nineteen per cent.) pneumonia is the chief cause of death and greatly increases the fatality. Other causes of death are cardiac failure, infection following injury, and suicide.

Treatment. — In warding off the development of delirium tremens in chronic alcoholics who have suffered injury or have developed pneumonia, one should withdraw the alcohol at once and attend particularly to nutrition and sleeplessness. Frequently repeated doses of ergot or the administration of apomorphin hypodermically (see p. 170) aids in this respect. The first indication for treatment is the establishment of proper *nutrition,* which requires frequently repeated administration of small quantities of liquid. If necessary, artificial feeding should be resorted to. Gastritis with nausea and vomiting may necessitate lavage. The second indication is to combat *insomnia,* for which purpose a combination of 3J grains each of chloral, potassium, and sodium bromide is most efficient, repeated every hour until sleep is secured. In case the cardiac condition will not permit the use of chloral, paraldehyde or chloralmide may be substituted. The patient should be confined in bed and watched constantly. If excitement increases to such an extent that the patient cannot be kept in bed, then the prolonged warm bath must be employed (see p. 140). Great excitement may necessitate its continuous use, combined sometimes with the use of chloral and the bromides or paraldehyde, or in its extreme cases, the use of hyoscine.

As already indicated, alcohol should always be withdrawn. In case the slightest evidence of cardiac weakness develops, one should not hesitate to make use of caffein, camphor, or camphorated oil, or in urgent states normal saline infusion.

Kokssakow's Psychosis

In 1887 Korssakow ' described a number of cases of apparent toxic origin and associated with polyneuritic symptoms, Which were characterized particularly by *a profound disturbance of the impressibility of memory, disorientation, and a tendency to fabrications of memory.* Later experience demonstrated that while this psychosis occasionally appeared in connection with other toxic states (see p. 134), it developed most often on the basis of chronic alcoholism. It also became apparent that the polyneuritic symptoms are not a constant accompaniment of the psychosis.

Etiology. — The intimate relationship of this psychosis to alcoholism has already been pointed out. Jolly regards it as a severe form of delirium tremens, while Bonhoeffer describes it as a chronic alcoholic delirium. It develops in three per cent. of the cases of delirium tremens. It is much more apt (eleven per cent.) to occur during the second or subsequent attacks of delirium tremens. Women appear to suffer in a proportionately larger percentage than men.

'Korssakow, Archiv f. Psychiatrie, XXI, 669; Allgem. Zeitsch. f. Psyehiatrie, XLVI, 475; Tiling, ebenda, XLVIII, 549; Uber alkoholische Paralyse und infektioese Neuritis multiplex, 1897; Jolly, Coariteannalen, XXII; Moenkemoeller, Allgem. Zeitschrift f. Psychiatrie, LIV, 806; Raimann, Wiener klin. Wochenschrift, 1900, 2; Elsholz, ebenda, 1900, 15; Heilbronner, Monatsschrift f. Psychiatrie, III, 459.

Pathological Anatomy. — There is an extensive destructive process involving the nervous tissue from the cortex to the peripheral nerves. The nerve cells present the usual signs of an acute process while the nerve fibres give evidence of varying degrees of destruction, especially in the region of the central convolutions, when there is a prolonged course of the disease. In the spinal cord there is an extensive atrophy of the fibres, particularly in the columns of Goll. Of particular importance are the numerous small hemorrhages, occurring especially in the central gray matter, where they are regarded as the cause of the oculomotor paralyses. The acute hemorrhagic polyencephalitis superior, described by Wernicke, according to Elsholz and Bonhoeffer, is frequently associated with Korssakow's psychosis. The above anatomical lesions, which are indicative of an extensive destruction of nerve tissue, in reality are only what one would expect to find in severe alcoholic intoxication.

Symptomatology. — The symptoms at the onset are similar to those of delirium tremens. But after the usual course of the delirium symptoms, disorientation continues, while the hallucinations, restlessness, and insomnia disappear.

The delirious experiences are not corrected, and in addition there develops a very striking disturbance of impressibility of memory (Merkfahigkeit). The symptoms sometimes follow a rapidly developing stupor with hallucinations, and they still more rarely develop gradually from the chronic alcoholic state.

In severe cases this disturbance of memory is so pronounced that the patients cannot remember for a few minutes or even seconds that which they have just experienced. They are conscious and understand what is said to them, yet they are wholly unable to put together their recent experiences or to form any picture of the course of events in their lives. They do not know what has happened in the past hour, although in the meantime they have washed and prepared for and eaten dinner and been visited by the physician, and, indeed, even if told all this, they cannot fit it into their memory and correct the defect. A few very striking impressions may be retained, but they are never connected with the events immediately preceding or following. The first result of this disturbance of memory is a *complete loss of orientation.* The patients have no conception of the time. They cannot tell where they are or those about them, and usually greet the physician as an old acquaintance, though they cannot recall the name.

While the memory is more particularly affected for events since the onset of the psychosis, yet it sometimes happens that there is a distinct loss of memory for events extending back several months or even years. They cannot tell you how they have been employed, or where they have been, or have lived during all this time. Some forget that they are married or have children. A few striking incidents may be recalled, but the time of their occurrence cannot be established. The lapses in memory are not only not recognized by the patient, but are very apt to be filled in with *falsifications of memory,* which are related by the patient with a feeling of absolute certainty. These falsifications may apply only to the lapses of recent date. The patients then relate visits which they have just had, or journeys which they have made, and give a detailed account of the good times they have had, while in reality for months they have been leading a wholly uninteresting and monotonous existence. These fabrications can usually be drawn out by questioning and influenced by suggestions. The fabrications are not always limited to mere filling the lapses of memory with ordinary experiences, but the patient may strive to amplify the incidents with altogether new and fictitious events. This latter tendency is pronounced only during the earlier stages of the disease. Indeed, the fabrication may extend to an intricate and fantastic falsification of the last ten years of the patients' lives, concerning which they relate all kinds of wonderful experiences. The apparent accuracy of these fabrications forcibly impresses one, together with the wealth of detail and the absolute certainty which they possess for the patient at the time. Although the facts are frequently altered, each time they are related as clearly and assuredly as if they had occurred only yesterday. Occasionally, expansive and depressive delusions are added, but these also tend to change rapidly and as suddenly appear and disappear. Sometimes hallucinations also occur at the beginning, which later disappear.

The function of the intellect outside of the disorders already mentioned is not particularly impaired. The patients show good judgment on other matters, understand facts presented to them, answer questions to the point, and know how to cleverly conceal the lapses in their memory. On the other hand, they do not possess a clear insight into their condition and are unable to employ themselves profitably. They can write letters well and carry out orders, but they become shiftless and lead a thoughtless and inactive life.

The *emotional attitude* at the onset is mostly anxious, but later it becomes one of indifference and apathy, though sometimes there is distrust and irritability, while in other cases a certain degree of good humor or elation exists. Usually the emotional attitude is also easily changed by suggestion into one state or another.

The *conduct* and *actions* of the patients after the subsidence of the delirium become orderly. The patients may complain a little about their surroundings, but they are mostly quiet. As a result of faulty memory they are always neglecting to attend to personal duties, or repeating what they have already done; hence the same questions are frequently asked, and numerous letters are rewritten. Delusions, if present, do not greatly influence the conduct.

The physical symptoms are usually those of alcoholic neuritis. These, however, may be absent. The extent of the symptoms also may vary considerably, but usually they are confined to minor paralytic signs, atony and reduced volume of certain muscle groups, especially in the legs; Romberg signs; sensitiveness of the nerves and muscles to pressure; more or less extensive anaesthesia, paresthesia, or hyperesthesia; loss, seldom increase, of the tendon reflexes; cystic disorders, some degree of ataxia; difficulties of deglutition and speech; and paresis of the facial nerve and especially paralysis of the eye muscles (abducens). The pupils are often unequal, and notched, and sometimes do not react to light. There is also tremor of the fingers, and frequently a history of epileptiform attacks. Furthermore, symptoms indicative of chronic alcoholism may be present, as nephritis, hypertrophy, or atrophy of the liver, icterus, ascites, and edema; also faulty nutrition, anorexia, and sometimes nausea.

Course. — Following the rapid development of the disease, the course is usually a long one. In some cases death ensues from paralysis of the heart or respiration. Not infrequently a rapidly developing tuberculosis leads to death. After a period of several months, there may be gradual improvement, with disappearance of the neuritic symptoms, a return of orientation and improvement of memory. In a small number of cases the improvement may, in the course of five to nine months, be sufficient to permit the patient's returning home, yet there regularly remains a considerable increased susceptibility to fatigue, uncertainty of memory, emotional apathy or irritability, weakness of will, and limited activity. Further indulgence in alcohol tends to quickly intensify these residual symptoms. Usually the disease terminates in a permanent dementia, which is particularly characterized by the persistence of falsifications of memory.

Diagnosis. — The conditions of excitement at the onset of the *post infection psychoses* may be differentiated by the fact that clouding of consciousness is much more pronounced, and hallucinations and illusions are more in the background; further, the alcoholic tremor is absent, the emotional attitude does not present the alcoholic characteristics, and finally the prognosis is distinctly more favorable. *Paresis* is distinguished by the usual history of a gradual onset. Pronounced neuritic symptoms with paralysis of the eye muscles and the alcoholic tremors speak for Korssakow's psychosis, while indications of aphasia, hesitating speech, marked paragraphia, and cerebral paralysis point to paresis. Again, the stupid or humorous emotional attitude of the alcoholic contrasts with the silly happiness of the paretic, while the only intellectual disturbance of Korssakow's psychosis is seen in the memory, which may not involve the more remote events of life, as in paresis. *Presbyophrenia* also is characterized by impaired impressibility of memory, loss of orientation and fabrication; but this disease occurs mostly in the senile period, may not be preceded by an alcoholic history, and is not accompanied by neuritic disturbances. Again, the activity of the patients is greater; they are communicative, often garrulous, trouble themselves about the environment, display a childish emotional state and a certain busyness, especially at night. The diagnosis may be difficult if the presbyophrenic patient has been addicted to excessive alcoholism.

Treatment. — During the early stages of the disease the treatment is identical with that in delirium tremens (see p.

182). The alcohol must be absolutely withdrawn, and the patient placed either in an institution or in a particularly satisfactory family environment, because of the great weakness of will displayed by the patients. Later in the course of the disease, it may be necessary to employ electricity, massage, and gymnastic movements in order to combat the muscular atrophy accompanying the neuritis. Some improvement of the memory disturbance may result from systematic mental exercises.

Acute Alcoholic Hallucinosis

This psychosis is characterized by the *sudden development of coherent delusions of persecution, based mostly upon hallucinations of hearing, with barely any clouding of consciousness.*

Etiology. — The etiology of acute alcoholic hallucinosis is identical to that in delirium tremens (see p. 172). Why one case should develop into delirium tremens and another into acute alcoholic hallucinosis is yet unknown. The various explanations offered for this by Bonhoeffer and others are not satisfactory. Acute alcoholic hallucinosis represents, in America, forty-five per cent. of the cases of alcoholic insanity committed to institutions, and occurs mostly in men of middle life, many of whom have been habitual daily drinkers for years. Mitchell, Types of Alcoholic Insanity. Amer. Jour, of Ins. Oct. 1904, p. 251. Symptomatology. — Occasionally, there are a few prodromal systoms, such as indisposition, headache, dizziness, insomnia, and irritability. The onset is usually sudden. The patients at first are disturbed during the evening or at night by indefinite noises, like shouting voices, cryings, and ringing bells. These *hallucinations* soon become more definite when they hear their own names called and numerous epithets. The patients then hear remarks about themselves, which appear to come from the next room or from fellow-workmen. These remarks are usually quite clear, and occasionally are heard in only one ear. The voices are recognized as those of an acquaintance, a chum, or a fellow-workman, but rarely as those of the immediate family, and consist of impreca-

tions and references to misdeeds of their past lives. They hear themselves called murderers, liars, and thieves. They learn that they are to be electrocuted, that the wife is unfaithful, or that the children have been drowned. They are laughed at because of their anxiety. At times they overhear long discussions concerning their welfare, in which various events of their past lives are rehearsed or an indictment for murder is read against them. Again, a group of men under their window discuss means of capturing them and bringing them to a public place for the purpose of having them lynched. All this is so very real to the patients that it is impossible to convince them to the contrary. Furthermore, it almost always happens that the voices are not spoken directly at them, but they only overhear what is being said among others about them. The content of these hallucinations is always of a depreciatory nature. Besides these numerous hallucinations of hearing, there are a few hallucinations of sight, especially at night. Strange and threatening forms appear before them, some crawling from under the bed, others creeping on the wall; brilliant specks come across the field of vision, and they may even see double. At times the food has a peculiar taste, and excites suspicion.

In connection with these various hallucinations there regularly develop pronounced *delusions,* mostly of a depressive nature. The patients believe that they are the center of attraction; every one about them watches and threatens them. Their every thought and action is known and commented upon. Passers on the street jeer at them, fellowpassengers on the trolley watch them closely, visitors in the factory are told all about them and stand and gaze at them, enemies shoot through the fence at them, and detectives in citizen's clothes follow them wherever they go. They are distrustful of their surroundings, are constantly on the alert for impending arrest, or they go into hiding, and refuse to leave their homes. These patients argue that they are condemned to die, and show considerable emotion. Fellowpatients refuse to speak to them because

they are implicated in the seduction of their wives. Sometimes they refuse to answer questions or associate with any one until brought to the court room for the supposed trial. At times they find consolation in prayer and in reading the Bible. These various delusions usually remain within the realm of possibility, and appear more like attempts on the part of the patient to explain the hallucinations. Occasionally, however, the delusions are of a fantastic nature and simulate those occurring in delirium tremens, sometimes also being associated with expansive delusions.

The *consciousness* is barely disturbed, there being only a slight dazedness. Yet at night, and at the onset, there may be a slight transitory delirium. The patients are mostly oriented, their speech coherent, and they are able to make an accurate statement of their symptoms, except occasionally in giving the correct time of their occurrence. They rarely possess clear insight, but they often realize that they are different, and frequently accuse their persecutors of drugging them or making them crazy. Others claim that they are only " nervous."

The *emotional attitude* at the onset is usually that of anxiety, but later in the course of the disease there is that characteristic mixture of anxiety and cheerfulness seen in delirium tremens, when the patients relate their frightful experiences with indifference, or perhaps laugh at the absurdity of their attracting so much attention. When not in fear, they are quiet, reserved, and in replying to questions are monosyllabic.

In *conduct* the patients may remain quite orderly, and not infrequently continue at work for days and even weeks. But even during this period peculiarities of manner develop as the result of their delusions. They become reserved, silent, and avoid acquaintances; later they often apply to the police for protection or hide under the bed, and some even attempt suicide. In our experience these patients are sometimes the most dangerous of the insane. They take the law into their own hands, purchase firearms, and assault those maligning their character or planning their destruction.

Physically. — The sleep is regularly disturbed. The appetite fails and there is a loss of weight. The reflexes are occasionally exaggerated, and tremor of the tongue and hands is often present, though not always. Occasionally, there are neuritic symptoms.

Course. — The course of the psychosis may be either *acute* or *subacute*. When acute, the duration varies from two to three weeks, with rapid disappearance of the symptoms, sometimes during a night. The prospect for a short course seems better the nearer the symptoms approach those of delirium tremens. Occasionally, *abortive forms* of acute alcoholic hallucinosis are observed, in which the patients for a few hours or a couple of days suddenly develop isolated transitory hallucinations, with anxiety, and a few persecutory delusions, such as, that they are to be poisoned, assaulted by fellow-workmen, or are watched by the police. In the subacute form the symptoms may persist from one to eight months, with numerous fluctuations, and then disappear gradually. The memory for events of the psychosis is usually excellent.

Diagnosis. — The differentiation between *delirium tremens* and acute alcoholic hallucinosis is by no means sharply denned. There are cases of the latter in which the orientation is markedly disturbed for only a short time, hallucinations of hearing are very pronounced, and there seems to be a definite delusional connection between the various individual morbid experiences, while, on the other hand, the difficulty of apprehension, the disturbance of the impressibility of memory, the presence of visual and tactile hallucinations, suggestibility, restlessness, and tremor give the stamp of delirium tremens. Provided they are not simply cases of undeveloped delirium tremens, may they not possibly represent a combination of delirium tremens and acute alcoholic hallucinosis, similar to those cases of delirium tremens occasionally seen in epileptics, paretics, hebephrenics, and manics? But usually the reten-

tion of a good orientation, the absence of restlessness and striking physical signs, the predominance of hallucinations of hearing with coherent delusions based upon them, and a more prolonged course are sufficiently distinctive evidences of acute alcoholic hallucinosis.

The differentiation from *dementia prcecox,* particularly the paranoid form, may be difficult, but in dementia praecox the onset is far more gradual: there is stupidity; looseness of thought; a lack of energy for work; peculiar conduct, such as, staring, impulsive acts, and catatonic signs. The hallucinations in dementia praecox are directed to the patient, while in the alcoholic psychosis the patient simply overhears what is said. The delusions involve mostly the physical and mental personality, which in the alcoholic psychosis are not involved. Finally, the emotional attitude is superficial, while in the acute alcoholic hallucinosis the anxiety is genuine and often desperate, except for the occasional appearance of the alcoholic humor. *Paresis* may be differentiated by the same signs in addition to the presence of pare tic physical signs and weakness of memory and judgment. Some cases of *manic-depressive* insanity may present some similarities to acute alcoholic hallucinosis, but they can be successfully differentiated by the previous history of the case, and by tendency to delusions of self-accusations, which are absent in the alcoholic condition.

Prognosis. — The outcome is usually favorable, as a large proportion of the acute cases recover. There is great danger of relapse with continued drinking, and subsequent attacks are more prolonged. Some patients have four or five attacks. The outlook in the subacute cases is not as favorable, as less than twenty-five per cent. wholly recover. In some cases there finally develops a condition of permanent dementia, with hallucinations and delusions.

Treatment. — The chief indications are the absolute withdrawal of alcohol, the administration of a nutritious diet, and incessant watching to prevent injury to self and others. The course of

the disease may sometimes be cut short at the onset by the use of hypnotics to overcome the insomnia and of the prolonged warm bath to ameliorate the anxiety.

Alcoholic Hallucinatory Dementia

This type of alcoholic psychosis, provisionally called alcoholic hallucinatory dementia (or alcoholic paranoia), is characterized by the sudden development of *numerous hallucinations, many depreciatory delusions of reference, influence and persecution, associated somatic delusions, and occasional change of personality, with some emotional anxiety and irritability, usually leading after a long course to moderate dementia.* It frequently represents the end stage of the acute alcoholic hallucinosis and as often follows delirium tremens.

Symptomatology.—The onset is sudden. If acute alcoholic hallucinosis or delirium tremens have preceded, the patients having become oriented and quiet, and having corrected at least a part of their delirious experiences, continue somewhat constrained and suspicious. Then *hallucinations,* particularly of hearing, develop again, and the patients complain of hearing threatening voices, that others are reading their thoughts, and that they are being influenced in various ways. They feel that they are being hypnotized, electrified, or chloroformed, are experimented upon when asleep; think that men are breathing on them, smearing mucus over them, changing their clothing, and creating disgusting odors about them. Comments are printed in the daily papers about themselves, and actors make allusions to them from the stage. Very often their delusions have a sexual content, when they claim that they have been assaulted, have their semen drawn off nightly, and that their Luther, Allgem. Zeitschr far Psychiatrie, LIX, 20, 1902.
organs are being shrunken up. These delusions are usually not elaborated, but remain unchanged from week to week, and are almost always expressed in the same phraseology. Witches and spirits are everywhere, assuming various forms, and constantly offering threats; everything is poisoned, and they cannot

escape the hypnotic influence. Occasionally, the delusions are still more fantastic and quite changeable. Expansive delusions may appear, but they also are limited in content, although they are fantastic. The patients' judgment concerning the surroundings, except in the severer cases, is quite good; they exhibit activity, converse with their associates, follow a daily routine, show a tendency to employ themselves, and are quite natural, in as far as their delusions are not involved. The memory shows no striking disturbances. Nevertheless, one can detect a considerable degree of mental weakness.

The *emotional attitude* at the onset is one of anxiety or irritability, impelling the patients at times to attempt suicide or attack their persecutors. Later, there regularly develops a more or less humorous attitude, manifested in witty and facetious remarks and rendering the suspicious and excitable patients more pliable and approachable. Physically, besides the alcoholic tremor, there are often present more or less severe neuritic disturbances.

Course. — The course of this disease, unless abstinence is enforced, is progressive. With persistent abstinence, the hallucinations and delusions slowly subside. In some cases they may entirely vanish, leaving the patient in a condition of simple alcoholic dementia. But usually they persist for many years, though steadily becoming weaker. Numerous fluctuations of the symptoms are characteristic; at times the patients express some insight into their condition; they think that they are sick, but they have no idea of how they came into such a state, and they are able also to associate in a friendly manner with their supposed persecutors; at other times they become excitable without apparent cause, complain of threatening hallucinations, and also become aggressive, but they are usually quieted without difficulty.

Diagnosis. — Alcoholic hallucinatory dementia may be distinguished from some of the *end stages of dementia præcox* by the history of the development of the disease, by the fact that the patients possess a greater emotional and intellectual activity, are more natural and approachable in conduct, and show the characteristic alcoholic humor. Furthermore, the symptoms do not progress if total abstinence is maintained, but rather tend to subside. There is, occasionally, a case of severe alcoholism, with pronounced catatonic symptoms. In such cases it would seem justifiable to assume that there is a combination of both diseases.

Alcoholic Paranoia

This form of alcoholic insanity comprises a *small group of chronic alcoholics who gradually develop a delusional state characterized particularly by delusions of jealousy.*

Symptomatology. — The family discord that naturally follows excessive drinking, together with the wife's aversion to sexual intercourse, and the increasing impotency of the alcoholic, is the nucleus about which the delusions of jealousy form. The tendency displayed by the alcoholic to lay the blame for everything upon some one else, naturally engenders the idea that the wife is unfaithful, and that the real cause of these difficulties lies in the fondness of the wife for other men or of the men for other women. Insignificant occurrences are regarded as important evidence of this infidelity: the assistance of some one in carrying a bundle, the fondness of a friend for their children, the voluntary implication of a neighbor in a family quarrel. The frequent clanging of a car bell means that the motorman is a correspondent. A side glance from a passer on the street, the arrival of an unusual letter, and even association with another man's wife are held as sufficient proof of the suspected misbehavior. Furthermore, the home and children are neglected. Patients have seen the wife enter the apartments of a neighbor, and from noises which they have heard are sure that she was guilty of adultery. Frequently, the children are disclaimed as those of other men, and hence must share in the abuse. Sufficient evidence of this is found in the fact that they have different colored hair or different dispositions. The saloon keeper is implicated, if he refuses to give them credit for liquor, or the coachman, if he happens to be amiss in any of his duties. Associated with these delusions of infidelity there may be delusions of poisoning.

These delusions of jealousy are by no means confined to married persons, but also exist in the unmarried when those persons with whom they are most intimately associated, the mother, sister, the paramour, and sometimes the clergy become the objects of their jealousy and assaults. These delusions are not elaborated and usually remain within the realm of possibility. The patients, however, state them coherently, oftentimes displaying considerable emotion, and, indeed, in this way they frequently convince chance acquaintances of the great injustice done. There are occasional *hallucinations of hearing,* when the patients hear peculiar noises about the house, such as a creaking of the door, whispering, rattling of the shutters, or suspicious sounds in another room. There may be a peculiar odor in the house, or an odd taste in the food, which is offered as proof that an effort is being made to poison them. This incites them to nail down the windows and to fasten the door in order to keep out the lovers.

There is *no clouding of consciousness.* In *actions,* the patients usually exhibit marked weakness; they bemoan their misfortunes while submitting to the injustice. At times the actions are entirely out of accord with their delusions, and this is especially true in cases of long duration. A man may live peaceably with his wife, whom he accuses of committing adultery night after night. Sometimes they are very irritable, and in fits of anger may be both aggressive and destructive. When under the influence of alcohol, the conduct of the patients is apt to be wholly-changed; then they become aggressive and threatening and, not infrequently, make murderous assaults upon their wives or the objects of their jealousy.

Course. — The course of the disease is usually progressive. The delusions seldom disappear permanently, though abstinence from alcohol often brings improvement, especially in conjunction with confinement in an institution. When removed from home environment, the delusions subside and patients are able to live very comfortably. In some patients the delusions subside and are denied; they desire to "let bygones be bygones "; " everything is past," and allow the inference that they have been mistaken. This apparent improvement, oftentimes accompanied by an alleged insight, influences one to yield to their importunities for release; but regularly the return to home surroundings, with an opportunity to secure alcohol, soon leads to recurrence of delusions.

Diagnosis. — It is often difficult to distinguish the delusions of infidelity expressed by the patient from actual occurrences and facts. The conduct of the alcoholic frequently results in an actual and permanent estrangement of the man and wife, which naturally smooths the way for adultery. One must rely in his judgment upon the grounds for jealousy offered by the patient. The positiveness with which the patient draws his conclusions from insignificant data, and the conviction with which he applies these to others, and finally the occasional relation of strange conclusions should leave little doubt as to the delusional origin of the ideas of jealousy. Indeed, under some circumstances we can come to the conclusion that a jealousy which appears to be justified by real circumstances, nevertheless, on account of its peculiar basis, must be regarded as morbid. This is especially clear when we observe how the patient disregards, with unconcern, the real, open adultery of the wife, while the delusion leads to passionate outbreaks. Delusions of infidelity may occur in the psychoses of the period of involution and occasionally also in dementia praecox. In general, the delusions are less apt to be fantastic in the alcoholic psychosis, and there are lacking the physical sensations, the hallucinations, and the nocturnal experiences which are encountered in the other psychoses. In addition to this, there is a striking contrast between the subsidence of the symptoms, the weakness of will shown by the alcoholic upon en-

forced abstinence, and his brutality and animosity when unrestrained. This psychosis is differentiated from *paranoia* by the lack of a stable systemization of the delusions and by the symptoms of chronic alcoholism.

Treatment. — In these cases the treatment is confined to enforced abstinence and careful watching or confinement in an institution to prevent assaults.

Alcoholic Paresis

This psychosis represents in the majority of cases a simple combination of the symptoms of chronic alcoholism with those of paresis. There is added to the defective memory the expansive delusions and the emotional deterioration of paresis, the hallucinations and delusions of infidelity of the alcoholic; while the speech disorder of the paretic is accompanied by the tremor and neuritic disturbances of the alcoholic. Epileptiform attacks also are particularly numerous. Usually the signs of alcoholism have existed for some time before the paretic symptoms develop. On the other hand, the initial symptoms may lead to such excessive drinking that the alcoholic symptoms develop.

Alcohol Pseudoparesis

There are included here severe cases of alcoholic hallucinatory dementia with more or less pronounced signs of Korssakow's psychosis, in which physical symptoms predominate, as, tremor, speech disorder, ataxia, paralyses, rigid pupils, and paralytic attacks. These cases are distinguished from true paresis by the history of their development, the predominance of the polyneuritic symptoms, the active hallucinations, and the more prolonged course, which leads to a simple alcoholic dementia and not to the absolute dementia and death that characterizes paresis.

B. MORPHINISM

The extensive use and abuse of morphin for its alluring effects place it second only to alcohol in the production of mental and physical wrecks.

Etiology. — The intolerance of pain among people of this age, together with the laxity of the physicians in dispensing analgesics, accounts in part for the extensive use of this drug. Being an ex-

pensive drug, its victims are limited to the better classes. Considerably over one-half of the patients are those who are best acquainted with its ill effects — physicians, dentists, and professional nurses. At least one-half of these patients are men. On the Continent it is claimed that seventy-five per cent. are men.

An important etiological factor is the defective constitutional basis, evidences of which in very many cases are earlier manifested by various neuroses, as hysteria. Individuals free from this hereditary taint usually succumb to the drug after its continued employment in persistent painful affections, as neuralgia, sciatica, rheumatism, headache, dysmenorrhea, and different forms of colic. The pleasurable feeling and the mental stimulus which supplement the analgesic effects are here the cause of its continuance. The majority of cases develop between the ages of twenty-five to forty years.

Pathological Anatomy. — In animals to which morphin had been administered for a prolonged period, Nissl has demonstrated a shrinkage of cortical neurones with an increase of the neuroglia.

Symptomatology. — *Acute Morphin Intoxication.* — The physiological action of morphin is to first produce an acceleration and excitation of the process of comprehension and a psychomotor retardation, which later passes into a befogged state, with changing fantastic hallucinations and an intense weariness in the psychomotor functions. Then ensues a quiet, pleasurable feeling, which acts as one of the strongest enticements for the habitue". For him it also produces a necessary stimulus for mental work, which cannot be accomplished by the exercise of the will power alone. There develops a metallic taste in the mouth, and sometimes rumbling in the bowels. Fortunately the drug fails to produce these pleasurable effects for all, owing to idiosyncrasies. Many after its exhibition suffer from a disagreeable fulness in the head, general feeling of discomfort, nausea, and colicky pains. Following the intoxication there is apt to be headache, profuse perspiration, and diminution in all of the secretions of the body.

Chronic Morphin Intoxication. — In the prolonged use of morphin the effects of acute intoxication disappear, and the individual obtains only the exhilarating and the quieting effects, which aid in endurance of annoyance incident to his work or his home life. The beneficial effects of this drug diminish with usage, and soon necessitate increased dosage, which may, in time, reach from thirty to fifty grains daily. The frequency of the doses must also be increased.

The character of the symptoms and the time of their appearance depend mostly upon the individual constitution and its powers of resistance. Some continue addicted to morphin throughout life without pronounced ill effect; others succumb in the course of a few months. In these the memory weakens, and the capacity for mental application diminishes. Difficult and exhausting work becomes impossible without its administration. Consequently the patients are either in a condition of exhilaration, stupidity, or nervous irritability, none of which are compatible with mental work. *Emotionally,* these patients exhibit many variations: they are sometimes dejected, irritable, cross, hypochondriacal; sometimes confidential, over-nice, with pronounced affectation; and occasionally anxious, especially at night. *Morally,* there is a pronounced change of character, noticeable especially in reference to their irresistible habit. They willingly submit to all sorts of depraved means in order to secure the drug. Finally all idea of personal responsibility vanishes. The home and the business suffer alike, and they fall into a state of apathy and indolence, with an absence of will power and energy. They are careless about the dress and the personal appearance. In *actions* they are apt to be sleepy during the day, and active and restless at night, reading, busying themselves about foolish trifles, and talking incessantly. They are also disagreeable, faultfinding, and obstinate to the extreme. Very many of them become addicted to alcohol, and other

drug habits. *Physically,* the sleep is much disturbed. The patients lie awake for hours, their minds busied with all sorts of fantastic ideas, sometimes accompanied by genuine hallucinations of sight. Disturbances of sensibility are usually present, such as paraesthesias and hyperaesthesias, especially about the heart, the intestines, and the bladder. There is usually an increase of the tendon reflexes. The movements are uncertain, tremulous, and sometimes ataxic. Occasionally there is difficulty in speech, also paresis of eye muscles (double vision and defective accommodation). The general nutrition suffers, and there is loss of weight. The skin is flabby and dry, due in part to the absence of normal secretions. The appetite, especially for meat, fails, though sometimes there is a ravenous appetite. Dryness of the mouth creates unusual thirst. In the circulatory system there is noticed palpitation, and slow, irregular pulse. The ringing in the ears, numbness, vertigo, and syncope, as well as the profuse perspiration and shivering, are attributable to vasomotor disturbances. The lack of sexual desires and impotence are prominent symptoms; in women there is amenorrhcea and sterility. The ensemble of these symptoms creates the picture of premature senility. Abstinence Symptoms. — The abrupt withdrawal of morphin in individuals who are addicted to large doses produces in the course of a few hours a characteristic train of symptoms called abstinence symptoms. These, according to Marme, are due to the action of oxydimorphin. The withdrawal even in milder cases is always attended with more or less disturbance. The patients become tremulous and uneasy, experience a tickling sensation in the nose and begin to sneeze; feel oppressed, complain of paraesthesias of different parts of the body, and are sleepless. The administration of hypnotics, especially chloral, at this time, only increases the excitement and aids in bringing about a delirious condition with hallucinations and dreamy confusion. In spite of precaution, however, a condition very similar to delirium tremens may appear.

This condition lasts but a few hours, or at most a few days. Occasionally there appears a condition of dazedness, with hallucinations and convulsive movements. *Physically,* the patients display involuntary movements, twitchings of the limbs, spasm of the diaphragm, paresis of the muscles of accommodation, tenesmus, paleness and flushing, vomiting, palpitation of the heart, fainting and collapse with heart failure, which is sometimes fatal. The secretion of saliva and perspiration, which during the ingestion of morphin has been diminished, now becomes excessive, and there is colliquative diarrhoea. Albumen is usually present in the urine. The duration and intensity of the symptoms depend upon the constitution of the patient, the duration of the habit, and the size of the habitual dose. The symptoms disappear gradually, except in the lighter cases, where they may vanish rapidly after a prolonged sleep. In the course of a few days, perhaps weeks, the patients begin to sleep and develop an appetite, but from this point convalescence progresses very slowly.

Course. — The rapidity with which the symptoms of chronic morphinism develop varies with the power of resistance of the individual and the quantity of morphin ingested; in some cases it requires a few months, in others several years. The duration also varies; some die within a year of inanition, heart failure, or in collapse, while others live for many years in spite of large and increasing doses.

Diagnosis. — The disease may be recognized by the varying emotional attitude; periods of mental freshness and unusual energy with a feeling of well-being, alternating with great weariness, stupidity, dejection, and irritability, and furthermore by the physical signs: the loss of sexual power, anorexia, myosis, and general muscular weakness, amounting in some cases almost to paresis. Scars from the hypodermic injections should always be looked for. The surest means of diagnosis is seclusion or close surveillance for a week, during which time the demand for the drug or some abstinence symptoms will appear.

Prognosis. — The prognosis is always very serious. Less than ten per cent. recover permanently; relapses are the rule. A few cases die from overdoses of the drug. The greater danger lies in cardiac weakness, which may lead to sudden collapse and fatal termination. The drug may be withdrawn with the proper precautions and the patients Buffer no ill-effects. Often, when the patients do not relapse into morphinism, they revert to substitutes, of which the most important are cocain, alcohol, chloroform, ether, and chloral. The treatment is preeminently unsuccessful in those with strong neuropathic tendencies.

Treatment. — The only successful method of treatment is complete abstinence. For this purpose the first requisite is isolation in a reputable institution. This method of treatment, however, cannot be safely undertaken in all cases, and especially where conditions of physical weakness are present, also during pregnancy, acute and severe chronic diseases. There are two methods of withdrawal, the gradual and the rapid, the latter of which requires the greatest skill and is by far the most efficacious. The former involves much time and patience, and is apt to create chronic and disagreeable traits which in the end are as difficult to eradicate as the habit itself. For these reasons only the rapid method is outlined here. It is necessary that the patients be placed in bed. In mild cases the drug may be withdrawn abruptly. Even in these the abstinence symptoms may appear. In cases where the dose has been large, the quantity is immediately reduced one-half, and after twenty-four hours to a nominal dose of one grain daily for several days, and in the course of two weeks entirely withdrawn. During the period of withdrawal the drug is best given in single daily doses in the early evening. If previously taken hypodermically, the drug should at once be changed to administration by mouth. Abstinence symptoms occur within the first thirty-six to forty-eight hours after the withdrawal of the drug and demand careful watching

on the part of the physician. To guard against these and to add to the comfort of the patient, alcohol in small doses with light nutritious diet may be given. Where there is impending collapse, faradization of the skin, injections of ether or camphor, the administration of hot coffee or hypodermic injections of strophanthus and strychnia are indicated, the last of which is often essential. If these fail, one always finds immediate relief in return to the usual dose of morphin. The greatest restlessness and insomnia often yield to the influence of ice packs on the head. If unsuccessful, the various hypnotics may be tried. The local pains may also be relieved by the application of ice. Purgation should be applied early; this, however, is contraindicated by pregnancy or an acute, serious, or chronic disease. Diarrhoea demands no special attention. Finally, it requires many months, and in some cases a year, to reestablish the former mental and physical health so that they are able to return to their old associations without fear of relapse. Even after being fully reestablished in health, it is necessary from time to time that the patients be subjected to close surveillance to ascertain if there is a return to the old habit.

0. COCAINISM

Cocain, in distinction from alcohol and morphin in its effects, is characterized by the great rapidity with which it produces profound mental enfeeblement and physical inanition. It is of rare occurrence to encounter symptoms of cocainism alone, because of the frequency of its complication with alcoholism and morphinism. For this reason it is difficult to draw a pure clinical picture of the disease.

Etiology. — The conditions giving rise to cocainism are similar to those encountered in morphinism. Most of the patients have a strong neuropathic basis, and many of them have previously been addicted to morphin. Early in the history of cocainism the habit arose from the substitution of cocain for morphin in the treatment of the latter habit, but at the present time most of the patients are physicians or druggists. The usual

method of administration is by the syringe, although it may be taken by insufflation.

Symptomatology. — *Acute Cocain Intoxication.* — Cocain in small doses produces moderate mental excitement, with a feeling of warmth and well-being, increase of pulse rate, and a fall of blood pressure. Its effects in the psychomotor field are similar to those of acute alcoholic intoxication: an excitement followed by paralysis. The patient is active, energetic, feels impelled to write, and is talkative. This condition is sooner or later followed by drowsiness. Large doses lead to delirious states with a tendency to collapse. Nissl has found in experiments upon rabbits that in the acute intoxication there is but a very slight alteration in the cortical neurones; *i.e.* a moderate disintegration of the chromophilic granules, some staining of the achromatic substance, and a moderate increase of the glia cells.

Chronic Cocain Intoxication. — In one accustomed to the prolonged use of the drug, there is a continuous mental state of nervous excitement with a flight of ideas, complete incapacity for mental work, lack of will-power, and defective memory. The patients are overenergetic, but their activity is planless; they are talkative and very productive, writing lengthy, meaningless letters, and evolving on paper impracticable schemes. They neglect their professional and home duties, also their personal appearance. In emotional attitude there is a variation between exhilaration with a pronounced feeling of well-being and great irritability and anxiety. They are very apt at times to mistrust their surroundings. At the same time they exhibit more or less indifference as to the legal consequence of their acts. The memory becomes defective and the judgment much impaired. *Physically,* the most prominent symptom is the profound disturbance of nutrition; the patients lose weight very rapidly, the normal expression changes, they look sleepy and tired, the skin becomes flaccid and pale. This is due in part to the fact that the drug supplies the place of nutritious food, for which they have lost all desire, and in part to excessive glandular action which makes a continuous drain upon the body tissues. There is muscular weakness and increased myotatic irritability, noted sometimes in the muscular twitchings. The pupils are dilated, but react normally, and there is tremor of the tongue. In the circulatory system there is slowness of the pulse, palpitation, and a tendency to faintness. In spite of increased sexual excitement, the sexual power diminishes. The sleep is disturbed, and occasionally interrupted by hallucinations.

Upon the basis of chronic cocainism there may develop a definite psychosis which bears close resemblance to the acute alcoholic hallucinosis.

Acute Cocain Hallucinosis. — Following a few days of irritability with anxiety and some restlessness, there appear suddenly hallucinations of different senses; the patients hear threatening voices compelling them to act strangely, and see moving pictures on the wall, which are filled with large and small objects. Characteristic of the hallucinations are the minute black specks moving about on a light surface, which are mistaken for flies, mosquitoes, and other tiny objects. This, according to Erlenmeyer, is an evidence of multiple disseminated scotoma. Peculiar sensations in the skin create the belief that they are being worked upon by electricity, being thrust with needles, or that poisonous material is being thrown upon them; but most characteristic is the sensation that foreign objects are under the skin, especially at the ends of the fingers and in the palms of the hands. The muscular twitchings, they believe, are due to the action of some poison. The hallucinations of hearing make them suspicious of their surroundings. Their thoughts are being read by means of some secret contrivance; they are being spied through holes in the ceiling. Some patients become so thoroughly frightened that they attempt to kill their supposed persecutors, or in despair may commit suicide.

A characteristic symptom is the silly delusions of infidelity. These are frequently obscene in character. Wives or husbands are accused of illicit relations, of receiving many love letters, of stealthily leaving the house and neglecting the family for immoral purposes, or of becoming known as public characters. In reaction to these ideas patients are usually vindictive and may even become aggressive.

The consciousness remains clear. There is good orientation, except in rare instances where the excitement is very great, or immediately following fresh injections of the drug. In emotional attitude patients are always dejected, excitable, irritable, and sometimes passionate. Occasionally they are reserved and reticent concerning their delusions. In actions they are usually very restless and unstable, though some may appear quite orderly. In the markedly delirious conditions which sometimes appear there is always great restlessness.

Acute cocain hallucinosis develops rapidly and may run its full *course* within a few weeks. The symptoms increase rapidly under the influence of single doses of cocain. The delirious state soon disappears after the complete withdrawal of the drug, sometimes within a few days, while the delusions may remain for weeks or even months. The coexistence of morphinism and cocainism in the same individual, which is of common occurrence, frequently leads to a combination of the symptoms. Morphinism alone seldom produces a rapid development of pronounced mental disturbance, unless in connection with cocainism.

Acute cocain hallucinosis is differentiated from acute alcoholic hallucinosis by its more rapid development, the greater severity of the symptoms, and by the fact that the delusions of jealousy appear earlier and as an acute symptom. The effect of a single dose of cocain during the psychosis produces an exacerbation of the symptoms, while in alcoholism it has little or no effect. Finally, the sensation of objects under the skin is characteristic only of cocainism.

The prognosis in cocainism is unfavorable for complete recovery. The symptoms of intoxication clear up after the withdrawal of the drug, but the power of resistance is profoundly affected, and few resist temptation for any great length of time.

Treatment. — The only successful method of treatment is complete abstinence. The rapid method of the withdrawal, similar to that employed in morphinism, is best. The withdrawal is usually attended only by unimportant symptoms, such as uneasiness, a feeling of pressure in the chest, with difficulty in breathing, also palpitation of the heart, and insomnia, and occasionally by a tendency to faintness which simulates collapse. If such emergency arises, it is necessary to employ stimulants, as alcohol, camphor, coffee, strychnia, etc. The insomnia may be combated with prolonged warm baths, paraldehyde trional, and also by a nutritious diet. An essential element in successful treatment is confinement in an institution, where it can be determined with certainty that the patient does not have access to the drug. Prolonged treatment with the employment of every possible means to fortify him against relapses is an important factor, which requires patience on the part of the patient and perseverance and tact on the part of the physician. If morphinism and cocainism coexist, cocain should be withdrawn first.

IV. THYROIGENOUS PSYCHOSES

The two forms of psychosis arising from disturbance of the thyroid gland are myxcedematous insanity and cretinism. They develop directly as the result of an absence of glandular activity, cretinism appearing in early childhood, and myxcedematous insanity in adolescence and later. Rightfully the symptoms accompanying Graves's disease belong in this group, but are not described because of their comparatively infrequent occurrence.

A. Myxedematous Insanity

The mental disturbance characteristic of myxcedema is that of a simple progressive mental deterioration accompanied by the characteristic physical symptoms of the disease.

Etiology. — The lack of glandular activity in the thyroid is supposed to be the exciting cause by failing to neutralize or care for some toxic product of metabolism. The gland in all cases is found atrophied or diseased. This is frequently the result of connective tissue increase, sometimes of colloid degeneration, and rarely of tuberculosis or syphilis of the gland.

Symptomatology. — The onset of the mental disturbance is gradual, with increasing difficulty of apprehension. The patients do not comprehend written or spoken language as well as formerly, and are unable to collect their thoughts. It takes them longer to perform ordinary duties, such as dressing, and they also tire easily. Memory for recent events becomes defective. The increasing difficulty in applying the mind and in performing even simple acts finally renders them completely helpless. There is no clouding of consciousness. At first they exhibit some insight into their defects, but later this gives way to indifference and stupidity, not only in reference to themselves and their condition, but also to their environment. They rarely express pleasure or pain, and very seldom give evidence of thought for themselves or their future. In emotional attitude it is characteristic for them to be anxious, dejected, and at times fearful. Sometimes they develop restlessness and moderate excitement with stubbornness. In rare cases there may appear conditions of confusion with hallucinations and delusions.

Physically, they present characteristic cutaneous and nervous symptoms. The skin becomes thick and dry, rough, inelastic, obliterating the characteristic lines of expression in the face, producing thick lips, broad nose, and deforming the hand and fingers. The mucous membrane is similarly involved, and the tongue is thick and unwieldy. The cutaneous change is most marked in the supraclavicular region, in the upper arms, and in the abdominal wall. The voice is changed, becoming rough and monotonous, and the speech is slow and difficult. The nervous symptoms consist chiefly of headache, vertigo, fainting, convulsive spells, and a fine tremor. Finally the skin and mucous membrane become anaemic and very sensitive to cold, menses cease, and temperature becomes subnormal. The blood changes vary; sometimes there is an increase of the red corpuscles, and at other times a diminution.

Course. — The psychosis is of gradual onset, and unless appropriate treatment is applied, progresses to advanced deterioration, extreme physical weakness, and profound disturbance of nutrition, the disease terminating fatally through the intervention of some intercurrent disease. Occasionally there are intermissions, and in a few cases marked improvement occurs in spite of the absence of treatment.

Treatment. — The administration of dried thyroids of the sheep, beginning at one and one-half grains, one to three times daily, may be regarded as a specific remedy in this disease. The dose is gradually increased, guarding carefully against intoxication symptoms, indicated by headache, dizziness, and irregular cardiac action. The improvement becomes evident within a week and increases very rapidly. The patients become active and show an interest in themselves and surroundings; they improve in memory and in judgment. The physical symptoms improve with equal rapidity. In the most successful cases the patients appear quite well at the end of two months, except for some lassitude, which persists for a long time. Not all cases recover through medication; the number of unsuccessful cases is difficult to ascertain at present. Relapses may occur.

B. Cretinism

Cretinism is characterized by a more or less high-grade defective mental development, associated with loss of function of the thyroid, and accompanied by definite physical symptoms.

Etiology. — The disease is mostly endemic in mountainous regions. In Europe the cases are most numerous in the Alps and Pyrenees; in America, in Vermont. Sporadic cases occur as the result of congenital absence of the gland or its atrophy during or following a fever, or in connection with goitre. The disease arises from an organic infectious material, and is in some way associated with disease of the parathyroid gland. It is unknown whether this infectious organism is the cause of an atrophy, a non-development, or disease of these glands, in this way producing a failure of mental development; or whether it is due to the direct action of the organism or its toxin upon the nervous system. Other important factors are defective neuropathic basis and unhygienic surroundings.

Pathological Anatomy. — The morbid anatomy is still doubtful. Asymmetries and dilatation of the ventricles of the brain and atrophy have been found, also hyperostosis of the cranium. The cortical neurones are deficient in number and processes, and are of the stunted globose form peculiar to idiocy and other forms of defective development.

Symptomatology. — The symptoms of the disease are first noticed during the first and second years, except in a few cases where the children are born goitrous. At that time they appear dull, stupid, indifferent, sleepy, and unable to care for themselves; have not learned to walk or talk, and are slow and awkward in their movements. The gland increases in size from the sixth to twelfth year in three-fourths of the cases; in the remaining it diminishes. Mentally, the patients fail to develop, presenting the symptoms of imbecility; they are dull, stupid, incapable of apprehending or of elaborating impressions, presenting about the capacity of a five-year-old child. They are rather indifferent and phlegmatic, and quite incapable of applying themselves to any work. A few cases present a condition of extreme stupidity. Their condition remains unchanged throughout life, except as interrupted by short periods of excitement, similar to those occurring in idiocy. This condition may form a basis for the development of other psychoses, especially manicdepressive insanity.

Physically, the long bones fail to develop in length, instead, becoming thicker. The head is large, and the neck short and thick. The nose is broad, and the ears are prominent, the skin is thickened as if padded, and in places, especially in the neck, hanging dependent in folds. The broad face, with heavy cheeks and eyelids, with thick lips and broad short nose, presents a very characteristic picture. The limbs are large and pudgy. The tongue is thick and clumsy in its movements. The hair is scanty, and dentition is late and the teeth poor. The speech consists of inarticulate sounds, which are loud, coarse, slurring, and stammering. The movements are unwieldy, the gait slow and cumbersome. Convulsions are rare. The sexual organs develop slowly, and in severe cases remain entirely undeveloped. Patients have little power of resistance, readily succumbing to intercurrent diseases.

Treatment. — The hygienic surroundings must be improved with special attention to drinking water. Many observers agree that it is advisable as a prophylactic measure to send children and families with cretinoid tendencies to the high mountains, which may bring about a complete recovery in children who already show some signs of disease. Potassium iodide in small doses seems to be beneficial. According to recent observation the administration of desiccated thyroid, if given early, may aid in preventing the development of the disease. After an extended duration the same drug may improve some of the physical symptoms, — thickness of the skin and amenorrhcea, — but the mental symptoms cannot be altered.

V. DEMENTIA Prjecox

Dementia Piuecox' is the name provisionally applied to a large group of cases which are characterized in common by a pronounced tendency to mental deterioration of varying grades. The disease apparently develops on the basis of a severe disease process in the cerebral cortex, but whether the process is always the same is by no means certain. Dementia fortunately does not occur in all cases, but it is so prominent a feature that the name dementia praecox is best retained until the symptom group is better understood.

Etiology. — The disease is one of the most prominent, comprising from fourteen to thirty per cent. of all admissions to insane institutions. As the name indicates, it is a disease of early life. More than sixty per cent. of the cases appear before the twenty-fifth year. This, however, varies in the different forms; in hebephrenia almost threefourths of the cases appear before the twenty-fifth year, in catatonia sixty-eight per cent., and in the paranoid only forty per cent. On the other hand, cases that cannot in any way be distinguished from hebephrenia have been observed in patients between fifty and sixty years. The disease in the younger cases seems to take the form of a simple gradually progressive deterioration; in the somewhat later periods, it assumes the acute and subacute forms with catatonic symptoms; while still later the more pronounced delusion formation appears. Kraepelin reports that in the hebephrenic form sixty-four per cent. of the cases are men, in catatonic and paranoid forms women slightly predominate; but in our experience men slightly predominate in the hebephrenic and catatonic forms, while in the paranoid form sixty-nine per cent. are women. Defective heredity is a very prominent factor, as it appears in about seventy per cent. of cases reported by Kraepelin, but in not more than fifty-two per cent. of our cases. It varies somewhat in the different forms, being far more prominent in the paranoid and equally less prominent in the catatonic and hebephrenic forms. Various physical stigmata are occasionally encountered, such as asymmetries and malformations of the skull, ears, and palate, puerile expression, strabismus, supernumerary nipples, general physical weakness. There is frequently an earlier history of deliria accompanying moderate forms of fever, of convulsions in youth, and great susceptibility to alcohol, as well as the absence of sexual impulses and their early or unnatural development. Besides the above evidences of a faulty endowment thirty-three per cent. of the patients previous to the onset of the disease have been only moderately bright. At least twenty per cent. exhibit mental peculiarities from early youth up, such as seclusiveness, affectation, eccentricity, precocious piety, impulsiveness, and moral instability, while seven per cent. have always been weak-minded. In women, child-bearing seems an important factor, as twenty-four per cent. of the female catatonics become afflicted during pregnancy, or at childbirth, but particularly the latter. This occurs in only nine per cent. of the female hebephrenics. In ten per cent. of the cases there is a previous history of some severe acute illness, particularly typhoid and scarlet fevers, from which time the patients have exhibited some change, as increased irritability, susceptibility to fatigue, and impairment of the full mental capacity. Head injuries precede a very small number of cases. Alcoholism, likewise, is an unimportant factor, but more than five per cent. of the male patients develop their disease while incarcerated in prison. These and the puerperal cases are particularly apt to develop into acute and subacute forms. Pregnancy favors the paranoid forms; and child-bed, the catatonic forms. Pathology. — The nature of the disease process in dementia praecox is not known, but it seems probable, judging from the clinical course, and especially in those cases where there has been rapid deterioration, that there is a definite disease process in the brain, involving the cortical neurones. This view is further upheld by the fact that in those cases which have been subjected to the most modern methods of research, anatomical lesions have been found which can be explained only upon such a basis. In a few cases this is a reparable lesion, but in most cases the impairment of function is permanent and progressive. This pathological basis finds clinical expression in the few cases that recover and the larger number that show a permanent mental defect. The means by which these assumed changes are brought about in the nervous system are no better known than those that exist in epilepsy and idiocy. The relationship of the disease to puberty, disturbances of menstruation, child-bearing, and climacterium, and the absence of every recognizable external cause, suggests first of all an autointoxication, which may be in some way related to processes *in* the sexual organs. Defective heredity, which exists in such a large percentage of cases, may be presumed to create a lessened power of resistance to the essential causes of the disease.

Finzie Vedrani, Rivista sperim.de freniatria, XXV, 1899; Christian, Ann. m6dico-psychol. 8, 9, 43,1899; Trcemmer, Das Jugendirresein (Dementia praecox), 1900; Serieux, Gaz. hebdomad. Mars 1901; Revue de psychiatrie, Juin 1902; Jahrmaerker, Zur Frage der Dementia praecox, 1902; Meeus, Bull, de la soc. de m6d. ment. de Belgique, mars-sept. 1902; Masselon, Psychologie des dements precoces, 1902; Stransky, Jahrb. f. Psych. XXIII, 1903; Bernstein, Allg. Zeitschr. f. Psych. LX, 554, 1903; Meyer, British Medical Journal, Sept. 29, 1906.

'In our experience in Connecticut the age of onset has been under 25 years of age in only 34 % of the cases; in the hebephrenic form 45 % develop the disease under 25 years of age, in the catatonic form 38 %, and in the paranoid only 11 %. The average age of onset in all forms is from one to four years earlier in the male than in the female patients.

Symptomatology. — In the field of *apprehension* there is usually very little disturbance. Ordinary external impressions are correctly apprehended, the patients being able to recognize their environment and to comprehend most of what takes place about them. Yet accurate tests show that very brief stimuli are not well apprehended. During the acute or subacute onset of the disease, apprehension is affected, and there is some disorientation. This may also appear during transitory stupor or excitement; but even in these conditions, and especially in the apparent stupidity and indifference which characterize the later stages of the disease, it is surprising to see how many things in the environment are apprehended. Indeed, it is not unusual to find that patients even notice changes in the physician's apparel, in the furniture, etc. Nevertheless, as the disease advances and deterioration appears, apprehension, as well as other mental phenomena, becomes perceptibly impaired.

The *orientation* is mostly undisturbed. Patients usually know where they are, recognize those about them, and are aware of the time. In stupor and in states of anxiety, the orientation may be considerably clouded, yet it is characteristic of dementia praecox that, even in spite of considerable excitement, the patients continue to apprehend well. On the other hand, the delusional form of disorientation may exist (see p. 28).

Apprehension is always more or less distorted by *hattucinations,* especially in acute and subacute development of the disease.-Occasionally, they persist throughout the entire course of the disease. They, however, tend to disappear in the end stages, though they occasionally reappear during exacerbations. Hallucinations of hearing are most prominent, next come hallucinations of sight and touch, the feelings of currents, of movements, and of influence. Hallucinations at first are distressing, and result in fear; but later they do not excite much reaction, except during exacerbations.

Consciousness is usually clear, but in conditions of excitement and stupor there is always some clouding of consciousness. It is, however, much less marked than one would judge from superficial observation, as the patients later are able to give some details of things that happened in the interval.

On the other hand, there is pronounced impairment of voluntary *attention,* which is one of the most fundamental symptoms. The controlling force of interest is altogether lacking, so that the presentation which happens to be the clearest and most distinct at any given moment is an accident of passing attention, never persistent enough to occasion connected activity. In spite of the fact that the patients perceive objects about them correctly, they do not observe them closely or attempt to understand them. In deep stupor and in the stage of deterioration it is absolutely impossible to attract the attention in any way. In the catatonic form of dementia praecox the presence of negativism inhibits all active attention. This becomes evident as the negativism gradually disappears. The patients emerging from

this condition are caught stealthily peeping about when unobserved, looking out of open doors or windows, and following the movements of the physician, but when an object is held before them for observation they stare vacantly about or close their eyes tightly.

There is a characteristic and progressive, but not profound, impairment of *memory* from the onset of the disease. Memory images formed before the onset of the disease are retained with remarkable persistence, — retention is good. Though their reproduction is increasingly more difficult, unusual stimulation or excitement may occasion the recollection of events long since supposed to be effaced by the advance of deterioration—recollection is not free. The formation of new memory images is increasingly difficult with the advance of the disease. Memory for recent events is poor. Events previous to the onset, especially school knowledge, may be recalled after the patients show advanced deterioration. Some few patients keep a careful account of the length of their residence in the hospital and elsewhere. Events during stupor and excitement are not remembered at all, or at most indistinctly.

The *train of thought* sooner or later in the course of the disease is profoundly disturbed by the appearance of a characteristic looseness and desultoriness, which has already been described (see p. 40). One finds even in the mild cases some distractibility, a rapid transition from one thought to another without an evident association, and interpolation of highsounding phrases. In severe cases there is genuine confusion of thought with great incoherence and the production of new words. In cases of the catatonic form especially, we meet with evidences of stereotypy; the patients cling to one idea, which they repeat over and over again. Besides, there is occasionally noticed a tendency to rhyme or repeat senseless sounds.

In *judgment* there appears from the onset a progressive defect. While patients are able to get along without difficulty under familiar circumstances, they fail to adapt themselves to new conditions. Owing to their inability to grasp the meaning of their surroundings, their actions are irrational. This condition of defective judgment becomes the basis for the development of delusions. The patients believe that they are the objects of persecution, and they may have delusions of reference and self-accusation. The lack of judgment becomes still more apparent in the silliness of their delusions. At first the delusions may be rather stable, but later they tend to change their content frequently, adding new elements suggested by the environment. Even relatively persistent delusions are constantly taking on new meanings. Furthermore, the delusions, which at first are of a depressive nature, later may become expansive and grandiose. In most cases the wealth of delusions so apparent at first gradually disappears. A few delusions may be retained with further elaboration from time to time, but they are usually expressed only at random. During exacerbations the former delusions, whether depressive or expansive, may again come to the foreground. In the paranoid forms, however, there persists from the beginning a great wealth of delusions, but these become more and more incoherent.

The disturbance of the *emotional field* is another of the characteristic and fundamental symptoms. There is a progressive, more or less high-grade, deterioration of the emotional life. The lack of interest in the surroundings already spoken of in connection with the attention may be regarded as one phase of the general emotional deterioration. Very often it is this symptom which first calls attention to the approaching disease. Parents and friends notice that there is a change in the disposition, a laxity in morals, a disregard for formerly cherished ideas, a lack of affection toward relatives and friends, an absence of their accustomed sympathy, and above all an unnatural satisfaction with their own ideas and behavior. They fail to exhibit the usual pleasure in their employment.

As the disease progresses the absence of emotion becomes more marked. The patients express neither joy nor sorrow, have neither desire nor fears, but live from one day to another quite unconcerned and apathetic, sometimes silently gazing into the distance, at others regarding their surroundings with a vacant stare. They are indifferent as to their personal appearance, submit stupidly to uncomfortable positions, and even prodding with a needle may not excite a reaction. Food, however, continues to attract them until deterioration is far advanced. Indeed, it is not unusual to see these patients go through the pockets and bundles of their friends for delicacies, without expressing a sign of recognition. This condition of stupid indifference may be interrupted by short periods of irritability.

Early in the disease, and especially during an acute and subacute development, the emotional attitude may be one of depression and anxiety. This may later give way to moderate elation and happiness. The latter, however, in a few instances prevails from the onset. Yet emotional deterioration remains a fundamental symptom.

Parallel with the emotional disturbances are found disturbances of *conduct,* of which the most fundamental is the progressive *disappearance of voluntary activity.* One of the first symptoms of the disease may be the loss of that activity which is peculiar to the patient. He may neglect his duties and sit unoccupied for the greater part of the day, though capable of doing good work if persistently encouraged. Besides this characteristic inactivity, there may appear a tendency to impulsive acts. The patients break out window lights, tear their clothing into strips, leap into the water, break furniture, throw dishes on the floor, or injure fellowpatients, all of which seems done without a definite motive. These states usually pass off very quickly, though in some this tendency may be more marked for a period of a few days.

The inability to control the impulses is also present in the stuporous conditions, and especially in the catatonic form of dementia praecox. Here each natural impulse is seemingly met and overcome by an opposing impulse, giving rise to actions directly opposite to the ones desired. In this condition, which is called *negativism,* the patients resist everything that is done for them, such as dressing and undressing, they refuse to eat when food is placed before them, to open their mouth or eyes when requested, or to move in any direction. In extreme conditions there may even be retention of urine and feces. This condition varies considerably in intensity at different times. It is not unusual to see the patients suddenly relieved of it, assume their former activity, talking freely and attending to their own needs, and again after an interval of a few hours or days relapse gradually into the negativistic state.

Still another condition is produced by the repeated recurrence of the same impulse, giving rise to a great variety of *stereotyped movements and expressions.* The verbigerations and mannerisms of the catatonic are explained in this way. The patients repeat for hours similar expressions, utter monotonous grunts, tread the floor in the same spot, dress, undress, and eat in a peculiar and constrained manner. While these symptoms vary considerably in individual cases, it is unusual not to find at least some of them present in every case.

Frequently also hypersuggestibility of the will and *automatism* are present, particularly in the stage of deterioration. The patients are not only very pliable, but they may show echolalia or echopraxia for longer or shorter periods. Some patients, however, never show these symptoms at any time during the disease.

One of the fundamental symptoms of the disease is the discrepancy or lack of uniformity between the emotional attitude and the content of thought. Thus, patients laugh and cry without apparent reason; they cheerfully refer to their attempts at suicide, and exhibit great anxiety or outbursts of passion upon the slightest provocation. Indeed this discrepancy between the ideation and the emotional attitude gives one the impression of *childishness.* The whole conduct shows many similar incongruities; the discrepancy seen between the feelings and the facial expression is called *paramimia;* such as, weeping on cheerful occasions, and laughing when sorrow should prevail; also the combination of laughing and crying, etc. There are many other symptoms, as mannerisms, eccentricities, and perhaps also the confusion of speech and the use of neologisms, which may be explained on the basis of a disruption of the natural connection between the processes of thought, feeling, and will. This loss of spontaneity frequently leads to the idea that the patients are *being controlled by the will of another.* They feel that their acts are not their own, but that they are compelled to do unnatural things. Hence some patients come to believe that they are being hypnotized.

The *capacity for employment* is seriously impaired. The patients may be trained to do a certain amount of routine work, but they utterly fail when given something new. A few patients display artistic abilities, as, for instance, in drawing or in music, but their efforts are characterized by eccentricities. They may show some technical skill, but their productions exhibit the absence of the finer aesthetic feelings.

Physical Symptoms. — *Attacks,* either of a syncopal or an epileptiform nature, are among the most important physical symptoms. These may occur frequently during the course of the disease or but once. They rarely involve alone single groups of muscles, or are apoplectiform in nature followed by more or less prolonged paralyses. Occasionally these attacks represent the first symptom of the disease. They occur in about eighteen per cent. of the cases and are twice as frequent among women as among men. In addition, hysterical attacks are also observed. There is still another type of convulsive movement, involving the muscles of the eye and speech, which is both characteristic and of frequent occurrence in dementia praecox. Some of these movements correspond exactly to the movements of expression; wrinkling of the eyebrow, distortion of the mouth, rolling the eyes, and those other facial movements which

are characterized as grimacing. These movements remind one of choreic movements and are quite independent of ideas and feelings. There may be associated with them smacking of the lips, clucking the tongue, sudden grunting, sniffing, and coughing. Furthermore, in the lips we observe very rapid rhythmical movements. More often there exists a peculiar choreiform movement of the mouth which may be described as an athetoid ataxia.

There is usually an increase of the deep reflexes as well as of the mechanical irritability of the muscles and nerves. The pupils are often dilated, particularly in conditions of excitement, and are occasionally unequal. Not infrequently sensibility to pain is diminished. Vasomotor changes, as cyanosis, circumscribed edema, and dermograph, may occur in all stages of the disease, but are most often met in the stuporous states. Excessive perspiration is sometimes present. The secretion of saliva is frequently increased. The heart's activity varies, sometimes being slowed, more often accelerated, but also sometimes irregular and weak. The menses usually cease or are irregular. The body temperature is often subnormal. In many cases there has been detected a diffuse enlargement of the glands, which sometimes undergo atrophy just before the onset of the disease. Exophthalmic goitre and tremor are sometimes present. Anemia and chlorosis are frequently observed. The sleep is apt to be much disturbed during the developmental stage, at which time there is also anorexia and the patients tend to take little nourishment; but later in the course of the disease the taking of nourishment may vary from absolute refusal of food to extreme gluttony. The body weight usually falls at the onset of the disease, and often to a marked degree, even in spite of the fact that the patients are taking a sufficient quantity of nourishment. On the other hand, the weight usually rises later and not infrequently rapidly and to a marked degree.

Clinically, the large group of cases comprising dementia praecox is divided into three smaller groups: the

hebephrenic, the *catatonic,* and the *paranoid,* each of which differs somewhat in the grouping, prominence, and course of the fundamental symptoms.

Hebephrenic Form

The hebephrenic form of dementia praecox is characterized *by the gradual or subacute development of a simple more or less profound mental deterioration.* An acute onset is rare.

This form represents in our experience fifty-eight per cent. of the cases of dementia praecox. The larger number of cases develop under twenty-five years of age. The first symptoms may appear at the beginning of puberty. The onset may be so insidious that the actual date cannot be placed. Some of these patients do not even come under the care of the physician until years after the onset of the disease.

The hebephrenic form should include a small group of cases which gradually develop a *simple hypochondriacal dementia.* The prominent symptom is a constantly increasing feeling of physical and mental incapacity, accompanied by all kinds of morbid sensations, which finally compel the patients to desist from any sort of activity. At the same time there develops an emotional indifference and general languor without hallucinations or pronounced delusions.

Symptomatology. — Usually the patients first complain of headache and insomnia, which are soon followed by a gradual change of disposition. They lose their accustomed activity and energy, becoming self-absorbed, shy, sullen, and seclusive, or perhaps irritable and obstinate. They may be rude and assertive, or perfectly indifferent. They become careless of their obligations, thoughtless, and unbalanced. They accomplish nothing, but rather sit about unemployed, apparently brooding, or they leave their work to go to bed, lying there for weeks without evident reason. Others, instead of this inaction, exhibit a marked restlessness, and continuous effort is impossible. They leave their work, stroll about or travel from place to place, especially at night. Others, with increased sexual passion, indulge in illicit and promiscuous intercourse.

During this period, which may extend through several months, remissions are common, when for a short time the patients improve greatly and may even appear natural. This period, on the other hand, may rather be characterized by alternating periods of depression and elation of increasing severity. Women usually show premonitions of the disease during the menses.

Sometimes the onset is characterized by a period of marked depression. The patients become apprehensive, dejected, sad, and reserved. They are troubled with thoughts of death, and sometimes suddenly attempt suicide, often in a peculiar manner. They are usually hypochondriacs, and complain of nervousness and weakness; they search quack medical literature and frequently ascribe their troubles to former masturbation. There is also a mistrust of the environment and a feeling that they are being watched, imposed upon, or badly treated. But most striking is the emotional indifference with which the patients express and defend their morbid ideas.

Many cases develop no further. The more severe cases at this time begin to show *hallucinations,* especially of hearing, and less often of sight. The patients are annoyed by strange noises, unintelligible voices, unfavorable comments upon their personal appearance; they hear threats and imprecations, music and singing, telephone messages, and commands from God. They may also see heavenly visions, crosses on the wall, dead relatives, frightful accidents, and deathbed scenes. Occasionally they smell various odors, especially illuminating gas and sulphur. They may experience various hyperaesthesias which lead them to believe that the head is double, that the throat or nose is occluded, that the genitals are being consumed, or that the bowels are all bound together.

At the same time *delusions* become a prominent part of the picture and are mostly of a *depressive character.* The patients believe themselves guilty of some crime, accuse themselves of being murderers, claim that they are lost, are damned, unfit to live, have practised self-abuse, and can never recover from its ill effects. They suspect their surroundings, detect poison in the food, are being worked upon by others, their thoughts are not their own, friends have turned against them and are trying to do them harm, some one is watching them constantly, and they are being harassed by various agencies. Women are followed by men who would ravish them. Later in the course of the disease, and occasionally from the onset, the delusions are *expansive;* the patients then regard themselves as prominent individuals: the President, the Son of God, the Creator, the possessor of the universe. They converse with God, are the Saviours of men, and possess all knowledge. Some patients are controlled by sexual ideas, fancying perhaps that they are betrothed to prominent individuals. Men believe themselves possessed of many wives, or regard themselves as the center of attraction for all women.

These delusions may be augmented by numerous *fabrications;* the patients claiming that they have been President for a century, chief commandant in various engagements, have been knighted, that they have been in heaven, have gained possession of the key of hell, have just returned from a visit to Mars. These fabrications, together with the delusions, gradually recede to the background. At first they become less numerous, less fantastic, then incoherent, and still more scanty, until finally, in the advanced stages of the disease, there remain only incoherent residuals of former delusions which may never be expressed except when elicited, or during excitement.

Some *insight* into their condition is often expressed at first by the patients. They are conscious that a change has come over them, and often complain that the head feels strange, benumbed, or empty. These ideas may be expressed in connection with somatic delusions, when they will claim that the brain is rotting, the memory failing, that they are different in every way, or are very much confused. But even this scanty insight gradually disappears as the disease progresses.

In those forms of the disease which develop slowly there is at first neither *clouding of consciousness* nor disturbance of orientation. In the acute or subacute onset, cloudiness and general disorientation may unite in the clinical picture with pronounced hallucinations and delusions, anxiety and restlessness, and incoherence of thought. The patients mistake persons, do not appreciate where they are, and are unable to record passing events. Physicians are regarded as enemies trying to kill them, working upon them with electricity, etc. They are confined in a prison for some grave offence, or are among the heavenly hosts, surrounded by saints.

The *train of thought* in the gradually developing cases is at first very little disturbed, the content of speech being both coherent and relevant; but later in the disease and with progressive deterioration there develops the characteristic looseness of thought and desultoriness, often combined with the use of neologisms and embellishments.

The *memory* at first suffers only moderately. Memory of earlier life and the chronological order of events is well retained for a long time. Some of the patients are able to tell with surprising accuracy the exact definitions in geography and many historical events almost word for word, as committed to memory years before. But with the progress of the disease there is an increasing impoverishment of the store of ideas. The impressibility of memory is retained, but the patients fail to make use of it, because there is a total lack of interest. Without this there is no incentive for observation and thought, and they fail to observe what is going on about them. As the disease progresses, there is increasing limitation of thought. For this same reason past experiences are seldom recalled, and so finally fade from memory; though it is not unusual for patients, in reaction to unusual stimulation, to recall events that seemed to have entirely passed from them.

The defect in *judgment* appears early, develops rapidly, and becomes profound. This may not be evident while the patient is confined at home, or during the early part of the residence in an institution, as long as his thought is employed with familiar facts, and his range for action limited. It becomes apparent, however, when he leaves the trodden path and attempts to adapt himself to new circumstances. He is unable to reason, to perform mental work, to recognize contradiction, or to overcome obstacles. The defect can also be seen in his tendency to formulate and hold to senseless, incoherent delusions.

In *emotional attitude* the most prominent and permanent feature is that of emotional dulness and indifference. Whenever we find emotional activity it is increasingly self-centered. At first there is usually more or less depression, with anxiety, peevishness, and often irritability. Exaggerated expressions of religious feelings are apt to be prominent, the patients being devout, praying frequently, reading their testaments, at first apparently in the spirit of penitence, but later because they are led by God or ordained to do some special work. The sexual feelings very often play a prominent role, particularly in those who have been addicted to the habit of masturbation. Thought may center about sexual matters, when they enjoy obscene literature, write long letters to acquaintances, and give expression to their lascivious feelings, masturbate, and solicit intercourse. Female patients are more apt to associate with their own sex. In both sexes these feelings are apt to disappear later in the course of the disease. Later in the disease the delusions, both expansive and hypochondriacal, are expressed without display of emotion. Patients fail to express emotion at the loss of friends, at the visits of relatives, or at an unusual supply of food, fruit, or candies. They live a very empty life, devoid of any cares or anxieties, and without thought for the future.

In *conduct* and *behavior,* the most characteristic symptom is that of childish silliness and senseless laughter. The voluntary activity is inconsistent and lacks independence. At one moment patients are increasingly headstrong, at the next as supremely tractable. They neglect their personal appearance, perform all sorts of outlandish and foolish deeds, such as prowling about all night, setting fire to buildings, throwing stones to break windows, and travelling about without evident purpose. They may even run away and secrete themselves, or as unexpectedly demand some one in marriage, forget their obligations, and finally are completely incapable of continued and comprehensive employment. A young man was found throwing stones into trees because the voices of evil spirits annoyed him. A student ran from his mates to a graveyard and covered himself with leaves in order to obtain aid in committing his ivy oration. A girl of fourteen attempted to stab her lover, believing him to be unfaithful. A young married woman solicited intercourse among gentlemen friends, even bringing them to her home for that purpose in the presence of her husband and children. The patients are very often seen to converse with themselves, sometimes aloud, while associated with this there is almost always silly laughter. This silly laughter is a very prominent and characteristic symptom. It is unrestrained, appears on all occasions without the least provocation, and is altogether without emotional significance. Besides these actions, mannerisms, such as peculiarities of speech and movements, eating and walking, are often present. A few of the mannerisms characteristic of the catatonic may prevail: echolalia, echopraxia, stereotyped expressions and movements.

The speech presents peculiarities indicative of looseness of thought and confusion of ideas. Their remarks may be artificial, containing many stilted phrases, stale witticisms, foreign expressions, and obsolete words. The incoherence of thought becomes most evident in their long drawn out sentences, in which there is total disregard for grammatical structure. The structure changes frequently, and there are many senseless interpolations. All this becomes even more apparent in their letters, which are verbose with frequent repetitions, while the handwriting is characterized by a marked lack or a superfluity of punctuation marks, shading of letters, and copious underlining.

Physical Symptoms. — During the onset of the disease the condition of general nutrition suffers. There is a loss of weight, and some patients even become emaciated. The appetite is poor. Patients eat sparingly or not at all, restrained by suspicion and fear, or because they are so directed by God. The sleep also is much disturbed, both by anxiety and distressing dreams. The pupils are occasionally dilated. The tendon reflexes may be exaggerated, and vasomotor disturbances may be present. The skin loses its normal healthy appearance, becoming dry and flaccid. The menses cease or become irregular. Later in the course of the disease the appetite returns and often becomes excessive. At this time the weight often rises rapidly, and the emaciated condition is frequently replaced by great corpulence. The menses also reappear and remain normal, and the evidences of muscular and nervous irritability disappear.

Course.—The course of the disease in the hebephrenic form is characterized by all sorts of variations. Suitable treatment during the active stages at the onset usually produces some improvement. But there develops later a condition of uniform dementia, which may be permanent, or interrupted by repeated exacerbations. Occasionally there develop conditions of pronounced excitement with mischievousness, talkativeness, clownish behavior, laughing, giggling, a tendency to sexual acts, and senseless wandering about. In other cases there develop profound clouding, with impulsiveness, greater incoherence of thought, dancing, smearing, destructiveness, and assaults. These conditions are usually of short duration. They may recur suddenly and without warning. The degree of mental defect increases from year to year, more especially following the transitory periods of excitement.

Of the cases that are admitted to insane institutions, about *seventy-five per cent, reach a profound degree of deterioration.* These patients are dull, indolent, apathetic, anergic, sluggish, and fail to apprehend the surroundings. They remain seated for hours wherever placed, are incapable of caring for themselves, are untidy, have to be dressed and undressed, and led to meals. At table they are slovenly, spattering and smearing themselves with food. They give but little evidence of voluntary activity. They seldom speak, are unproductive and mute; occasionally they may be seen to laugh sillily or repeat to themselves some unintelligible word or syllable.

Their attention is attracted with difficulty and held only for a short time. External objects usually fail to make an impression upon them. Questions are apparently uncomprehended, seldom exciting intelligible answers. These are usually monosyllabic and irrelevant. Simple directions, however, may be correctly carried out. Relatives and acquaintances may not be recognized. Bits of former knowledge are retained in many cases for a long time, such as historical and geographical facts and the ability to solve problems in arithmetic. In this respect the patients often surprise one. One of my patients was able to name the islands of the Pacific and give the names of their sovereigns. Another, who for two years had been mute, unable to care for himself, untidy, sitting through the day with bowed head, entirely unmindful of his surroundings, recognized a college mate, straightened up with an air of dignity, and laughed at some college jokes. In the course of time even such relics of former mental activity disappear, and we have nothing left but the unproductive vegetative organism. A few patients retain some remnants of mental activity, but they are quite unbalanced, silly, and present the residuals of hallucinations and delusions. Instead of the extreme stupidity and indolence some patients continue restless and talkative, producing an incoherent babble with silly laughter. During the periods of transitory excitement these patients are very apt to be aggressive, breaking windows and attacking fellow-patients, to masturbate shamelessly, pull out their hair, and fre-

quently show homicidal tendencies. Usually it requires several years before the patients reach this stage of dementia. In cases with an acute onset it may appear within a year.

In about *seventeen per cent, of the cases the degree of deterioration is not as far advanced.* These patients, after the subsidence of the more acute symptoms, show a certain amount of mental activity and are capable of some employment under supervision. They are oriented and have a certain amount of insight into their mental incapacity, but lack mental energy and the power of application. They have little interest in the surroundings, no care for their own livelihood, and no thought for the future, but are contented to live and be cared for. In conduct they are apt to present many mannerisms.

The judgment is weak and memory defective. Important events may be retained, together with school knowledge, but memory for events subsequent to the onset of the psychosis is very poor, while they are quite incapable of acquiring additional knowledge. The hallucinations and delusions of the various stages of the disease for the most part entirely disappear. While retained in a few cases, they are of little importance to the patients, rarely influencing their behavior. As in the other grades of dementia, so here, there is a tendency for the deterioration to increase as the patients advance in age. This is especially noticeable following short periods of excitement, which are apt to be coincident with menstruation. At these times the patients show motor restlessness, with great irritability and sometimes violence, with a reappearance of former delusions and hallucinations, talkativeness, silly behavior, and incapacity for employment. The delusions are more apt to be expansive, changeable, and incoherent, but at times there may be verbigeration and repetition of single phrases. The actions are usually purposeless.

A *few of these cases leave the institution apparently recovered,* but upon reaching home the patients fail to employ themselves profitably. They spend

much time in reading, evolving impractical schemes, and pondering over abstract and useless questions. Or, if employed, they show a lack of interest, are unbalanced, and unable to advance in their profession or occupation. Later their field of thought becomes more circumscribed and their relations with the outside world correspondingly meagre. They become seclusive and so much disinterested in intellectual work that they pass their time in purely machine-like action, engaged in gardening or transcribing.

Finally in about *eight per cent, of the cases the symptoms of the disease entirely disappear, leaving the patients apparently in their normal condition.* Not all of these cases should be regarded as perfect recoveries, because in some instances there have been recurrences in later life, followed by deterioration. In still other cases there has been a stunting of mental development. The patients have been unable to realize their ambition. Young men and women whose academic or collegiate courses have been interrupted by the psychosis find themselves unable to enter into active business or professional life. These patients are able to care for a farm or a small business where there is little demand for intellectual work. In this way we lose sight of the mental shipwreck following dementia praecox, because enough mental capacity is retained to permit them to maintain the battle of life in their chosen narrow field.

Catatonic Form *(Catatonia)*

The catatonic form of dementia praecox is especially characterized *by stuporous states with negativism, hypersuggestibility, and uniform muscular tension; excited states with stereotypy and impulsiveness; leading in most cases, with or without remissions, to mental deterioration.* This form comprises in our experience about eighteen per cent. of the entire group of dementia praecox.

Pathological Anatomy. — Alzheimer, in fatal cases of acute delirium which he believed belonged to catatonia, has described profound changes in the cortical neurones of the deeper layers. The nucleus was much swollen, its membrane wrinkled, and the cell body shrunken, with a tendency to disappear. In the glia there was an increase of fibres which fastened about the cell in a peculiar manner. Nissl, in all prolonged cases of catatonia, has demonstrated extensive changes in the cells, which vary considerably in degree as well as kind. Even in cases where there appeared to be no atrophy in the cortex, he found a number of cells which had undergone degeneration. In the deeper layers of the cortex very large glia cells were found which normally appear only in the outer layers. Elsewhere the cortex contained glia cells with slightly stained cell bodies and large pale nuclei with small vesicles, which were in close approximation to the degenerated nerve cells, not only at the base of the cell body, like the satellite cells, but also surrounding it. This pathological lesion and the type of glia cells are not peculiar to catatonia, but they are found to a striking degree in the deeper cortical layers in this disease. Symptomatology. — The onset of the psychosis is usually subacute, with a condition of mental depression quite similar to that observed in the hebephrenic form. The patients for several weeks before the onset may have appeared unusually quiet, serious, or even anxious, complaining of difficulty of thought, of headache, or of peculiar sensations in the head. Besides this, they may have suffered from insomnia and loss of appetite, and have left their work because of nervousness and general ill health. Gradually the patients show great anxiety, and express fear of impending danger. Their religious emotions become more prominent, and *hallucinations* and *delusions* appear. A voice from heaven directs them to do all sorts of things. One patient is commanded to spit to the right, and another to convert sinners. There is a vision of Christ on the cross, the Virgin Mary appears, faces are seen at the window and pictures on the wall, spirits hover about, some one speaks from the radiator, and there is music in the next room. They hear their children cry for help. Some one calls their name, and they hear their own thoughts. Little

birds speak to them. Specks of poison are detected in the food; sulphur fumes are set free about them; some one pulls at their hair, injects water into their limbs, or applies electricity to them.

The *delusions* are usually of a religious nature, are incoherent and changeable from day to day. The patient is persecuted for his sins, a priest has come to anoint him before he dies. God has transferred him to heaven, where he is surrounded by angels. He no longer needs food, as Christ has forbidden him to eat. He is eternally lost, is possessed of the devil, has caused destruction of the whole world; all are dead; he is surrounded by spirits, his children are lost, the wife false, his body has been transformed into mules' hoofs, his hands into claws, his brain has been drawn off, and while hung to a cross, his limbs and body have run away like molten metal. The delusions may later become expansive, though they are occasionally expansive from the onset. The patient then believes himself transformed into Christ, has all power, can create worlds, has lived for thousands of years, possesses all knowledge, can cast out evil spirits, is a millionaire, owns railroads, etc.

During the earlier stages of the disease some peculiarities of movement and action appear, particularly *constraint,* which may increase to a state of muscular tension. The patients assume constrained attitudes, holding the arms in awkward positions, as in the form of a cross, etc., standing or walking in an awkward manner, all of which may be symbolical of their ideas. One patient stood for hours with hands behind him and head thrown back, staring fixedly at the ceiling, and another lay in the form of a cross upon the floor. In some there is a tendency to execute rhythmical movements, such as rolling the head from side to side, or expectorating at stated intervals in a fixed direction.

In this period of depression the *consciousness* is somewhat clouded, orientation is slightly disturbed, and the patients do not apprehend clearly what goes on about them. They may know that they are at home or in an institution,

but they fail to appreciate the mental condition of their fellowpatients, mistake those about them for friends and acquaintances, or they claim that everything is changed and that they cannot understand the mystery of it all. Some believe themselves translated to heaven, that they are in a cloister, or in a foreign city.

Thought is loose and somewhat desultory and reasoning is difficult. The *memory* for remote events is well retained and impressibility is surprisingly good. Although the physician may be mistaken for Christ or some one else, he is always remembered. Occasionally genuine falsifications of memory are seen.

The *emotional attitude* is at first quite in accord with the delusions and hallucinations. The patients are sad, dejected, anxious, complaining, irritable, distrustful, and sometimes threatening; when interfered with, they are very apt to become violent. Occasionally sexual excitement leads to masturbation and obscenity. Later they lose their early anxiety, become indifferent or contented with their environment, and the delusions are expressed without emotion. Some patients are even cheerful and happy, or ecstatic.

The disturbances in *conduct* and *actions* are very striking. The patients cease work and lie listlessly about; they laugh without apparent reason, indulge in excesses, neglect themselves, and sometimes utter threats. Many patients pray constantly and devote much time to attending church services; not a few attempt suicide or assault friends or relatives without reason.

Following this preliminary period of the disease, which in most respects is quite similar to that in the hebephrenic form, the more characteristic catatonic symptoms appear; namely, the *catatonic stupor* and the *catatonic excitement.* In at least one-third of the cases these symptoms appear at the very onset of the disease.

The *catatonic stupor* is chiefly controlled by the symptoms *negativism* and *automatism. Negativism* often occurs first in the form of mutism, when the patients refuse to speak. They begin by speaking low, breaking off in the midst of a sentence or answering in monosyllables, then they may whisper unintelligibly, and finally refuse to speak altogether. Some patients in this condition may be persuaded to write or sing answers to questions. When addressed they remain with closed eyes or staring fixedly at some distant object, apparently paying absolutely no attention to the physician. Even shaking patients, pinching them, or prodding them with a needle fails to elicit a response, except when in pain; then the lips may become more closely pressed together or the patients may move away indifferently.

Further evidence of negativism is seen in the *obstinate* and *persistent resistance* which the patients make to every attempt at handling them. They resist being put to bed and being taken out, dressing or undressing, moving forward or backward, opening the eyes or closing them. The active resistance is well demonstrated by suddenly withdrawing the hand which has been placed against the patient's forehead, when it springs forward with a jerk. The physical origin of this resistance becomes more apparent in those cases in which the desired action is only elicited by commanding the patient contrariwise. One may get a patient to open his eyes by urging him to close them tightly, to lower the hand by telling him to lift it, etc.

Even the most *natural impulses are resisted,* as seen in their stubborn refusal to wear shoes or stockings, in the tendency to sit on the floor rather than in a chair, or to sleep under the bed and not in it, and go to the closet by the longest route. They prefer to eat another's food, and some persist in crawling into the beds of others. Finally the refusal of food and the retention of urine and feces are evidences of more extreme negativism. The former may last for months. The absence of food for a week will not overcome this disinclination to take food voluntarily. It is not unusual for this form of negativism, as well as the others, to appear and disappear suddenly. Sometimes the patients will begin to eat if transferred to another

ward, or will remain in bed if given a different bed. The urine and feces may be retained until there is marked distention. In a few cases it is necessary to overcome this by catheterization and enemata.

There is usually associated with negativism an unusual uniformity of the *muscular tension* which is exhibited in several ways, especially in the extraordinary uniformity of position maintained by the body or its various parts. In this condition patients maintain the same position for weeks and even months. The usual position is on the back, with limbs stretched out, the eyelids closed with the eyeballs rolled upward and inward, or with the eyes open staring fixedly in the distance, the face mask-like with lips slightly closed and at the same time protruded. The hands are very often clenched, as if there were permanent contractures, the fingers producing pressure marks on the palms. Plates 1 and 2 represent two stuporous catatonic patients. The boy rigidly maintained this uncomfortable position for weeks, with his head thrown far backward, eyes tightly closed, and face mask-like with protruded lips. While in this condition he required daily feeding by nasal tube. The woman maintained this same position for over four years without a known voluntary attempt to change it. The body and head are slightly bent forward with the eyes staring directly in front of her, the lips protruded, the arms flexed, and hands so tightly clenched that cotton must be placed in the fists to prevent pressure sores. While in bed she lies straight upon the back with knees strongly adducted and arms drawn closely to the chest, but with the fists in the same constrained position. During this long period it has been necessary to feed her by spoon. Others lie rolled up like a ball, with head thrown forward and knees drawn to the chin. In the extreme condition these patients may be rolled about or lifted and laid across some object without movement, as rigid as a piece of wood. Muscular tension is not evenly distributed, but is most frequently seen in the hands, arms, face, and lower

limbs. The gait is often influenced by this condition, some patients being unable to move at all, falling rigidly to the floor when raised to their feet; others walk stiffly, with unbent knees, on tiptoes, or on the outer side of the feet with the body bent forward or backward. The movements are usually slow and constrained. Sometimes the counter impulses seem to be suddenly overcome and the movements become rapid.

The *hypersuggestibility* is seen especially in *catalepsy,* and less frequently in *echopraxia* and *echolalia,* the latter of which are usually of short duration. In the echolalia and echopraxia the patients simply repeat in a wholly mechanical and monotonous manner what they may happen to hear or see done in their presence. They imitate or mimic every act of some person in their environment. Questions asked are only repeated. The condition of catalepsy is well seen in the patient depicted on Plate 3. She had been placed in this awkward and very uncomfortable position, which she maintained until relieved. The feet are separated, drawn backward, and elevated so that the toes barely touch the floor; the arms are elevated and drawn backward; and the head is extended as far as possible.

These disturbances of the will become evident when one requests the patient to protrude his tongue, in order that it may be punctured with a needle. Although he sees the needle and comprehends that you are threatening him with it, yet upon request he shoots out his tongue without hesitation, and will repeat the experiment as often as you command him. He frowns when pricked, but is unable to suppress the impulse released by the command.

These apparently opposite states of negativism and hypersuggestibility may pass directly from one into another during the stage of stupor. Absolute silence suddenly gives way to loud and unrestrained shouting or to incessant prattle; the patients awake from the stupor and talk as if nothing had happened, and again in a few hours relapse into their former stuporous state. Sometimes these changes can be brought about by mere suggestion. Such changes are quite characteristic of catatonia.

Interrupting the stupor or following it, and sometimes even preceding it, we have the *catatonic excitement,* which is characterized by *impulsive actions* and *stereotyped movements.* The condition of excitement usually develops rapidly and often follows the initial condition of depression already described. The patients suddenly leap from bed, tear their clothing, break the furniture, race about the room, shouting or singing, throw themselves upon the floor, rotating the head from side to side, breathing rapidly, churning saliva in the mouth, or making a peculiar blowing sound. They may run about the house for hours at a time, striking the bed or the wall in a certain place. While lying in bed the body may be swayed regularly back and forth, or the bed tapped at a certain place at regular intervals In walking they are apt to assume peculiar attitudes. One patient stood for hours against the wall in the form of a cross, repeating, "the Father, the Son, and the Holy Ghost"; another, holding his nose tightly with his hands, uttered a monotonous grunt for hours at a time. Mingled with these movements are seen numerous impulsive movements when the patients jump about from one object to another, pounding themselves, knocking their heads against the wall, wringing their hands, jumping up and down on the bed, and stamping on the floor. All of these most varied movements are carried out with great strength and recklessness, without regard for the surroundings or themselves, and are for the most part purposeless and impulsive. In the midst of their ceaseless tramping about the room they may suddenly grab at the clothing of the physician or assault a fellow-patient. During this excitement the patients are very untidy and filthy, expectorating in the food, smearing with feces and food, urinating in the bed and clothing, and even washing themselves with urine. Sexual excitement very often accompanies this condition.

Mannerisms in facial expression and speech are especially characteristic of these catatonic states. Accompanying speech there is a peculiar gesticulation, winking of the eyes, senseless shaking and nodding of the head, and drawing of the muscles of expression. The voice assumes a peculiar intonation or may quiver. The manner of speech may be scanning, rhythmical, or explosive. The content of speech is often quite characteristic, consisting of a series of senseless syllables repeated in a fixed measure or rhyme. Words or short sentences are likewise repeated; the words may be clipped or the last syllable drawn out. Usually these expressions bear no relation to the trend of conversation. One patient, when asked how he felt, repeated for three minutes, "I see you, I see you."

Another common disturbance is the *inconsequential answering of questions.* The patients react to every question but not according to its sense. The answers are generally irrelevant, though occasionally they have more or less remote reference to the question as though the desired information was avoided. The following is an example: —

How do you feel this morning? "It is a fine morning." Did you sleep well? "It was a cold night." Who is this lady (indicating a nurse)? "The lady with the black clothes" (dressed in white). What is her name? "Clara Swanson" (the name of a fellow-patient). How many windows are there in the room? "Three" (four). How many of us are there in the room?" Three " (four). What day of the month is it?" September 35" (October 5). How much money have I here? "Two dimes " (a quarter). How much now? "Two dollar bills" (one dollar bill), etc.

Such responses in a medico-legal case would be very suggestive of simulation, but their apparently close relationship to negativistic states should in such cases lead one to search for other negativistic signs.

In their voluntary speech genuine desultoriness is often seen (see example, p. 40). Neologisms, the repetition of senseless expressions, and the use of sentences that are wholly devoid of connection are frequent, while at the same time the patient affects lisping and grunting, or speaks in a falsetto voice. Agrammatism is sometimes present, in that the patients seem unable to construct sentences and use only infinitives in speaking.

Verbigeration is also a frequent symptom in the catatonic excitement as well as in the stupor. It consists in the use of many motor expressions, the tendency to stereotypy, and the repetition of similar impulses. The patients will repeat for hours and even days at a time senseless expressions, or single syllables, usually in the same monotonous manner, though sometimes modified by shrieking or singing them. Verbigeration is especially noticeable in the voluntary writings of the patient, which are made still more striking by excessive underlining, shading, and addition of symbols.

Catatonic stupor often passes abruptly into catatonic excitement and *vice versa.* The excitement is more apt to precede. Sometimes one state replaces the other for only a few minutes or hours. The degree of stupor or excitement varies considerably in individual cases.

During the stage of catatonic stupor and excitement, the *consciousness* is somewhat clouded, but the patients seldom lose their orientation completely. In spite of the fact that they seem quite unconscious of and unable to comprehend their surroundings, the patients will awake from a condition of stupor and give the names of those about them, telling the day and the month, and showing surprising knowledge of what has happened within their limited range of observation.

Partial *insight* into the conditions of stupor and excitement is frequently expressed by the patients, when they refer to their peculiar acts as foolish, but say they could not help doing them. Others say that they felt compelled to do what was requested, that they could not remain quiet until it was done, or that they are commanded by God; but whatever the explanation, it is apparent that their peculiar acts are distinctly impulsive and not the outcome of reasoning.

The *emotional attitude* during these

distinctly catatonic states exhibits no striking disorder. They are mostly indifferent as to their delusions and conduct. Threats make no impression upon them. Provided negativistic symptoms are not present, they will not wince when threatened with a burning match or an open knife, and will not even wink when the eye is approached with a needle. Occasionally there are observed changeable states of childish petulancy, irritability, or silly elation and ecstasy.

Physical Symptoms. — In some cases elevated temperature, varying between one hundred and one hundred and two degrees during the acute onset of the symptoms, may persist for two or more weeks. Cyanosis, dermography, and localized sweating often occur. Convulsive attacks are also encountered in a few cases, mostly at the onset. There is loss of weight during the stage of depression. This becomes more prominent during the stupor and may reach extreme emaciation in spite of forced feeding. Later, sometimes beginning during stupor, the weight rises. During the stage of deterioration the patients usually become quite fleshy. During stupor the skin is cold and clammy, the heart's action slow and feeble, and the bowels constipated.

Course. — The usual course in the catatonic form is depression and stupor, followed by excitement, passing into dementia. In a few cases the stupor is immediately followed by dementia without the intervention of the characteristic excitement. Occasionally the excitement precedes the stupor and may even appear at the very onset of the disease.

A prominent feature in the course of the disease, which rarely appears in other forms of dementia praecox, is the *remissions*. Remissions for a few days or a few hours occur in almost all of the cases. The consciousness of the patients becomes perfectly clear. They apprehend and remember events, are quiet and rational, and often express a feeling of illness. At these times close observation discloses a certain constraint in manner and actions, an inconsistent emotional attitude, and a lack of full appreciation of their previous condition. These brief remissions occur most frequently in the states of excitement and are both less frequent and less complete in stupor. In at least twenty per cent. of all the cases, the remissions are long enough for the patients to seem to have completely recovered. Yet, in these cases, one often detects peculiarities which indicate that recovery is not complete, such as irritability, seclusiveness, and forced, affected, or constrained manners. A relapse usually occurs within the first five years, though it may not come within fifteen years.

The outcome in *fifty-nine per cent,* of the cases is ultimately *pronounced mental deterioration*. In these cases, the stupor and excitement disappear and the hallucinations and delusions become less prominent, but the patients give numerous evidences of dementia. They are stupid and indifferent, and have lost their mental activity. They are able to comprehend simple questions, but they lack mental initiative. The memory is defective, the judgment poor, and they are unable to acquire new knowledge. They have no regard for themselves, their personal appearance, or their future. They remain contented wherever they happen to be, and never express any desires. They are wholly unfit for intellectual employment, as they have no idea of how to work. Upon questioning, and in a few cases voluntarily, delusions and hallucinations are expressed; the former are usually expansive but quite incoherent, and without effect upon the conduct of the patient.

Some of the patients are very inactive, remaining stupidly in one place most of the time, sometimes muttering to themselves, but taking no interest in their surroundings. Other patients are active, restless, and unbalanced. In both of these groups, and especially in the latter, we find *mannerisms*. The movements lack freedom, are constrained and peculiar; the patients walk on tiptoe, along cracks, or with bent limbs, with head thrown forward and with cramped hands. The head is usually held in peculiar positions. When sitting, they always assume fixed positions, shaking or nodding the head at regular intervals, making a blowing noise with the lips or grunting. They pass to meals only through certain doors, or perhaps backwards. The mannerisms are especially marked in dressing and at table. They may eat with great rapidity, filling the mouth to its fullest extent before swallowing. Others eat very deliberately, waiting a certain interval between mouthfuls, perhaps counting three, each bit of food being prepared and carried to the mouth in a certain definite manner. Many patients eat with their hands, others hold the knife and fork in some peculiar fashion. One of my patients refused to eat unless he had been allowed to stand on his head and crawl under the table. Similar mannerisms are evident in speech and writing. In speech, neologisms may prevail, especially during the transitory periods of excitement, when in addition there may be a genuine word-jumble.

The deterioration gradually deepens, particularly following the short periods of excitement, which appear in most cases. At these times the patients are restless, irritable, and threatening, and express delusions of persecution. The speech, in addition to shouting and laughing, shows marked confusion. Impulsiveness also is prominent, as seen in the destructiveness, aggressiveness, and even homicidal attempts.

In twenty-seven per cent, of the cases the dementia is of a lighter grade. Here the patients return to clear consciousness, are quiet and orderly, able to return home, and in a few cases resume their former occupations. But a profound change in character has occurred; their former mental vigor does not return, they are listless, dull, and lack energy and endurance. Their judgment is defective. They are cleanly and orderly in conduct except for a few catatonic mannerisms. Some of the patients are very quiet, seclusive, distrustful, or self-conscious; while others are somewhat childish and silly.

These cases not infrequently present *periodical attacks of excitement* very similar to those exhibited in manic-depressive insanity. These attacks are of short duration, not more than a few days or weeks, but the intervals vary greatly. The patients become loquacious, distractible, less accessible, are elated, and have a pressure of activity in which the movements are mostly purposeless, stereotyped, and characterized by impulsiveness. These periodical attacks may not develop until after several years have elapsed. There should also be included here a series of cases in which there is a regular alternation between brief periods of excitement and brief intervals. In women these attacks seem to bear some relation to the menses *(menstrual insanity).* The patients begin to laugh much, to wink their eyes, and to wander about; then there suddenly develops an extremely active excitement. The weight falls rapidly, sometimes five to eight pounds in twenty-four hours. The improvement comes almost as rapidly, although toward the end of the attack there is a slight diminution of the dazedness and activity. The patients become clear and orderly, but for a time continue very quiet, apathetic, and rather stupid, and usually fail to gain an insight into their condition, although they may be able to recall several incidents of their psychosis. The weight is regained rapidly. These attacks may recur at intervals of one to three weeks for a long time. In the greater number of these cases the intervals become shorter, but in either event there ultimately develops a condition of profound dementia.

About thirteen per cent. of the cases seem to recover. Some of these patients manifest slight peculiarities in conduct and a change in character which is apparent only to those closely associated with them. A number of these cases later in life suffer from another attack, terminating in dementia.

Unfortunately, it is impossible to determine what cases will recover, what cases will have long remissions or will become deteriorated. This much can be said, however, that those with an acute development, also those in which the stupor or excitement is very pronounced, are more apt to have a remission. Marked improvement is not a fa-

vorable indication, provided that with the clearing of consciousness, there is not a corresponding improvement in the emotional attitude; if senseless delusions are expressed without corresponding effect or excitement; if mannerisms and stereotypy persist; and finally, if there is a recurrence of periods of excitement. Prolonged stupor of itself does not necessarily indicate deterioration, as patients have remained in stupor from three to five years.

The fatal termination of the catatonic cases usually occurs as the result of some intercurrent disease, of which tuberculosis is the most prominent.

Paranoid Forms

In both the hebephrenic and catatonic forms of dementia praecox delusions are characteristic, but they tend to fade within a short time. In the paranoid forms of the disease, on the other hand, *delusions and usually also hallucinations persist for many years, although there are evidences of a more or less rapid deterioration while consciousness remains clear.* The paranoid forms, comprising twenty-two per cent. of the entire group of dementia praecox, consist of two groups of cases.

First Group *(dementia paranoides).*—This group is characterized by the persistence of numerous incoherent and changeable delusions of both a persecutory and an expansive nature associated with a moderate degree of excitement, and a rather rapidly developing dementia.

Symptomatology.—The onset of the disease, as in the other forms, follows a period of headache, malaise, and insomnia with a rapid loss of energy and often irritability. The patients act peculiarly, are unusually devout, seem depressed and anxious, and remain alone. Very soon they divulge a *host of delusions,* almost entirely of persecution; people are watching them, intriguing against them, they are not wanted at home, former friends are talking about them and trying to injure their reputation. These delusions are changeable and soon become *fantastic.* The patients claim that some extreme punishment has been inflicted upon them, they have

been shot down into the earth, have been transformed into spirits, and must undergo all sorts of torture. Their intestines have been removed by enemies and are being replaced a little at a time; their own heads have been removed, their throats occluded, and the blood no longer circulates. They are transformed into stones, their countenances are completely altered, they cannot talk, eat, or walk like other men, etc.

Hallucinations, especially of hearing, are very prominent during this stage; fellow-men jeer at them, call them bastards, threaten them, accuse them of horrible crimes, and numerous slanderous telephone messages are overheard. Occasionally faces and forms are seen at night, or a crowd of men throwing stones at the window. Foul vapors may be thrown into their bedding.

The patients show *agitation;* they are anxious, restless, quarrelsome, and emotional. They laugh, cry, and sing. The *orientation* is not disturbed. In conduct, they may perform all kinds of serious and outlandish acts, attempting suicide, assaulting persons, and committing arson.

The *emotional attitude* soon changes and becomes more and more exalted. At the same time the delusions become less depressive and more expansive and fantastic. The patient in spite of persecution is happy and contented, extravagant and talkative, and boasts that he has been transformed into the Christ; others will ascend to heaven, have lived many lives, and traversed the universe. They have the talent of poets, have been nominated for President, and have represented the government at foreign courts. These delusions may become most florid, foolish, and ridiculous. A patient may say that he is a star, that all light and darkness emanate from him; that he is the greatest inventor ever born, can create mountains, is endowed with all the attributes of God, can prophesy for coming ages, can talk to the people in Mars; indeed, is unlike anything that has ever existed.

Associated with these variegated and ever changing expansive delusions there are delusions of persecution almost as absurd and extreme, but expressed without corresponding emotion. Patients smilingly complain that they have been deprived of their limbs, have been pierced with thousands of bullets, and been thrown into hell, where they were exposed to furnace flames. Suggestions for many of these delusions may be obtained from pictures on the wall or from reading. The hallucinations also become more extreme. Angels descend from heaven and commune with them daily, God also talks to them, the President directs their conduct, beautiful visions are displayed at night which are full of meaning.

These patients are usually talkative and express freely their many delusions. Some of them fill hundreds of sheets of paper trying to describe them. At first they are quite coherent, but later there is such a wealth of ideas loosely expressed that it is difficult to follow them. They wander aimlessly about from one delusion to another, and show frequent repetitions of the same ideas. Questions, however, are answered in a coherent and relevant manner. Later in the course of the disease the speech becomes more and more difficult of comprehension, because of the number of peculiar phrases and neologisms to which they attach special significance and freely repeat. The writings likewise become more and more unintelligible.

The patients rarely possess *insight* into their condition. The *consciousness* usually becomes somewhat clouded, especially later in the disease. Orientation as to place is least disturbed, but people are soon mistaken and often designated as celebrated personages, and all conception of time is lost. Patients recognize relatives and can give a fairly clear statement as to where they are. They may recall some past knowledge, but they soon become unable to use it in reasoning and utterly fail to follow long conversations. They cannot apply themselves to any mental work. The patients show an exaltation of the ego with heightened feelings, they are self-conscious, with an important manner, and demand special attention. In *emotional attitude* they are almost always exalted,

rarely depressed, although a few patients show restlessness, some irritability, and occasionally some passion, often in connection with the menses. Increased sexual excitement is also common. Some patients are able to do some mechanical work, but need supervision because of their capriciousness and fickleness.

Physical Symptoms. — There is very little physical disturbance except the loss of weight and insomnia at the onset, faulty nutrition, and occasionally increased vasomotor irritability with easy blushing and blanching.

Course. — The course is progressive without remissions. The signs of mental deterioration may appear within a few months, and are usually well marked by the end of two years.

The patients may for a long time retain clear consciousness and partial orientation, but the content of thought becomes thoroughly incoherent and there is a lack of energy and plan in their activity, which incapacitates them for all mental application. While active and somewhat interested in their environment, they still display a self-conscious serenity. From this stage of dementia there may be no further progress for a number of years. Occasionally transitory exacerbations of excitement or depression occur. Finally there may be periods when the patients disclaim their delusions and refer to them as foolishness, but at the same time they do not regain clear insight.

Second Group. — There is provisionally grouped here a larger series of cases which are characterized by *fantastic delusions usually accompanied by numerous hallucinations which are more coherently developed and expressed for a number of years, when they either become incomprehensible or disappear altogether, leaving the patients in a condition of moderate dementia.*

Symptomatology. — The first symptoms to appear are those of despondency with some self-accusation. The patients are troubled with thoughts of death and religious doubts; they are unusually devout, and seek religious advice. They fear that they have done

wrong, have committed some crime, or are suffering the penalty of self-abuse. Coherent *delusions of persecution* develop gradually; people watch them, peculiar actions are noticed, acquaintances are less friendly, and children on the street jeer and laugh at them, perhaps mimicking their manners. Strangers on the street turn and stare. In public places, in the cars, and at the church, they observe peculiar acts which refer to them. They believe themselves libelled by the newspapers. They understand these mysterious occurrences and will shortly expose the offenders and bring them to justice. Affairs at home are unsatisfactory; the children are different, and the husband or wife is unfaithful. *Hallucinations,* especially of hearing, rarely of sight, are prominent at this time, aiding in the elaboration of the delusions. Enemies take advantage of their confinement by standing below the window, calling them all sorts of names, announcing that they are to be imprisoned, that they have committed murder, and are to be put to the rack. Voices are heard from the walls and from under the floor, stating that they are wretches and outcasts of society. Very often the noises really heard, such as the blowing of whistles and the ringing of bells, are misinterpreted in accord with their delusions. They complain that the food contains poison which they can taste, they suspect phosphorus in the tea and detect kerosene on the clothing. They notice that their clothing is changed, buttons are missing, there is a rip in the coat and a pocket torn. Objects in *their* surroundings are changed in order to confuse them. *Delusions of physical influence* become particularly prominent. Many common somatic sensations, such as twitching of individual muscles, headache, specks before the eyes, pain about the heart, and cramp in the bowels are all evidences of such influences wielded by their enemies. The explanations of these somatic sensations are often most fantastic. An itching of the foot is sufficient evidence that a poisonous powder has been blown into their shoes, pain in the back indicates that they have been shot there while asleep, a frontal headache is the result of poisonous vapors, which are set free in the room at night in order to destroy their intellect. A tremor of the fingers is produced by means of electric currents sent through the air. Something is placed in their food to create sexual excitement. Their persecutors employ the most varied means in producing physical discomfort. All known agencies are mentioned, as, magnetism, hypnotism, X-rays, telepathy, and electricity. Organs of the body are removed and then replaced out of order, and the intestines are shrunken. It is quite characteristic for the patients to refer to these physical changes by some invented names, such as, ugly duberty, snicking, lobster cracking, etc. Others complain that their minds are influenced, their thoughts are gone, they have no control over their thoughts, which, in spite of themselves, are always evil. They attribute the origin of such thoughts to others. Frequently they complain of "drawing of the thoughts," and they may say that they don't know whether their thoughts are their own or suggested by some one else. Sometimes their thoughts become audible (double thought), especially when reading. Their thoughts are known to the whole world.

Ideas of *spirit-possession* are often a prominent feature. Here the enemy enters and takes possession of the body, causing the bones to crack and the head to rattle; obscene remarks proceed from the stomach; their ears are filled by all sorts of noises made by these spirit-possessors. They cause the testicles to fall and the throat to dry up.

In connection with the delusions of influence there develops in almost all cases more and more pronounced *expansive delusions*. These are as variegated and fantastic as those of persecution. The patients have been awarded a prize for bravery and now rule the country, possess beautiful dresses, and are betrothed to the king, etc. God daily appears to them and gives them a blessing. They have recently been intrusted with millions which they are to invest in mining. They have consummated an immense trust, of which they are president.

All of the many delusions expressed by the patients are at first coherent, and may be partially systematized; but in the course of a few years, they tend to become somewhat incoherent, and at the same time the hallucinations become more agreeable.

The *consciousness* during the development of these delusions, and for a long time afterward, perhaps years, remains clear, and the patients are oriented. *Thought* is coherent, but centers about the delusions. The patients are able at first to offer some basis for the delusions, to refute objections, and to show some "method" in their ideas; but later, as deterioration appears gradually in the course of several years, thought becomes confused, and the delusions incoherent, contradictory, and changeable. There is rarely *insight* into the disease. Many patients appreciate that they are not normal, but their defects and ailments are rather regarded as the work of their persecutors.

The *emotional attitude* is at first one of depression, with anxiety and combativeness, but later this gives way to a certain amount of happiness and cheerfulness, with considerable egoism. There may be transitory outbreaks of anxiety as well as of irritability. In some cases stuporous states have been observed.

The *conduct* is mostly in accord with the delusions; the patients are suspicious, journeying about to get rid of their enemies, applying to police for protection; or, taking the matter in their own hands, they attack supposed persecutors or attempt to expose them through the papers. Others for self-protection contrive a sort of armor for themselves, place metals in their shoes or wires in their clothing to divert the electrical currents, etc. In accord with expansive delusions they may decorate themselves in fantastic costumes, adorn themselves with badges, assume a superior air, and use highflown language.

Furthermore, during the course of the disease peculiarities of conduct develop, such as, grimacing, striking gesticulations, mannerisms in eating, walking, and speaking, as well as signs of negativism or of stereotypy.

Course.—The duration of the disease extends through many years. It is sometimes possible to discern certain stages in its development: at first a change of disposition, then a prominence of delusions of persecution, later the appearance of delusions of grandeur, indicating the onset of deterioration, and finally the fading away and entire collapse of the delusions. Remissions in the symptoms may occur. The *outcome* is always deterioration. The rapidity with which the dementia develops varies greatly. Usually some signs of dementia appear within two or three years. On the other hand, there are cases which deteriorate within a few months, and there are others which do not dement for a number of years.

In some cases the delusions gradually fade, are never expressed, are forgotten or wholly denied, and at the same time there appears some insight. But in all these cases there still remains some impairment of memory and judgment, apathy, and a loss of the characteristic energy and activity. Or the delusions and hallucinations may be retained, while the patients become quite indifferent to them, and rarely complain of persecutions or show agitation. They are usually capable of employment, and sometimes are even industrious, the former " Pope " becoming a trusted farm-hand, and the " queen " a good seamstress.

More frequently the outcome is characterized by an increasing confusion of thought, when the delusions become more and more incoherent and unintelligible, while the peculiarities of conduct increase with a tendency to occasional states of excitement and impulsiveness. If the deterioration advances further, the patients may reach a stage of silly, quiet dementia.

Diagnosis of dementia precox. — There are not only no pathognomic signs of dementia precox, but even some of the more characteristic signs of the disease, such as, negativism, automatism, stereotypy, and mannerism, occur in other diseases; for instance, paresis, senile and other organic psychoses, as well as in some of the infection psychoses, and even in manic-depressive and epileptic insanity. Hence the diagnosis must rest on the entire picture and not upon any single symptom. While it is possible that different disease processes may exhibit at times similar groups of symptoms, it is altogether improbable that these same diseases will at all times resemble each other, both as regards the manner in which the symptoms develop, their course, and their outcome.

The slowly developing cases of hebephrenia must be distinguished from *acquired neurasthenia.* This differentiation depends especially upon the presence of signs of dementia, the silliness of the hypochondriacal ideas, especially sexual hypochondria, faulty judgment, emotional apathy, and the fact that the patients do not improve with quiet and relaxation. The emotional apathy of the hebephrenic stands out in contrast to the increased emotional irritability of the neurastheniac. Finally, any evidences of hallucinations, of automatism, or stereotypy distinctly indicate dementia precox (see also p. 155).

The differentiation of dementia praecox, occurring in middle life, from *paresis* in which the physical symptoms have not yet appeared, may be quite difficult. The catatonic symptoms that occasionally occur in paresis — catalepsy, mutism, verbigeration, and stereotypy — are by no means as varied and characteristic as in catatonia; while the general incapacity and genuine weakness of will is more prominent in contrast to the eccentricities and the unruliness of the catatonic. Furthermore, the mental deterioration in paresis is apt to be more rapid and more profound and characterized by greater disorder of the apprehension, orientation, and impressibility of memory, while these faculties in comparison with the emotional stupidity and the weakness of judgment in dementia praecox are retained for a relatively long time, although they may be temporarily overpowered by negativism. The appearance of definite hallucinations and of persistent mannerisms speaks for dementia precox. The speech disturbances of the paretic may be closely simulated by the mannerisms

of dementia praecox; even epileptiform and apoplectiform attacks may occur in dementia praecox. In such doubtful cases one must depend upon the lymphocytosis in the cerebrospinal fluid as determined by lumbar puncture and the microscopic examination of the fluid (see p. 103).

In the acutely developing cases of dementia praecox, the clouding of consciousness and the confusion of speech often render it difficult to distinguish *amentia.* Here one must depend upon the presence of negativism, stereotypy, and automatism. If the latter are present in amentia, they are not marked. In amentia, the patients are more natural in their acts, less constrained, and not silly and eccentric. The orientation and impressibility of memory is far more disturbed in amentia than in dementia praecox. The amentia patient, in spite of his best efforts, is unable to solve long mental problems, loses the thread in long conversations, and indulges in incoherent reminiscences, yet he is able to answer some questions rapidly and to the point. On the other hand, the dementia praecox patient answers in a silly manner or perhaps not at all. Again at times he surprises one by his correct conversation, and his thoughtful, bright remarks, or he even solves a difficult problem and recalls correctly historical and geographical facts. In amentia the emotional attitude is exceedingly changeable from depression to exaltation and *vice versa,* while in dementia praecox, even during excitement, a certain emotional stolidity and apathy prevails. The amentia patient may not have a very accurate knowledge of the surroundings, yet he attends to and watches what takes place; but in dementia praecox the patient exhibits remarkably little interest in those things that he comprehends well. Finally, in amentia there is always a history of some exhausting etiological factor, which only occasionally antedates dementia praecox.

Beginning cases of catatonia may be mistaken for *epileptic befogged states,* particularly when an epileptiform attack has occurred. The negativism of the catatonic contrasts with the anxious re-

sistance of the epileptic, while orientation is much more disturbed in the epileptic. Silly answers to simple questions and rapid and correct obedience to commands speaks for catatonic. In epileptics an anxious or ecstatic emotional attitude prevails. The epileptic is much more apt to make frequent assaults and attempts at escape, while the impulsive acts of the catatonic are purposeless and manneristic.

The greatest difficulty arises in distinguishing the *depressive phases of manic-depressive insanity* from the periods of depression which one encounters at the onset of the hebephrenic and the catatonic forms. The early appearance of many hallucinations and senseless delusions, especially ideas of physical influence, and the retention of a clear consciousness speak for dementia precox, as well as an emotional attitude which does not correspond to the depressive character of the delusions. The catatonic patient remains quite indifferent during the visit of a relative, while in manicdepressive depression the feelings are apt to be intensified. Hypersuggestibility of the will may exist in both conditions, but a manic-depressive patient will not upon request protrude his tongue for the purpose of having it perforated with a needle. The uniform lamentations that sometimes occur in manic-depressive depression are the expressions of a persistent and overwhelming feeling of sadness, and not the result of a senseless persevering impulse. The conditions of negativism of the catatonic and of anxious resistance and retardation of the manic-depressive are at times distinguished only with difficulty. In the former there is uniform, rigid, and stubborn resistance to every passive movement, and if pain is produced by pricking the eyelid, there is a simple withdrawal without effort at defence; while in retardation the passive movements are mostly permitted. In case the retarded patient shows some resistance he does not persist in returning his hand to the same position, and if one threatens to approach him he utters an outcry, shrinks back, or defends himself. Voluntary movements in catatonic stupor are rare, but when executed are carried out without delay, and at times even rapidly, except when these movements are made by request, then there is always delay. In retardation, all voluntary movements are carried out very slowly. There is sometimes a certain resistance due to apprehension and fear, but this is active.

The differentiation between *manic-stupor* and catatonic stupor is quite difficult and depends upon the characteristic happy temperament, distractibility of the attention by the environment, the susceptibility to command, the accessibility to conversation, and finally the occasional purposeful and frolicsome character of the movements of manic-stupor in contrast to the silliness, indifference, insusceptibility, and the senseless impulses of the catatonic stupor.

The excitement of the catatonic is to be distinguished from *the excitement of the manic phases of manic-depressive insanity.* In the catatonic excitement the clouding of consciousness is less marked than in the manic excitement, the patients being partially oriented, even in the greatest excitement, while in the extreme manic states there is complete disorientation. On the other hand, the speech of the catatonic who has less motor excitement is more senseless and difficult to follow than that of the manic who has extreme motor excitement. The catatonic speech abounds in verbigerations and stereotyped expressions and is free of comments upon the surroundings, while the speech of the manic presents the characteristic flight of ideas, and is centered upon, or drawn largely from, the immediate surroundings. Also attention is readily distracted by the surroundings, while the attention of the catatonic cannot be. The emotional attitude of the manic is exalted, frolicsome, and irritable, while that of the catatonic is silly, childishly happy, and indifferent. The movements of the catatonic are purposeless, frequently repeated, in contrast to the pressure of activity of the manic, in whom the movements are always purposeful, related to the surroundings, dependent upon ideas, impressions, and emotions, and always ap-

pearing in new forms. In catatonia there is no parallel between the excitement in speech and that in movement; for instance, the patient may be extremely productive, lying quietly in bed, or he may be extremely active and not utter a word. The increased activity of the catatonic is more apt to be limited to one corner of the room or of the bed, while that of the manic is limited only by his confines, and in addition to this the individual movements of the catatonic tend to be manneristic, stilted, unnatural, and associated with silly impulses; those of the manic, natural and more comprehensible.

The *extreme excitement* of the *paretic* may resemble closely the catatonic excitement. In addition to the history of the development of the disease, the age, and the physical signs, paresis may be recognized by the more profound clouding of consciousness, the greater disorientation, and disorder of the impressibility of memory.

Dementia praecox, especially where there have been hysterical attacks, must frequently be differentiated from *hysterical insanity.* The latter fails to show the desultoriness, the weakness of judgment, the indifferent emotional attitude, and the similarity and purposelessness in the conduct of the dementia praecox patient. All of these symptoms stand in contrast to the shrewdness, capriciousness, slyness, keenness, tyranny, and the purposeful obstinacy of the hysteric. Finally, pronounced hallucinations and delusions favor dementia praecox. But there is still a large number of cases, which present at the outset clear symptoms of hysteria, but which later show unmistakable evidence of the deterioration of dementia praecox. The very same condition may exist in manic-depressive insanity, in epilepsy, in paresis, and in brain tumor, which would favor the view that in constitutionally defective individuals the early stages of these diseases may resemble very closely the picture of hysteria.

The distinction of the paranoid forms of dementia praecox from pure *paranoia* depends upon the lack of system, the rapid development of fantastic delu-

sions commencing with prominent hallucinations; while in paranoia the onset is very gradual, sometimes extending over one year with only a few hallucinations. The delusions in dementia praecox are extremely fantastic, changing beyond all reason, with an absence of system and a failure to harmonize them with events of their past life; furthermore, the delusions of physical influence are very prominent. In paranoia the delusions are largely confined to morbid interpretations of real events, are woven together into a coherent whole, gradually becoming extended to include even events of recent date, while contradictions and objections are apprehended and explained. In emotional attitude the dementia praecox patients soon show clear and marked changes, — depression or silly elation, sexual excitement, and remissions; while in paranoia the emotional attitude is uniformly natural, the demeanor is almost normal, and the patients are capable of occupation for a long time. In paranoia there may be partial remissions when the patients react less actively to the delusions, but the delusions never disappear.

In the absence of history of the early life and of the psychosis, *imbecility* may be confused with the end stages of dementia preecox. The recognition of dementia praecox then depends upon the presence of exacerbations in which dementia praecox signs appear and occasional utterances which evince extensive earlier knowledge.

Treatment. — Our meagre knowledge of the causes of the disease restricts the indications for treatment to the individual symptoms. The cases which develop acutely or subacutely demand careful watching in order to prevent self-injuries and suicidal attempts. Unless this can be accomplished with the aid of a sufficient nursing force at home, it is best that the patient be sent to a hospital. Cases of the hebephrenic form with gradual onset can be much more safely cared for at home. At the onset in all forms of the disease the patient must be placed in a quiet and restful environment, free from all irritating circumstances, and in the charge, if possible, of a judicious nurse. It is usually advisable that the patient should not be in charge of a member of the family. In the acute and subacute cases, bed treatment should be regularly prescribed.

The *insomnia* is best combated by the simplest measures, as hot baths upon retiring, warm liquid nourishment, or the hot or cold pack. If the patient does not secure six or seven hours sleep by the simple remedies, one may resort on alternate nights to sparing doses of some hypnotic, as, trional, veronal, somnos, chloral, or paraldehyde. These drugs should not be given for long periods without being alternated. Conditions of *excitement* are always best controlled by the prolonged warm bath (see p. 140), at first preceded by a preliminary dose of hyoscine hydrobromate -*fa* to 35-grain, or scopalamine hydrobromid in the same dosage. The extreme excitement sometimes encountered, especially in the catatonic form, may not yield to the prolonged warm bath, in which event one can often successfully employ hot or cold packs (see p. 321). These packs, however, are not applied without some risk, and usually require the supervision of a physician. But in the employment of any sedative it must be borne in mind that the remedy is not curative, and, therefore, it is not advisable to employ high doses in order to wholly curb the excitement. If it seems essential to secure quiet where these other measures have failed, one may occasionally resort to a hypodermic of hyoscine hydrobromate q with morphine sulphate grain. If the excitement is still unabated, nothing remains but confinement in a padded room with careful watching. Simple persuasion on the part of a well-trained, tactful nurse or physician often succeeds in bringing about quiet, at least temporarily; but this requires great patience, a kindly disposition, and selfcontrol.

While the condition of *nutrition* demands careful attention during the early stages of the disease, it becomes particularly urgent during the stuporous states. The patient should eat a liberal quantity of easily digested food. In order to estimate the state of nutrition such cases should be regularly weighed at least once a week. During stupor with refusal of food, the patient should not be permitted to go without food and water for more than three days. If the patient is illy nourished, one should resort to feeding by stomach or nasal tube at the end of thirty-six hours. The patient may be fed artificially two or three times daily, the total amount aggregating two quarts of milk with six raw eggs, and, if need be, an ounce of olive oil, varying quantities of meat juice, and stimulants, particularly whiskey.

The excretory functions must be daily watched, particularly during the stuporous states, when patients retain the feces and urine. During the acute manifestations of the disease, frequent high flushings of the lower bowel with normal saline solution are well recommended.

During the periods of despondency at the onset of the disease, in addition to the bed treatment already referred to, the patient should be given an opportunity at times during each day to leave the bed for short periods and exercise. Furthermore, simple methods of occupying the mind, at the same time affording some diversion, as, reading, playing games, needlework, etc., should be a part of the daily routine. Friendly encouragement, with a frank discussion of the various delusions and hallucinations, persistently carried out by a kindly and tactful nurse and physician, is not the least important feature of the treatment, and must not be overlooked.

As the more acute symptoms improve and the fear and increased activity subsides, the patient may then be allowed to leave the bed for longer periods, but at the same time the graduated exercise and mental application should be increased. The whole effort of the physician should then be directed to developing remaining mental capacity and preventing further mental defect. This requires a considerable amount of specialized attention in the individual cases in order to prescribe means that at the same time are adapted to the patients' needs and traits and also are suited to their environment. Very many patients improve sufficiently so that they are able to return to their homes or to their full liberty. But in advising this, one must not overlook the possibility of exacerbations, and in women the possibility of pregnancy, and the resumption of excessively burdensome home cares. The cases exhibiting advanced grades of deterioration must be kept under surveillance. An essential feature of the care of these mental shipwrecks is healthful employment, preferably out of doors.

VI. DEMENTIA PARALYTICA (Paresis)

Dementia Paralytica, or *general paresis of the insane, is a chronic psychosis of middle age, characterized by progressive mental deterioration with symptoms of excitation of the central nervous system, leading to absolute dementia and paralysis, and pathologically, by a fairly definite series of organic changes in the brain and spinal cord, probably the result of some toxin, in the origin of which syphilis is most often an important factor.*

Etiology. — The disease is unknown among the uncivilized nations and is most prevalent in western Europe and North America, hence, it seems to be a disease of modern civilization. In America, the disease comprises from five to eight per cent. of the admissions to insane institutions, but in some European cities, notably Berlin and Munich, the paretics average thirty-six to forty-five per cent. of the male admissions. The disease is somewhat more prevalent in large cities and manufacturing centers, while it is relatively rare in farming communities. The proportion of male to female paretics is 1 to 3. 9 to 7. This disproportion has recently gradually decreased. Negresses show a striking tendency to the disease; in Connecticut, the negress paretics are ten times more prevalent than the female white paretics. Women suffer more often from the depressive form and least often from the agitated form, and in them the disease lasts longer. Our average age of onset in one hundred and seventy-two cases is forty-two years. Kraepelin in two hundred and forty-nine cases finds that it occurs preeminently in middle life, as eighty-one per cent. of the cases occur between thirty and fifty years, the disease rarely appearing before twenty-five or after fifty-five years of age. The average age of onset in our women was two years younger than in men, and one-third of the women became afflicted between thirty and thirty-five, while one-fourth of the cases occurred after fifty years. Kraepelin, however, finds that the onset in women averages later. In our experience, the onset is earlier in syphilitic and alcoholic women. Our natives are slightly more prone to paresis than our foreign-born.

Voisin, Traits de la paralysie gSndralc des alidads, 1879; Mendel, Die progressive Paralyse der Irren, 1880. Mickle, General Paralysis of the Insane, 2. ed. 1886. v. Krafft-Ebing, Nothnagels spezielle Pathologie u. Therapie, Bd. IX, 2,1894. Ilberg, Volkmanns klinische Vortrage, 161; Binswanger, Deutsche Klinik, VI, 2, 59, 1901.
» Diefendorf, Brit. Med. Jour., No. 2387, p. 744. Wollenberg, Archiv. f. Psy., XXVI, 2. Gudden, ebenda. v. Krafft-Ebing, Jahrb. f. Psy., XIII, 2 u. 3. Oebecke, Allgem. Zeitschr. f. Psy. , XL. Hirschl, Jahrb. f. Psy., XIV, 321. Bar, Die Paralyse in Stephansfeld, Diss. , Strassburg, 1900.

Recently a number of cases of *juvenile paresis* have been reported occurring between the ages of ten to twenty years in which hereditary paresis, syphilis, and alcoholism are prominent factors. Clinically, the juvenile form is characterized by simple deterioration of three to four years' duration with numerous paralytic attacks, choreic disturbances, and paralyses.

The disease afflicts chiefly the unmarried, and among the women especially prostitutes; in our experience prostitutes are forty-five per cent. more prone to the disease than other women. Married women are usually childless. Not infrequently the disease occurs in man and wife; sometimes tabes is present in one and dementia paralytica in the other and paresis occasionally exists in the parents. The male paretics come from all classes and from most profes-

sions and trades, though the disease is more prevalent among hotel and saloon keepers, quarrymen, carriage and hack drivers, bakers, sailors, hostlers, mechanics, masons, salesmen, and clerks, and least prevalent among farmers, servants, and factory employees. Defective heredity is comparatively insignificant, except in juvenile paresis, as it occurs in only fifty per cent. of cases.
Alzheimer, Allgem. Zeitschr. f. Psy., LII, 3. Thiry, De la paralysie progressive dans le jeune Age, 1898. Hirschl, Wiener Klin. Wochenschr., 1901, 21. v. Rad, Archiv f. Psy., XXX, 82. Mingazzini, Monatsschr. f. Psy., Ill, 53. Frolich, Uber allgemeine progressive Paralyse der Irren vor Abschluss der koerperlichen Entwicklung, Diss., 1901.
Among the causes of the disease, *syphilis* is statistically the most prominent. Its prevalence varies, according to various authors, from one and six-tenths per cent. to ninetythree per cent., but most observers place it between thirty-four and sixty-five per cent. In our experience it existed in fifty-two per cent. Gudden in the *Charitt,* and Kraepelin at Heidelberg cannot establish a clear history of syphilis in more than thirty-four per cent. of male paretics. In other psychoses, we find syphilis in but five and five-tenths per cent. of the cases. Therefore, there seems to be some relationship between syphilis and paresis, a view which receives further support not only by the experiments cited by KrafftEbing, in which nine paretics inoculated with syphilis failed to develop secondary syphilic lesions, but also by the clinical observation that paretics infected with syphilis during the disease do not show secondary manifestations. This latter is now doubted by Marchand, Gabiana, and Garbini, who have reported seven cases in which paretics developed syphilis. Other apparently significant facts are the infrequency of paresis in women of the better classes and Catholic priests, its frequency among prostitutes, and the occurrence of paresis in man and wife. Other important causes are *excessive alcoholism,* which existed in sixty per cent. of our cases, head injury twenty-three per cent.

, and mental shock. Finally, a factor which cannot be overlooked is the ensemble of modern life with its restless overactivity and insufficient relaxation, coincident with the struggle for existence in large cities, and the common excesses in eating and drinking.

Pathology. — In view of the uniform course of the disease leading to dementia and nervous paralysis, accompanied by a general and extensive destructive process, involving not only the central nervous system, but also the general vascular system, and to a limited extent the internal organs of the body, it seems probable that we have to do with a toxic process. There exist symptoms of excitation of the neurones, their rapid destruction, gradual sclerosis, occasional exacerbations of the symptoms, and the possibility of a regeneration of the neurones, all of which can be reproduced by experimentation upon test animals with any toxic material which causes a destruction of the neurones. These anatomical facts are wholly in accord with the clinical observations; namely, the gradual onset, great clouding of consciousness, rapid or gradual deterioration, and marked remissions, some of which almost approach complete recovery. The vascular lesions and the broad extent of the process indicates that the toxin reaches the neurone by means of the blood vessels. The involvement of the kidneys, heart, and the entire vascular system, the fragility of the bones, the alternate loss and increase of the body weight, ending at last in great emaciation, all speak for the profound general disturbance of nutrition of which the mental are obviously the most severe, but not the only symptoms.

The sudden and high elevation of temperature, as well as the prolonged subnormal temperature, and finally the paralytic attacks, judging from our experience in eclampsia, myxedema, and uremia, can best be explained by intoxication arising from disturbance of metabolism. Viewed in this light, the pathology of paresis resembles that of myxedema, diabetes, osteomalacia, and acromegaly, except that in these diseases the toxin does not involve the nervous tissue.

The character of the toxin and the sources from which it arises are questions still in doubt. Syphilis cannot be the sole cause of paresis, as long as it does not exist in more than thirty-four to sixty-five per cent. of the cases. Furthermore, paresis, anatomically, is not a simple syphilitic process. Again the late manifestations of syphilis arise within a comparatively short time after primary symptoms, while paresis does not develop until ten or more years have elapsed after the initial lesion. Taking into consideration all of these facts, the only acceptable view is that in a considerable number of cases *syphilis somehow produces a profound change of metabolism which in turn gives rise to a toxin, which secondary product is the direct cause of the pathological changes characteristic of dementia paralytica.* Other apparent etiological factors, as, alcohol, head injury, lead, and excesses, may bear a similar causal relation to this disturbance of metabolism.

Pathological Anatomy. — The pathological changes here enumerated can, as a whole, be regarded as pathognomic of this disease. Hyperostoses and exostoses of the *cranium* with, but more especially without, thickening of the tables, are occasionally present. The dura is usually adherent to the calvarium in places. Pachymeningitis interna and hematoma are common. The false membrane is almost always situated on the vertex over the frontal, parietal, or temporal lobes, and is of varying thickness, from a thin, almost imperceptible rust-colored membrane, to a thick, firm, white membrane, with small or large, fresh or partially absorbed clots.
Nissl, Monatsschr. f. Psy., IV, 413; Allgem. Zeitschr. f. Pay., LX, 215. Nacke, ebenda, LVII, 619. Cramer, Handbuch der pathol. Anatomie des Nervensystems von Flatau-Jacobsohn-Minor, 1470, 1903.
The *pia* is thickened, whitish, and translucent along the vessels, and especially over the vertex of the frontal and parietal lobes and the first three temporal convolutions, and rarely over the occipital lobes. The internal surfaces of

the frontal poles are often adherent. The leptomeningitis is always more intense over the poles of the frontal lobes. The Pacchionian granulations are usually increased in size. The pia over the atrophied convolutions and broadened fissures often contains blebs filled with serum. The *convolutions* are atrophied, especially in the frontal lobes. In these portions the cortex is narrow and often strongly adherent to the pia, tearing upon its removal. In the other portions of the cortex, and in the basal ganglia, the atrophy is much less marked. The *ventricles* are dilated, and the choroid plexuses may contain many cysts. The *ependyma* especially of the fourth ventricle, and the inner walls of the lateral ventricles, present granulations, which give the usual glistening surfaces a frosted appearance. These granulations are composed of an increase of neuroglia, which in many cases has undergone hyaline degeneration. The weight of the brain is regularly below normal, and in some cases of long duration may be reduced to nine hundred grammes. The average weight is eleven hundred and sixty to thirteen hundred grammes.

Microscopically, nerve cell changes of varying intensity are found in the cortex. None of these cell changes are pathognomonic for paresis. Many, especially the *acute alteration* (see Plate 4, Figure 2), apparently represent a destructive process, while in others, as, for instance, the chronic change — *cell sclerosis* — (see Plate 4, Figure 5), the cell may persist for some time. Furthermore, in cells giving evidence of sclerosis, there may also appear evidences of a superimposed acute change. The *grave alteration* (see Plate 4, Figure 3) apparently leads to absolute destruction of the cell. Undoubtedly also the acute and the chronic changes can terminate in a destruction of the cell. Of all the cell changes only the acute alteration involves uniformly the entire cortex. Both the extent and the intensity of the destructive processes are apt to vary. There is least involvement of the occipital lobe, especially in the calcarine area, and of the central convolutions, particularly the precentral. Furthermore,

in a disease area, normal cells may be found lying side by side with altered cells. In all cases there is involvement of the greater portion of the cortex, but only in the severe or prolonged cases are all of the cortical cells diseased. The *nerve fibres* in the cortex and corona suffer atrophy in proportion to the extent of the degeneration in the cortical neurones. Where the clinical course has been prolonged and the neurones are much degenerated there remain but a very few normal fibres. Similar destruction of the nerve fibres may be found in senile dementia and epileptic insanity, but it is not as far advanced as in dementia paralytica.
Binswanger, Die Pathologische Histologic der GrosshirnrindenErkrankungen bei der allgemeinen pregressiven Paralyse, 1893. Nissl,
As the result of the degeneration of the nerve cells and their processes, there is an atrophy of the cortex, which in extreme cases may shrink to one-half its normal width.
Archiv f. Psy., Bd. 28, S. 989. Heilbronner, Allgem. Zeitschr. f. Pay., Bd. 53, S. 172.
Fici. 4 Fin.-i
Pr.AtK 4
F'g. 1 — Normal large pyramidal cell. Fig. 2 —Acute alteration in deme lytica. Fig..'!— Grave alteration in dementia paralytica. Fin-4 — Pli crowded about a vessel in dementia paralytica. Fig. S — Chronic cell dementia paralytica. Fig. ii — Rod-shaped cell in dementia paralytica

Fiti. ti ntia paransma cells change in

This degeneration may be more marked about the vessels. The remaining cells are no longer arranged uniformly, but are turned in all directions, either closely pressed together, as seen in Figure 3, Plate 5, or surrounded by areas composed only of sclerotic tissue and vessels with thickened walls. Figure 3 should be compared with the normal cortex as represented in Figure 2. *This anatomical picture is most characteristic of paresis.* The cell changes already described may be found in other conditions, but in none do all the elements of the cortex suffer to such a profound degree as here. In senile dementia, idiocy, and even in dementia precox, many cells and fibres are destroyed, but the general conformation of the remaining elements is undisturbed. This distortion with the presence of scar tissue is present to a recognizable extent in dementia paralytica, even when the process is not far advanced.

In the areas of degeneration there may be a considerable increase in the *neuroglia tissue,* in which spider cells take a prominent part, appearing especially in the deeper cell layers of the cortex and about blood vessels. This great increase of spider cells may be seen in Figures 5 and 6, Plate 5, in comparison with Figure 4, which represents the neuroglia present in the normal cortex. The increase in neuroglia does not necessarily correspond to the destruction of nerve cells, as normal nerve cells are often surrounded by considerable neuroglia, and, on the other hand, in some areas all the nerve cells may have disappeared without an appreciable increase of the neuroglia.

Vascular lesions in the cortex form a prominent part in the microscopical picture. The vessels are increased in number and their walls thickened, as may be seen in Plate 5, Figure 3. Some of the vessels are dilated, a few totally obliterated, and others show small aneurisms; but the characteristic feature of this vascular change is the infiltration of the perilymph spaces with ordinary lymph cells and particularly *plasma cetts* (see Plate 4, Figure 4), the latter of which may be regarded as distinctive of paresis, since they are rarely found in other disease processes. Furthermore, the prevalence of these cells stands in rather definite relationship to the extent of the disease process. They are most prevalent in the acute stages of the disease and later may disappear. Another form of cell, distinctive of paresis, is the *rod-shaped cell* first described by Nissl (see Plate 4, Figure 6). The cell is long and narrow, sometimes curved, with a clear nucleus and one or more nucleoli. These cells are found in large numbers mostly in proximity to blood vessels and lying parallel to the long axis of the large nerve cells.

In addition to the finer microscopic changes in the cortex, one occasionally finds *small areas of softening,* which are discernible by the readiness with which either the superficial layers of the cortex or the entire cortex are detached from the white matter. Gross *focal lesions,* such as one might expect to accompany paralytic attacks, are rarely encountered. On the other hand, Lissauer, Starlinger, and others have pointed out that in the cases with circumscribed paralyses, hemianopsia, word blindness, and aphasia there really are present corresponding definite circumscribed disease areas in the cortex with recognizable secondary degeneration in the corona, basal ganglia, pons, and cord.

The *basal ganglia,, central gray matter,* and *cerebellum* also present degeneration of the nerve cells and fibre tracts. Weigert has demonstrated an increase of neuroglia in the granular layer of the cerebellum, with a destruction of the Purkinje cells and their processes. The cranial nerve nuclei Starlinger, Monataschr. f. Pay., VII, 1; Storch, ebenda, IX, 401.

Fig. 1 — Cerebral cortex In idiocy. Fig. 2—Normal eerebral cortex. Fig. 3 — Cerebral cortex in dementia paralytica. Fig. 4 — (Ilia in normal cerebral cortex. Fig. 5 — Glosis witb presence of spider cells in cortex in dementia paralytica. Fig. li — Showing the relation of spider cells with vessel walls in deep layers of cerebral cortex in dementia paralytica. of the medulla show similar changes to those seen in the cortical cells.

The *spinal cord* ' is involved to a greater or less extent in almost all cases, the most important lesion being degeneration of the fibre tracts in the posterior and lateral columns. Degenerative changes are occasionally found in the peripheral nerves. In the internal organs vascular changes are so frequently found that they seem to bear a definite relationship to the disease process. Of these, atheroma of the aorta and arteritis of the vessels of the liver and kidneys are the most prominent.

Symptomatology. — From the onset of the disease there is increasing diffi-culty of *apprehension* of external impressions. Patients are unable to grasp clearly and sharply the character of the environment. Later they mistake persons, fail to recognize former well-known objects, and overlook important details. Attention is maintained with effort. Long and complicated sentences are not comprehended, and they often miss the connection of things. Customary duties are performed with difficulty and often incorrectly. Thus, there develops a *clouding of consciousness;* the patients live a dreamy existence, as if constantly under the influence of liquor. This condition of torpor is an important diagnostic sign. Later the disorientation increases. The patients may answer questions quite correctly and upon superficial examination seem to conduct themselves in accord with their environment; but at the same time they neither know where they are, with whom they are speaking, nor the significance of what is taking place about them. They fail to recognize the season or the time of day. A patient may say that it is summer while leaning upon a hot radiator and looking out upon a snow-covered landscape. This condition finally reaches one of absolute disorientation, when the patients cannot perceive or elaborate any external impressions. Westphal, Allgem. Zeitschr. f. Psy., Bd. 20-21. Westphal, Archiv f. Psy., H. I. , Bd. 12. Westphal, Virchow's Archiv, Bd. 39. Fuestner, Archiv f. Psy., Bd. 24. 1.

At the onset of the disease there is usually an *increase of the sense of fatigue.* The patients tire easily at their accustomed duties and require more frequent and longer periods of rest. *Hallucinations* play an unimportant part. In the greater number of cases none appear, but in some cases there exist for some time very many hallucinations of all senses. Again the clinical picture may be very like that of the acute alcoholic hallucinosis. Hallucinations of sight are often present in patients with optic atrophy. Hallucinations of touch in connection with delusions of influence are not infrequent.

The *defects of memory* are very characteristic and are among the most prominent of the mental symptoms. The memory at first becomes defective for recent and passing events. This defect is sometimes keenly appreciated by the patients, who complain of and sometimes devise means for correcting it. Later, memory becomes progressively more defective. The memory is especially defective in the temporal arrangement of experience, and the patients fail to recall the time of the occurrence of events. They cannot inform you when the mail arrived, when they had breakfast, or when they last saw you. These patients may live so completely in the present moment that they may ask several times a day where they are, how long they have been there, or if they have ever seen you before. The early events of life are comparatively well retained for some time, the patients being able to tell of their occupation, former places of residence, and events of their childhood. This remote memory also suffers late in the disease, and here also the time element is the first to be affected. Dates of marriage, births of children, and important events are completely forgotten. Finally they are unable to recall the place of birth and even the names of their parents and children. Lapses of memory, when definite periods of time are completely forgotten, may occur following epileptiform or apoplectiform seizures.

The *store of ideas* undergoes a progressive impoverishment, terminating in a complete destruction of all the mental possessions. The rapidity of this process varies with the intensity of the disease and the power of resistance as well as the intelligence of the individual. The more intelligent resist longer, and the most frequented paths of thought are retained longest. As memory fails, its place in the intellectual life is often made good by the *imagination*. As real reminiscences disappear, invention runs riot. Whatever enters the mind is related as genuine; stories, or what may have been told them by another, become a part of their own experience. The patient relates that he was in a terrible railroad accident last night, in which

a dozen were killed; he led the troops at San Juan; yesterday he had a conference with the British ambassador. He has captured a hundred beautiful women from a Turkish harem, and discovered a new and inexpensive motive power for automobiles. These dreamlike *fabrications* are most pronounced in cases of optic atrophy. Very often such fabrications are used in filling in the gaps in recent memory. They can be brought out and influenced by suggestion on the part of the listener. The patient may be somewhat dubious at first when expressing these absurd reminiscences, but at the next interview all doubt will have disappeared. This susceptibility of the memory to external influences is a part of the general susceptibility of thought of the patients. Their ideas are never firmly grounded, and fail to exert a lasting influence upon their thoughts and actions. Any accidental impulse suffices to distract and lead them into another channel.

Impairment of judgment is another very prominent symptom. It may be the first to call attention to the disease. Objects of former criticism now fail to arouse comment. The former conservative principles which have made their business life a success are lost sight of, and new plans lack unity and system. Weighty obstacles are overlooked and senseless schemes produced with perfect serenity. Business and social standards are completely disregarded. Their conceptions have no bearing upon the environment, but center almost entirely about themselves, so that they come to live in a sort of dream world, in which everything depends upon their own ideas and wishes. The *formation of delusions*, which partially results from this defect of judgment, varies much in different cases. In some there are but few delusions, but in most cases the delusions form a prominent feature in the early stages of the disease. These delusions are transitory, unstable, without system, and show confusion and incoherence. They are characterized by vagaries, senselessness, numerous variations, and contradictions. It only rarely happens that for short periods the delu-

sions are stable and uniform like those of paranoia.

It is not unusual at the onset for the patients to express some *insight* into their mental disease, complaining of their failing memory, irritability, and increasing difficulty of thought. Later, with increasing deterioration, all genuine insight disappears. The patients then usually exhibit a feeling of well-being; they claim that they never felt stronger or more vigorous mentally. At times during the course of the disease the patients may make various hypochondriacal complaints, but even then they fail to recognize the real physical symptoms of the disease.

The *emotional life* shows a profound disturbance. At first there is usually increased irritability. The patients are easily disturbed at home and work, are sullen, peevish, and apt to show considerable passion at trifling annoyances, and completely lose control of themselves. On the other hand, they may show an unusual insensibility to the claims of others, indicative of the deterioration of the finer feelings. They then fail to show sympathy at the suffering of their children, are indifferent to immoral surroundings, and do not take their wonted pleasure in reading or professional pursuits.

The emotional attitude is much in accord with the character of the delusions; it is elated with expansive, or dejected with depressing delusions. Later the emotional tone becomes very unstable, and there are frequent and abrupt changes. In the midst of laughter they may break out in a storm of tears, or misery may give way to silly happiness. These changes of emotion may be brought by simple suggestions or by raising or lowering the tone of voice, or even by the expression of the face. A patient lying on the floor, complaining that he had lost all his organs, that he had no blood and could not breathe, when tickled in the ribs and asked how he felt, exclaimed, beginning to laugh, "I am feeling fine; come and see me again." In the demented forms of the disease, where there may be only a few delusions, no especial emotions are shown, the patients being in a condition of simple joy or irritable dissatisfaction most of the time.

There is a profound *change of disposition;* the former stability and independence of action give way to progressive weakness of the will power. The patients become very tractable, but occasionally may be extremely stubborn. Early in the disease they are led to indulge in all sorts of excesses and sometimes persuaded to deed away property. When angered and determined to commit an assault upon some one, they may be easily influenced to desist by a simple suggestion. A patient about to leap from a third-story window because of fear, was readily prevented by the suggestion that it would be better to go down and jump up. Any impulse that arises may be acted upon without reference to the extreme difficulty of its accomplishment. One patient is said to have stepped out from a second-story window for the purpose of picking up a cigar stump.

In *conduct,* the patients show a disregard for the demands of custom and law, are unconstrained, and often commit grave offences into which they have no insight. As a reason for such conduct, they often say that they acted so because it happened to come into their minds. The social restraints normally imposed upon one by the environment never interfere with the carrying out of their wishes. They are quite reckless of personal safety, and occasionally injure themselves severely in their foolhardy actions. In conditions of great clouding of consciousness or in advanced deterioration there are sometimes present some symptoms characteristic of the catatonic form of dementia praecox, such as catalepsy, verbigeration, negativism, and stereotyped movements; but these are transitory and change more readily and frequently than in catatonia.

Physical Symptoms. — The physical signs of the disease, in both the motor and the sensory fields, are as extensive and profound as the psychical. These may appear either before the mental symptoms or not until dementia has become well advanced; usually they are coincident.

Of the sensory symptoms, *headache* is often the first to appear, accompanied by a feeling of pressure as if the head were being held in a vice, together with ringing in the ears and dizziness. The *special senses* at first give evidence of excitation, which later subsides into a state of insensibility corresponding closely in degree to the stage of deterioration. Some patients have difficulty in the recognition and localization of objects held before them, which by Fuerstner is ascribed to involvement of the occipital cortex. Word blindness and asymbolism are often observed. Hemianopsia occasionally follows apoplectiform or epileptiform attacks. Optic atrophy is found in five to twelve per cent. of the cases. Disturbances of the senses of taste and smell have also been observed by some, especially the loss of the sense of taste for saline solutions. The disturbance of the cutaneous sensations is quite often prominent; at first there may be all sorts of uncomfortable sensations, burning or drawing sensations, rheumatic pains, etc. Hence, many patients are for a long time regarded as neurastheniacs. In some cases there is an increased sensitiveness to cold. Later *analgesia* appears, which may be so pronounced that needles can be thrust entirely through a limb without pain. Finally, the patients may pull out their hair, disturb an open wound, draw out their toe-nails, and persist in mangling their own flesh.

Of the motor symptoms *paralytic attacks,* mostly epileptiform or apoplectiform, are very important, occurring in from forty-six to sixty per cent. of cases. The attacks may be very light, consisting only of a transitory dizziness with perhaps an inability to speak. Attacks of this sort are often the first symptoms to call attention to the disease. Occasionally the attack consists of a suddenly developing aphasia lasting several days, unaccompanied by paralysis. In the *epileptiform* attacks, which may be either of the Jacksonian or of the ordinary type, confusion or stupidity may usher in the attacks, which begin with a fall to the floor, loss of consciousness, and convulsive movements, usually in one limb, extending gradually to the others. Clonic movements predominate and are often synchronous with the pulse. Convulsive movements may be confined to a single group of muscles or to one limb. The duration of the attack is from one to several hours, but sometimes clonic movements of varying intensity continue in one or more limbs for days. A condition similar to status epilepticus, where there are from twenty to one hundred attacks daily, may persist for days, often terminating in death. During the attacks the temperature is often febrile, the urine frequently contains albumen, and there may be retention of urine and feces, as well as paralysis of the muscles of deglutition. The fatal termination is usually due to aspiration pneumonia. The attacks pass off slowly, sometimes leaving the patients in a condition of confusion. In the earlier stages of the psychosis, these attacks leave the patients in a condition of more profound deterioration, and sometimes also with signs of transient aphasia, hemiplegia, hemianopsia, convulsive movements, or areas of anaesthesia. *Apoplectiform attacks* often occur, and may be the first important sign of the disease. In these attacks there is the usual loss of consciousness and stertorous breathing, with occasional high elevation of temperature, accompanied by hemiplegia and aphasia. In some attacks there is no loss of consciousness, simply the sudden appearance of transitory paralysis. Transitory sensory disturbances can similarly appear; as, severe paresthesias, anaesthesias, or defects of vision. It is a distinguishing feature of these apoplectiform attacks that the paralysis disappears quickly and without evident residuals. Other somewhat similar attacks, occurring in the course of the disease, are those in which there is a sudden development of extreme confusion, with motor restlessness, difficult speech, flushing of the face and body, vomiting, and high temperature. These last from a few hours to a few days and pass away quickly, leaving the patient in his former state.

The frequency of the apoplectiform

and epileptiform attacks depends somewhat upon the character of the treatment. They may result from emotional disturbances, excesses in eating, and especially from an accumulation of feces in the rectum, but they frequently appear without evident cause. Bed treatment, regularly, reduces their frequency. They occur most often in the demented form of the disease.

Motor disturbances of the eye include transitory paralysis of single muscles (eighteen per cent. of the cases) and rarely complete ophthalmoplegia. Differences of the pupil occur in about fifty-seven to eighty-three per cent. of the cases, immobile pupils in from thirty-four to sixty-eight per cent., and sluggish reaction to light in thirty-five and five-tenths per cent. (Argyll-Robertson pupil).

The *muscles of the face* lose their tone, the nasolabial fold and other lines of expression disappear, and the countenance becomes expressionless. This washed-out, expressionless character of the countenance is well represented by the group of three paretics seen in Plate 6. Lack of tone in the muscular system is also seen in their slouching and inelastic attitude. There is also a loss of control of the muscles, giving rise to incoordination, noticeable mostly when the mouth or eyes are forcibly opened. A fine tremor of these muscles is almost always present. The voice loses its characteristic tone and becomes monotonous. Tremor of the tongue, which may be either finely fibrillary or coarse and retractive, is a constant sign. In advanced cases there is often a rolling of the tongue about the mouth as if it were a quid. This in some cases has been explained by the presence of areas of anaesthesia in the mucous membrane. Gritting of the teeth is occasionally associated with these movements of the tongue, or may be present alone.

Disturbances of *speech* are among the most characteristic symptoms. They are either aphasic or articulatory. Transitory *aphasia* often appears after paralytic attacks. Paraphasia, which may appear at the same time, is more persistent and sometimes lasts several months.

Word blindness and word deafness are rarely encountered. There is occasionally agrammatism, as seen in the misuse of infinitives and omission of conjunctions. There may be an elision of syllables, as in the use of elexity for electricity, or a reduplication of syllables, as electricicity, and finally there may be tendency to repeat syllables, forming a genuine word clonus, as Massachusetts-etts-etts-etts.

Disturbances of *articulation* are more frequent. They may follow paralytic attacks, but more often occur independently of them. As the result of difficulty in movement of the lips and tongue frequent pauses are made between syllables or words — *hesitating speech* — and when accompanied by a fall in the tone of voice produce a *scanning speech.* Gliding over the poorly articulated sounds gives rise to an indistinct and *slurring* speech. These difficulties lead to the substitution of words or syllables similar in sound but more easily pronounced, or to the elision of difficult syllables. Many patients, in their efforts to overcome these difficulties, stutter and produce an *explosive speech.* The patients often appreciate the difficulties of speech, but are ready to explain them by dryness of the mouth or loss of teeth. Speech disturbances are readily observed in ordinary conversation. The test words and phrases, if used, should be introduced into long sentences, because, if the attention is concentrated upon single words, they may be pronounced correctly. Words and phrases used for this purpose are: electricity, national intelligency, methodist episcopal, ninth riding Massachusetts artillery brigade, etc.

The central and ataxic speech disturbances are best elicited by asking the patients to read aloud. Writing usually shows defects similar to those noticed in speech, but they are proportionately more prominent (Plates 7 and 8). Patients, on the other hand, who speak clearly may produce on paper an unintelligible muddle of words and syllables. In advanced cases there is complete agraphia (Plate 7, Figures 2 and 3). The patients are then able to make but a few unintelligible marks, and may even give up without making a sign. The handwriting is characterized by irregularities caused by the tremor, excessive pressure on the pen, and carelessness. The irregularities are more extensive than in the case of the senile, whose lines show the effect of a fine regular tremor.

Ataxia appears first of all in those finer movements such as are employed by skilled workmen. Later the more delicate movements in locomotion, such as turning about quickly, become ataxic. The clothing cannot be readily buttoned, the gait becomes unsteady, swaying and shuffling. In from sixteen to twenty-four per cent. of the cases of paresis there are tabetic signs; such as, loss of reflexes, ataxia, Romberg sign, paralysis of the rectum and bladder, and occasionally girdle symptoms, lancinating pains, and crises. In from six to eight per cent. of cases, genuine tabes antedates for several years the appearance of the paretic symptoms *(ascending paresis* or *tabo-paresis).* In about fourteen per cent. of the cases of paresis there are evidences of involvement of the lateral column of the cord, as shown by the spastic paralyses. In many cases spastic and tabetic symptoms are variously combined. Intention tremor may be present, and in a few cases choreiform movements are marked enough to simulate Huntingdon's chorea. Later in the course of the disease the patients become bedridden and often develop contractures and muscular atrophy. The body also tends to assume a curved position with a fixed tension of the muscles of the neck so that the head is thrown forward and the body does not rest upon the bed throughout its entire length. During this stage of the disease there is occasionally noticed convulsive movements of the individual muscle groups, especially during active and passive movements, but also when the muscles are at rest. Cotton, Amer. Jour. of Insanity, Vol. 61, p. 581. Gaupp, Uber die spinalen Symptome der progressiven Paralyse, 189S. Torkel, Besteht eine gesetzmassige Verschiedenheit in Verlaufsart und Dauer

d. progressiven Paralyse nach d. Charakter d. begleitenden Rmaffektion? Diss., Marburg, 1903.

The pressure of the spinal fluid, according to Schaefer, is increased in two-thirds of the cases from normal (40 to 70 millimetres) to 150-380 millimetres. Furthermore, he finds that the albumen is increased and contains serum albumin, while the normal fluid contains only globulin. The microscopical examination of fluid shows a lymphocytosis (see p. 103). The *tendon reflexes* are usually exaggerated, sometimes so markedly that the entire body shakes when the tendon is struck. Frequently the exaggeration diminishes, and in twenty to thirty per cent. of the advanced cases the reflexes are lost. In eighteen per cent. of the cases there is a difference in the two sides. The loss of the patellar reflexes is usually associated with immobile pupils and myosis. The Babinski reflex is often elicited in connection with spastic Schaefer, Allgem. Zeitachr. f. Psy., LIX, 84.

symptoms. The electrical irritability of the muscles is increased at first, but later diminished. Disturbances of the bladder are often present, both retention and incontinence, the latter usually being the result of the former. Sluggishness of the bowels may extend to obstinate constipation. Finally in the end stages there is paralysis of both sphincters. The sexual power may be increased at the onset, but later it is diminished. The *vasomotor disturbances* consist of erythema, persistent blushing of the skin, rush of blood to the head, dermographia, and cyanosis. The so-called *trophic* changes, acute decubitus, increased fragility of the ribs, and othematoma, stand in close relation to the vasomotor changes, and are of frequent occurrence. Furthermore, there is a loss of vitality and of the power of repair in all tissues, so that a very trifling injury may lead to an extensive lesion. Acute decubitus once started is difficult to heal.

The *temperature* during the course of the disease is mostly normal, except toward the end, when it is apt to be subnormal. A striking peculiarity is the excessive elevation of temperature with trifling disturbances, such as mild bronchitis, overdistention of the bladder, or obstinate constipation. There is often a rise of temperature during paralytic attacks, and finally, as already mentioned, there may be short periods of a few hours or more of an excessively high temperature apparently without adequate cause, j

The *sleep* is usually somewhat disturbed during the first stage and more so during the second, where there is motor excitement, but in the last stage the patients are sluggish and may sleep much of the time. This varies, however, as in some cases the patients may, from the onset, show a tendency to sleep continually, while in other cases insomnia persists throughout the whole course. The *appetite* suffers at first and during excitement, but later the patients eat well. The condition of *nutrition* is poor until excitement subsides and deterioration is well advanced, when there is usually an increase in weight, which may last until death. Sometimes loss of appetite and impaired nutrition coexist, leading to extreme emaciation. Occasionally albumen and sugar are present in the urine. The *blood changes* consist of a moderate and progressive anaemia, in which the fall in haemoglobin is most marked, a progressive increase of the polymorphoneuclear leucocytes reaching its highest point during the terminal state, and a transitory leucocytosis accompanying paralytic attacks. D'Abundo has called attention to an increased toxicity of the blood, and Idelsohn finds that the blood of paretics in a considerable proportion of cases inhibits or prevents the growth of cultures of bacteria.

The mental and physical symptoms enumerated above represent in general the clinical picture. The grouping of the individual symptoms, however, varies widely in different cases. This has led to the recognition of four types of cases: the *demented, expansive, agitated,* and *depressive,* each of which presents a somewhat different course from the onset. The deviations from these types deter many from the acceptance of this differentiation, but its value becomes apparent in a considerable number of cases where one is able to forecast the future duration of the disease and the character of many of the symptoms.

The demented form, because of the simple deterioration, unaccompanied by many delusions and hallucinations, its rapid course without remissions, and the relative frequency of its occurrence should be regarded as the type of the Diefendorf, Amer. Jour. Med. Sciences, Vol. 126, p. 1047. Capps, Amer. Jour. Med. Sc, 1897.

Idelsohn, Archiv f. Psy., XXXI, 64a disease. The clinical picture of megalomania, which has been and still is, by some, regarded as the prototype of the disease, has in recent years become less and less prominent, until it is now encountered in less than twenty-five per cent. of cases.

Demented Form *The demented form is characterized by gradually progressive mental deterioration without prominence of either hallucinations, delusions, or great psychomotor disturbance.* Transitory periods of delirious excitement, of anxious unrest with hypochondriacal ideas of depression, delusional states, or periods of megalomania may occur in this picture, but they are insignificant when compared with the rapid advance of profound deterioration.

The *onset* of this form is very gradual. The symptoms at first may resemble those of neurasthenia; patients complain of inability to apply themselves to work, loss of energy, indefinite pains, feeling of pressure in the head, and irritability. They are forgetful and flighty, at times drowsy, and at others somewhat confused. Soon mental deterioration becomes apparent in the inability to explain their actions, in errors of judgment, failure of memory, and absence of the usual moral feelings. *Their* work is irksome, and they occasionally fall asleep over it. They forget to go to meals, make mistakes in figures, and overlook important matters. They are usually good-natured, tractable, are easily led astray, and often drink to intoxication. In some cases, however, they become obstinate and self-willed. The household suffers, dinner is uncooked or improperly seasoned, and the children are neglected. Patients are reckless and may even act in opposition to established precepts. The *consciousness* soon becomes clouded and the patients fail to thoroughly comprehend their environment, lose account of time, get confused as to place, and mistake persons. They may even get confused in their own home and not recognize friends and relatives.

Transitory hallucinations and *delusions* may appear, but the latter are very weak, childish, and easily influenced by suggestion. Occasionally there are weak attempts at *fabrication*. During the early stages there may be some anxiety with weeping and praying, and frequently also an increased irritability, some sexual excitement, aggressiveness, and assaults; but the characteristic *emotional* change is a progressive deterioration of the feelings. The patients become increasingly dull and apathetic. They are perfectly contented wherever placed as long as the simplest needs are satisfied; such as, food, drink, and tobacco. They have a complacent smile when addressed, greet strangers very cordially, and are friendly with every one. Often at first there is some *insight,* when the patients complain of slowness of thought and failure of memory, but the increasing deterioration obscures this feeble capacity. On the other hand, they may express a feeling of well-being and perfect confidence in their business capacity.

The *capacity for work* suffers soon. The patients become careless in their duties, forget engagements, allow letters to go unanswered, go to work at all hours, and finally stay away altogether. A few patients may struggle along with their work, realizing and worrying over difficulties and frequent errors, while others neglect their occupation to look after all sorts of unnecessary and unprofitable affairs. They may become restless, wandering aimlessly about, indulging in excesses or committing petty crimes. They lack will power, are easily led astray, are unable to care for themselves, forget when to go to meals, and neglect their personal appearance. On the contrary,

some patients are inaccessible, repulsive, and surly, answering questions as if angry, rebuffing friendly advances, and opposing without reason anything desired of them.

A few patients, in spite of an advanced stage of deterioration, present a good demeanor. They greet one correctly, and appear perfectly at ease in talking about themselves, but at the same time are disoriented, and are unable to give any coherent account of their lives. The patients usually enjoy a good appetite, sleep well, and are the picture of health. The mental deterioration may have been so gradual and so unobtrusive that the friends and relatives fail to appreciate the profound degree of deterioration exhibited.

This form of dementia paralytica embraces forty per cent. of the cases admitted to institutions. Paralytic attacks occur in almost one-half of the cases. Remissions are less frequent than in the other forms. The duration in almost half of the cases does not extend beyond two years. In eighteen per cent. of the cases death ensues within the first year, and it is very rare that the disease lasts five years.

Expansive Form *The expansive form is characterized by great prominence of expansive delusions, a prolonged course, and greater prevalence of remissions.*

The *onset* is usually gradual, with change of character, difficulty of mental application, signs of failing memory and judgment, increased irritability, and, in addition, such physical signs as fainting spells, transitory speech disturbances, syncopal attacks, and headaches. Occasionally the onset is quite sudden.

Following these prodromal symptoms, there may first develop the picture of the depressed type with delusions of persecution, self-accusation, and anxiety, but usually from the onset there is a condition of excitement with elation, and grandiose delusions, during which transitory states of depression with weeping may occur. In case there have been signs of despondency and illness, these then disappear and the patients

gradually — occasionally suddenly — develop a marked feeling of well-being; they are bright, affable, talkative, and energetic. They busy themselves with new and elaborate schemes for getting wealthy, stake out property, and draw designs for wonderful machines. They are busy from early morning to late at night, soliciting patronage, ordering large quantities of material for building and for other purposes. The numerous expansive delusions at first are within the range of possibility and may appear attractive to the unsuspecting, but soon pass into the realm of absurd imagination, reminding one very much of the prattle of children. These, with the restlessness, present the characteristic picture of *megalomania.* The patients claim never to have felt better in their lives, can lift tons, can whip the best man on earth, have the strength of a thousand horses, and can move a train.

They believe their English the best; they speak as fluently several other languages; their voice is clear and distinct and can be heard for many blocks, because of its excellent qualities. They have the inspiration to write a book; can compose beautiful poems; can deliver an oration on any subject. They associate only with the most cultured people; only the genuine blue blood courses through their veins; they are going to build a marble mansion at Newport, and have a floating palace. Business is flourishing; they are making a "mint of money," have several gangs of men working for them, and still there is more work than they can attend to; besides their regular business, chickens are being raised by a special method at an enormous profit; they have secured rich gold claims in Nevada, which are doubling in wealth daily.

Formerly they were brakemen, but now run the fastest and finest train in the world from New York to Chicago without a single stop, allowing none but millionnaires to ride; besides a profitable law business, they are now engaged in writing a novel which will startle the world, and for which they have received priceless offers from publishers in this country and in Europe. A ship carpenter developed wonderful power in his eyes, so that he could detect defective wood in a vessel by simply standing in the hold and looking outward, and for this reason he was appointed detective of a marine insurance company, and had travelled all over the world inspecting vessels. He had become so wealthy that all the banks in the state were in his possession.

A seamstress had devised a new method for cutting dresses, which had won her world-wide fame, having been called to all of the courts of Europe because of her wonderful success. She herself could cut and sew a hundred dresses a day, and had under her five hundred girls, all of whom used gold thread. She could sew on a thousand buttons a minute. A jockey had discovered a new way of breeding and training runners, and now from his Kentucky ranch was supplying every circuit and handicap with winners.

The utter absurdities which increase from day to day are proof of the increasing mental weakness. The delusions abound in contradictions and become more incoherent, the product of a more dreamy ingenuity. The patient now drives the largest engine in the world, drawing a thousand palace cars, all lined with gold and trimmed with pearls, which encircles the globe every twenty-four hours, stopping only at New York, San Francisco, Calcutta, Paris, and London. He now has formed a chicken trust to extend over the whole earth, and will reconstruct the social system of the world, so that only the Chinese will be employed in hatching the eggs. Another has a most wonderful herd of cattle, whose horns are forty feet high, whose eyes are diamonds, whose feet are gold, and each cow produces five hundred pails of milk in twenty-four hours, the patient himself milking a thousand a day.

The patients are the most beautiful beings that ever lived. They have married seven hundred millionaires, have twenty thousand children, all of whom have gold slippers and gold dresses; they themselves wear only diamond trimmings; they can fly away in the air

to a world where there is a castle ten thousand miles long filled with lovely people who do nothing but amuse themselves. They are not human, but divine; can create a universe, visit all the stars, have sent Christ to Mars; whatever they touch turns to gold. They know all sciences, are the greatest physicians in existence; will build a hospital of marble twenty stories high, provided with a bar for the doctors, where the choicest wines and the best Havana cigars will be supplied; and there will be a dissecting room, with a huge ice box, where ten thousand bodies can be kept all the time.

They will build a tunnel through the earth and bring all the Chinamen here to work. One patient said that he was going to build towns; that he had been to Washington to see the President, that he wanted six thousand billion gunboats, one million bomb-shell boats, one million marines, and that he would cross the ocean and blow up all of the countries and bring the people out west and put them on farms; that he would blow up the Queen's buildings, and that he would give each one of the marines two bags, and each would have to go two times in order to bring away the silks and diamonds.

These delusions are almost entirely self-centered. They may change rapidly, each day new and extravagant ideas appearing, which are filled with the most glaring contradictions. In women the tendency to expansiveness is less marked. Transitory *hallucinations* of sight and hearing are. occasionally expressed, but they never take a prominent part in the disease picture.

Consciousness is somewhat clouded during the development of the megalomania. There is usually disorientation for time, places, and persons, — the patients are too much absorbed in their numerous ideas to note the surroundings or to take account of time. Later they become acquainted with the place and a few of the persons, but they rarely know the month, day, or the year. The *content of thought* is centered entirely about self and the many varied delusions. At first it is usually coherent, although at times,

in connection with great psychomotor restlessness, there may be incoherence, distractibility, and sometimes flight of ideas. The patients are usually talkative, and may produce a continuous stream of delusions. Incoherence of thought is more evident in their letters.

The *emotional attitude* corresponds closely to the content of the delusions; the patients are cheerful, happy, hopeful, contented, and exalted. Everything in the environment is pleasing; they are in luxurious quarters, have the best of food, plenty of servants, fine clothing, fast horses, and are associated with the finest men in the world. It often happens that for a short time, a few moments or hours, rarely days, they lose spirits and become depressed, complaining of confinement, and expressing hypochondriacal delusions, or weep bitterly because of harassing persecutions. Even when most miserable it is often possible by suggestions to reestablish the feeling of well-being, showing the great instability of the emotional condition. Increased irritability is always present, manifesting itself upon the slightest provocation. Disagreements or doubts relative to their superiority or immense wealth may arouse anger or even an aggressive attack. Later in the course of the disease the patients are usually in a uniform state of quiet cheerfulness in spite of their bedridden condition with filthiness, paralysis, and even contractures. The paretic on his deathbed, when asked how he feels, often drawls out with some animation, "Fine, fine."

In the *psychomotor field* excitement predominates from the onset and may reach an extreme degree. At first the patients are restless, bustling about on new and important business, remaining up until late at night, devising plans, writing many letters, and travelling about from place to place. They are very talkative and make confidants of every one they meet. For short periods in the course of the disease they may develop extreme restlessness, with insomnia, complete clouding of consciousness, recklessness, aggressiveness, and impulsiveness. They shout from fear, mutilate their own bodies, and rush about blindly diving into any obstacle. It is impossible to attract their attention or to get coherent answers. They fight off imaginary enemies and shout threats and curses. These conditions of excitement rarely last longer than a few hours or days, and disappear gradually, usually leaving the patient in a state of more profound deterioration.

In *actions* the patients soon become foolish and show a lack of judgment and moral obtuseness. They develop bad habits, smoke or swear, enjoy telling obscene stories, seek the company of lascivious women, and become disorderly in dress and careless in appearance. They may assault or commit thefts, but every action shows an absence of plan, recklessness, and utter disregard for others. When confronted with their observed behavior, it is all denied with perfect serenity.

As the disease advances, the activity is limited to the production of unintelligible letters and plans, scribbling on paper, and collecting useless rubbish. The patients are happy and contented throughout it all, invariably asserting with brightening countenance that they are feeling fine. They may be heard mumbling to themselves, "millions," "fine horses," "beautiful women," "grand mansions," — mere relics of former ideas which now represent the last traces of their intellectual life.

The expansive form comprises from fifteen to sixteen per cent. of the paretics. The duration is more prolonged, less than one-third of the cases dying within two years. Some cases even live fourteen years. Remissions occur in onethird of the cases, which in part accounts for the prolonged course. It sometimes happens that the expansive form passes over into the depressive, and *vice versa,* and this may take place several times, simulating the picture of manicdepressive insanity.

Agitated Form *The agitated form is characterized by a relatively sudden onset with a condition of great psychomotor excitement and delirium, and the presence of the most extremely expansive delusions, great clouding of consciousness, and a short course.* The usu-

al prodromal symptoms are lacking and there rapidly develops *extreme megalomania.* A change of disposition is often noticed for a time previous to the sudden outbreak. The patients rapidly become very energetic, and express a pronounced feeling of well-being. They are born again, possess the ambition and the strength of ten thousand men; could cany an ocean vessel or fly to the moon in a second. They have acquired all knowledge, can educate a thousand men an hour, teaching them to speak every known language. They themselves are Gods, Gods over God, have created God and the universe; have been everywhere from the heights of heaven to the depths of hell. They are now establishing a new method of reckoning time; by their decree the days are to be one thousand hours long, the weeks are to contain one thousand days, and the years ten thousand months. They know how to create animals, and by a new formula man shall be increased a hundred-fold in size and shall have a third eye. The world moves and stands at their command. They are interested in all wars and have marshalled huge armies. Their wealth is fabulous, more than any one man ever possessed before. All quantities are reckoned in the ten thousand billions; they own ten thousand billion houses; ten thousand billion cows; ten thousand billion acres of land, etc. Their houses are built of Italian marble, with gilded domes set with diamonds, the floors are of onyx, the furniture, pure gold, and the hangings, the finest fabric, trimmed with pearls and sapphires. Their ideas become more and more expansive, and finally seem even to surpass the bounds of imagination.

In the midst of these megalomanic delusions, one occasionally encounters the most extremely *pessimistic ideas* which are sometimes hypochondriacal. The patients claim that they are suffering untold misery from sharp pains in the back; some one entered the room at night and disembowelled them, so that the following morning they could not go to stool; miles of fine electric wires have been placed in the flesh, about the limbs and completely filling the skull,

through which electrical currents are nightly applied, causing the flesh to burn. There may be some *insight* into the failing memory and the defective nutrition, which leads them momentarily to fear that they are suffering from cancer of the most malignant type, but at the same time one is assured that they are undergoing a process of purification which will leave them healthier and mightier. Sometimes they are perplexed at their own stupidity for allowing themselves to be confined in a hospital instead of going to Europe to consummate a deal by which millions would have been made. *Hallucinations* of sight and hearing may be present, but are not prominent, and fail to influence greatly the clinical picture.

The *psychomotor condition* is one of great restlessness, showing occasional impulsive movements. The patients are talkative, sing, laugh, shout, and prattle away like children over their innumerable plans and many pleasures. They are constantly in motion, going from one thing to another, working in a planless way on various schemes, scribbling unintelligible letters to millionnaire friends, issuing commands to military staffs, and sending cablegrams to the different crowned heads. They have no care for themselves, neglect personal appearance, forget about eating, smear their dresses or the walls with the food placed before them, masturbate, and expose themselves indecently.

Thought is usually incoherent, and there is often observed a flight of ideas. *Emotionally,* there is a marked irritability, and interference quickly leads to outbursts of passion, with cursing, threats, and aggressiveness; but elation predominates. *Physically,* the condition of nutrition suffers profoundly, and there is a great loss of weight, because of the small amount of food ingested and great restlessness. The temperature may be subnormal.

A few cases of the agitated form may be characterized as galloping paresis. *These cases present an extreme grade of excitement and profound clouding of consciousness, leading within a few weeks or months to fatal collapse.* It sometimes represents the end stage of the agitated form and occasionally also of the depressed form. The patients are completely confused, unable to comprehend the surroundings or to respond to questions. They are noisy, shouting and singing, producing an unintelligible babble, with many repetitions of syllables or purely inarticulate sounds. The restlessness is extreme, the patients being in constant motion, pounding the bed or wall, forcing the legs up and down, running about the room, slapping their hands, waltzing to and fro, and bruising themselves extensively by their reckless movements. Insomnia is extreme and food is refused, or if taken, cannot be retained, and the patients are wholly unable to care for their personal needs. The weight falls rapidly, the temperature becomes slightly elevated, and the heart's action feeble and irregular. Epileptiform and apoplectiform attacks are frequent. Within a few days or weeks the restlessness subsides into a condition of stupor, in which the movements are uncertain and tremulous. The temperature becomes elevated as the result of infection from the various wounds or acute decubitus, the mouth is filled with sordes; profuse perspiration and diarrhoea appear, which with heart failure lead to death.

The agitated form represents about eleven per cent. of the paretics. Remissions occur in one-fourth of the cases. Paralytic attacks are frequent. The duration in more than two-thirds of the cases is less than two years.

Depressed Form *This form is characterized by despondency and depressive delusions which prevail throughout the whole course of the disease.*

The *onset* in this form is insidious. The patients notice their failing memory, decreasing power of application, greater weariness upon exertion, and change of disposition. The persistent headaches, the numerous pains, and failing memory lead them to consult one physician after another. They worry about themselves and soon become *hypochondriacal.* They claim that they are suffering from a complication of diseases and that they can never recov-

er. During this stage they are not infrequently regarded as neurastheniacs, hypochondriacs, or hysterical patients.

But their hypochondriacal complaints sooner or later become entirely senseless. They then complain that the scalp is rotting away, the skull is filling in with bone, causing the brain to shrink, the mouth is filled with sores, the sense of taste is lost, the throat is clogged up, so that the food passes up into the brain, the stomach is melted away, and the intestines are so paralyzed that excrement has been accumulating within them for many months, the kidneys have been moved, so that water passes directly through their bodies. They claim that they are dead, the blood has ceased to circulate, and they have turned to stone. The testicles have dried up and their manhood has disappeared; a false passage has formed so that the " vital fluid " passes out of the rectum. In connection with these ideas they are constantly fingering different parts of the body, especially the face and sexual organs. They may sit for hours with hands on their throat for fear feces will pass into the mouth, or may he abed as if dead, claiming that they would fall apart if moved.

Delusions of self-accusation are usually associated with these hypochondriacal ideas and occasionally predominate in the clinical picture. The patients believe themselves great sinners, that they have committed the unpardonable sin, must die on the cross, have stolen property, and injured then-children. They have caused the death of a friend by negligence, and every one knows that they are murderers. They persist that they have always been impure and have led many astray. A patient moaned for months because he had not provided his family with sufficient food and was being held up to the whole world as an example and must suffer the penalty of death. Very often *fear* develops in connection with these ideas of self-accusation, when the patients are in terror because they are being constantly watched, expecting at any moment to be imprisoned or carried away to the scaffold; or they dread personal injury and

abuse. *Delusions of persecution* are usually accompanied by *hallucinations* of hearing, when they suspect plots against their lives and complain that their families are being outraged. They are being regarded as desperadoes on whose head there is a high price. The troops have been summoned to escort them into exile. They hear themselves slandered by a crowd of men outside, or overhear intrigues against them. Others threaten them. Hallucinations of the other senses are infrequent.

The *consciousness* soon becomes much clouded. There is considerable disorientation; friends are mistaken, and time is confused. Occurrences in the surroundings have reference only to themselves. The bathing of others suggests to their minds that they have polluted their fellow-patients, and the preparation for the morning walk signifies that the whole company are getting ready to attend their public prosecution. At the table others are deprived of food on their account. In this condition they develop great anxiety with restlessness; pace back and forth in their rooms, moaning and groaning, sometimes uttering single expressions, as "death," " destruction," pick at their finger-nails, pull out their hair, and are unable to eat. Every unusual sound frightens them and causes them to shudder and shrink back farther into their rooms. Finally they cannot be persuaded to leave the bed, but lie huddled up at one side, with the head buried in the clothing. In this condition they may attempt suicide or mutilate their own bodies; one patient tore through the anal sphincter into the vagina with her hand.

Extreme anxiety with restlessness does not exist very long at a time, usually only for a few hours or at most a few weeks. It may appear and disappear suddenly. In the interval the patients are not as agitated but yet are despondent and seclusive. The depressive delusions are retained but they show far less emotion. The mental depression is not always uniform, as one occasionally notices emotional indifference, and even transitory periods with a feeling of well-being and of elation. When deterioration is well advanced, expansive delusions occasionally appear.

More or less prolonged *stuporous states* appear at times during the course of the disease, when the patients become mute, lying abed in one position oblivious to the surroundings, refusing nourishment, and allowing the feces and urine to pass unheeded. Requests are carried out slowly or wholly ignored. The patients appear indifferent, but at times they display some emotion, or they may show some anxiety. Hallucinations and illusions may be more or less prominent or entirely wanting. Consciousness is usually clouded. These states may last several months.

The depressive form of dementia paralytica comprises one-fourth of the cases, and appears rather late in life, mostly after forty years of age. Remissions occur in less than twelve per cent. of the cases, while paralytic attacks occur in twenty-five percent. This type is one of the severer forms, as over seventy per cent. die within two years.

Course of dementia paralytica.—Dementia paralytica may be divided into three stages: the stage of onset, the stage of acute symptoms, and the terminal stage of dementia. The lines of division are very indefinite, as the first stage may very quickly pass into the acute stage, when the symptoms remain in abeyance for a few years; or the case may be one of apathetic deterioration from the onset, devoid of any prominent symptoms indicative of definite stages. The terminal stage is apt to be prolonged. In it the patients are dull, stupid, apathetic, entirely indifferent to their surroundings, unable to care for themselves, or occasionally expressing incoherent fragments of former delusions. They sit unoccupied save for the taking of nourishment, to which they often have to be helped. The physical symptoms in this stage advance to general paresis of all of the muscles, necessitating confinement in bed. Sensation is greatly impaired, muscular atrophy and weakness become marked, and finally contractures appear. In the end patients become nothing more than vegetating organisms. The course of the physical symptoms by no means correspond to those of the mental symptoms. On the one hand, there are cases in which speech disturbances and incoordination may antedate for a long time the appearance of faulty memory or judgment, and on the other hand, the mental symptoms may appear first.

The two important factors in the course of the disease are *paralytic attacks* and *remissions*. The attacks may appear at any time during the course, producing an unexpected progress in the deterioration or even a fatal termination. They may usher in the disease, being followed by a condition of advanced deterioration, but more frequently occur during the terminal stage. These attacks accompany chiefly the demented and the expansive forms.

Remissions are most often encountered in the agitated and expansive forms and very rarely in the demented forms. The improvement, which is usually rapid, appears only during the earlier stages of the disease. Both the physical and mental symptoms show marked improvement; the consciousness becomes clear, the content of thought coherent, and the delusions and hallucinations disappear. The patients often look back upon their psychosis as a sort of dream, without clear insight. In the course of a month or two they may have improved so much that, as far as the limited associations of the institution permit, they appear perfectly well. When at liberty, however, it is apparent to their friends that they have lost their former mental energy; they tire easily, and are changed in disposition. Yet they are usually eager for employment and disregard the advice of the physicians to exercise care. Some of the patients are able to engage successfully in their former occupation and support their families. In other cases the remission is only partial; the patients become clear and coherent, while the expansive and depressive delusions disappear; but there still remains a tendency to excessive activity, with a desire to enter into uncertain business ventures, to be lavish with money, careless in personal appearance, and irritable and fretful in disposition. The duration of the remission seldom lasts over three or four months, but in some cases it extends over three or more years.

Diagnosis. — During the early stages of paresis, there may be considerable difficulty in distinguishing *acquired neurasthenia* (see p. 153).

The depressive form of paresis is distinguished from *melancholia of involution* by the evidences of mental deterioration: weakness of judgment, moral instability, failure of memory, defective time orientation, silliness and incoherence of the delusions, and presence of physical signs. The melancholiac shows a greater prominence of self-accusations and good orientation, except in cases with many hallucinations and delusions. The intense apprehensiveness of the paretic is less persistent than that encountered in melancholia, and is occasionally relieved by short periods of moderate but distinct feeling of well-being. The melancholiacs have their good days, but they never show elation.

The *depressive phases of manic-depressive insanity* are distinguished by the absence of any signs of mental deterioration and by the presence of retardation among the motor phenomena. In the stuporous states the manic-depressive patient takes some notice of and partially apprehends his surroundings, although he takes no part in them; he shows some anxiety and discomfort when threatened with a needle and seldom moves voluntarily and then slowly, while the paretic is partially disoriented, does not react when threatened with a needle, and occasionally moves freely and even restlessly, and usually presents characteristic physical signs.

The *manic phases of manic-depressive insanity* are differentiated from the expansive and agitated forms of paresis by the absence of mental deterioration. The paretic is unable to recall correctly recent events, and especially the date of their occurrence. His delusions are more extreme, fantastic, and contradictory; his emotional attitude is variable, and dependent upon the surroundings and suggestions, and he is more pliable. The manic, on the other hand, is more alert and quick in apprehending when hi attention can be attracted; he shows an accurate memory; his delusions are less often contradictory, are expressed with less assurance and more facetiousness; and he is seldom contented and is less pliable. In conditions of extreme excitement, the orientation and the coherence of thought is more disturbed in paresis.

It often happens that periods of excitement at the onset of the disease are mistaken for *delirium tremens,* especially where early paretic symptoms have escaped notice in an alcoholic (see p. 183).

Dementia prœcox is usually differentiated by the absence of the characteristic physical signs, good orientation, and the presence of catatonic features (see p. 270). The socalled catatonic symptoms, if they occur in paresis, are accompanied by a greater disturbance of memory and greater insensibility and cloudiness than what one encounters in dementia praecox. In case these distinguishing features cannot be determined, on account of negativistic signs, then one has to depend upon the presence or absence of physical signs. The presence of simple difference of pupils, increased reflexes, moderate tremor, and, indeed, even attacks of dizziness and of an epileptiform nature, are not conclusive for paresis. If a patient with such symptoms is uncertain and helpless in simple figuring tests, is unable to orient himself as regards time and to readily recall early experiences, and is easily influenced in action and feeling, provided it is not the mechanical response to stimuli, then the condition is more indicative of paresis. The states of dementia in paresis lack the tendency to adornment, the mannerisms, the occasional exacerbations, and the persistent stupor, negativism, and refusal of food. In the paretic excitement, there may occur impulsive and stereotyped movements; but they are not accompanied by the irrelevant and incoherent speech of the catatonic, and furthermore, the excited paretic is not oriented to the extent that the catatonic usually is. In the paranoid forms there is neither the paretic inability to comprehend the surroundings nor the permanent feeling of wellbeing, hallucinations are much more frequent and expansive delusions develop more

slowly, while the paretic does not show the delusions of influence so common in paranoid dementia. The late cases of dementia precox, in which despondency may predominate, are distinguished by the susceptibility to external influences, such as commands, and by the impulsive restlessness or stupor with resistiveness. Ultimately the diagnosis may rest upon the examination of the cerebrospinal fluid.

The differentiation of paresis is apt to be most difficult in those diseases in which there are extensive cortical lesions, particularly *cerebral syphilis* (see p. 331), arteriosclerotic insanity (see p. 338), and *senile dementia. Senile dementia* may be recognized by the age at onset, the more prolonged course, comparative poverty of delusions, and absence of characteristic motor symptoms.

Cases of *cerebral tumor* occasionally present mental symptoms similar to those in the demented form of dementia paralytica. The chief point of differentiation, in case no focal symptoms exist, is the presence of the cupped optic disk.

Prognosis. — The prognosis of the disease is decidedly unfavorable. Death occurs in the vast majority of cases within two years; the length of life, however, varies in the different forms. A few cases survive five or six years. One case of eighteen years' duration has been reported. There are, however, some cases of so-called *arrested paresis.* Undoubtedly not a few of these cases were never paresis at all, but rather belonged to the group of organic psychoses characterized by extensive degenerative changes in the cortex, especially syphilitic, which during life are differentiated only with great difficulty. Again, there is a possibility that some of these cases represent a group of cases still undifferentiated, which at the onset present the characteristic mental and physical symptoms of paresis, but later subside into a condition of dementia with possibly a few delusions and the residuals of the former physical signs. It cannot be positively stated that some of these are not paretic cases which fail to run the usual fatal course. It is still a mooted question whether patients may

not even recover from paresis. In the first place, Tuczek reports a genuine case of paresis, confirmed by autopsy, with a remission of twenty years. Again, Alzheimer has found in paretics, dying during a complete remission, the characteristic paretic lesions. When one considers that these remissions often cannot be distinguished from genuine recoveries, except for the later recurrence of the disease, it at once becomes apparent that a complete subsidence of all mental symptoms may occur, which, extending through a series of years, encourages the belief that recoveries are possible. The immediate causes of death are paralytic attacks, pneumonia, and intercurrent diseases, sometimes septicaemia following infection from wounds, sometimes suffocation caused by food entering the air passages; but the usual manner of death is from marasmus and heart failure. The patients become emaciated, the muscles atrophy, the heart weakens, the pulse becomes imperceptible, and life gradually flickers out.

Treatment. — The treatment of the disease is mostly *symptomat1c.* In cases where there is a history of probable syphilitic infection the intensified mercurial treatment is justified by the small number of reported cures. It consists in the intramuscular injection of mercuric salicylate in albolene, beginning with J grain twice weekly and increasing to 1J grains, administered for six weeks, and then an interval of six months during which general tonics are pushed. Following this, another period of similar mercurial treatment. Some prefer the injection of bichloride of mercury, to J grain daily, given for six to eight weeks, repeated after an interval of six months. All other specific methods of treatment have fallen into disuse.

Collins, Med. Record, Vol. 9, p. 125. Dana, Jour. Amer. Med. Ass'n, May 6, 1905.

It is of utmost importance that the patient be submitted to forced rest, with removal from business and uncomfortable surroundings, and the establishment of a suitable daily routine in the physical and mental life. Quiet and tractable patients in good circumstances may be treated at home, but others usually require sanitarium or hospital treatment. Suitable rest and relaxation cannot be procured at the fashionable health resorts with the numerous " cures" and attractions.

Next to rest, there should be outlined a simple nutritious diet, including abstinence as regards alcohol, coffee, tea, and tobacco. A carefully planned daily routine, including exercise in the open air, and carefully executed hydrotherapy with gentle massage, is of importance.

The conditions of paretic excitement are best relieved by the bed treatment and the use of the prolonged warm baths (see p. 140). At the first application of the bath, it may be necessary to give preliminary doses of hyoscine. If the excitement is extreme, forced feeding or hypodermoclysis with normal saline solution (see p. 139) given twice daily should be employed. The conditions of extreme anxious restlessness and agitation should also be treated with the prolonged warm bath and if necessary the use of the hypodermoclysis, but not infrequently these patients fail to yield to any form of treatment, when all that remains to be done is to watch the patient carefully to prevent injuries and to maintain nutrition.

Where the warm bath is inaccessible, the cold packs may be substituted, which in the hands of several American physicians seem to give excellent results. The packs to be effective must be properly applied. The partial pack usually suffices to bring about the desired result, applying it to the lower extrm ities, or to the arms. In the whole pack a large and heavy woollen blanket is spread upon the mattress, and over it is laid a coarse linen sheet, well wrung out in water of a temperature from sixty to seventy degrees, so placed that the patient can lie at the junction of the middle, and right third of the sheet. When the patient is in position, with the arms elevated, and provided with a wet turban, the right portion of the sheet is drawn across the body and tucked. The arms are lowered to the side and cov-

ered with the left portion of the sheet, which is drawn across the body and securely tucked, especially about the neck and feet. The patient is then covered with several woollen blankets. The duration of the pack should be from one-half to one hour, and may be followed by brisk rubbing with alcohol. The duration of the partial pack may be more extended than that of the whole pack. When the patient falls asleep in it, it is not necessary that it be removed until he awakes. There is no harm in an immediate renewal of the partial pack. It should be remembered in the application of these partial packs, as well as in the whole packs, that all air must be excluded from in under the cover of woollen blankets, for which purpose many use a final covering of rubber cloth or oil silk.

In the last stages of the disease, extreme cleanliness is most essential in order to prevent bedsores. The bedclothing must be kept dry, clean, smooth, and free from crumbs, and the body frequently cleansed with cold water. Alcohol or hardening applications are better withheld, and instead the skin should be carefully rubbed with cocoa butter. Frequent changes of the position of the body every hour, day and night, aid greatly in preventing the occurrence of acute decubitus and hypostatic pneumonia. Acute decubitus, once formed, is very obstinate and should be treated surgically like an ulcer. Where there is a marked tendency to the formation of acute decubitus and also where it does not heal readily, the best method is to keep the patient continually in the prolonged warm bath. The *nourishment* during this stage must be liquid, in order to prevent choking. Daily percussion of the lower abdomen to detect distention of the bladder and observation of the condition of the bowels is also necessary. In case there is paralysis of the bladder, the patient should be regularly catheterized, followed by a washing of the bladder with a saturated solution of boracic acid. Finally, the mouth should be kept thoroughly clean. The paralytic attacks may yield to ice packs on the head or to amylene hydrate (thirty to

sixty minims) or chloral hydrate, the former of which may be given by subcutaneous injections in a five to ten per cent. solution. If immediate action is demanded, chloroform may be employed.

VII. ORGANIC DEMENTIAS

The term is here used in a limited sense, applying only to those psychoses that are associated with organic disease of the central nervous system, and includes cerebral gliosis, Huntingdon's chorea, multiple sclerosis, cerebral syphilis, tabetic psychoses, arteriosclerotic insanity, brain tumor, cerebral trauma, and cerebral apoplexy.

Gliosis of Cortex. — This disease, described by Fuerstner, presents numerous tumorlike accumulations of glia in the superficial layers of the cortex with the formation of small cavities and atrophy of the nervous tissue.

The course of the disease is chronic, the mental symptoms may be of sudden onset with convulsions and irritability, but later there develops a progressive deterioration with failing memory, accompanied by disorder of speech, optic atrophy, and often tabetic symptoms. *Diffuse cerebral sclerosis,* in which there is an extensive increase of the supportive tissue, is accompanied by progressive dementia.

Huntingdon's Chorea. — The mental symptons of Huntingdon's chorea are distinctive, consisting usually of a progressive dementia with faulty memory, weak judgment, paralysis of thought, apathy, and irritability. Patients are unstable in employment. Suicidal attempts are not infrequent, and occasional homicidal tendencies are encountered. Hallucinations and delusions are infrequent, but if present are unaccompanied by emotion. Anxious states, outbreaks of anger, restlessness, sometimes develop. The choreic movements are intensified by any mental excitement.

Fackkm, Archiv f. Psy., XXX, S. 138.
Zinn, Archiv f. Psy., XXVIII, S. 411.
Diller, Am. Jour. Med. Sciences, Dec., 1889, April, 1890.
Hallock, Jour. Nerv. & Ment. Dis., 1898.
Sinkler, Med. Rec., XLI, p. 281.

Physically the choreic movements of

Huntingdon's chorea differ from those of acute chorea in that they are less extensive and less frequent. They involve the entire trunk, limb, head and face, and are jerky, at times quick, but often sluggish. The speech becomes hesitating, indistinct, and indecisive, while the writing is rapid and hasty. The voluntary movements are rendered uncertain, yet it is surprising to observe how advanced cases maintain their equilibrium in walking. The arms, head, and trunk may be drawn into various awkward positions, the patient still keeping on his feet. The accompanying photographic group (Plate 9), of three cases of Huntingdon's chorea, shows the rapidly changing attitudes of these patients who were trying to look at the photographer. As the disease advances, general muscular strength wanes, until in the end stages the patients become bedridden. The deep tendon reflexes are usually exaggerated, and the muscle irritability increased. Sensation does not suffer. Epileptiform and apoplectic attacks rarely occur.

The *course* of Huntingdon's chorea is slowly progressive, leading in the greater number of cases to considerable dementia in the course of ten to thirty years. The mental symptoms usually appear coincidently with the first of the choreiform movements, but they may not appear for years; indeed, the writer knows of one case of Huntingdon's chorea of fifteen years'standing in which the individual still conducts successfully a large and lucrative law practice. While the underlying mental process is one of progressive dementia, as described above, the onset of the mental symptoms may be sudden and of a manic character; occasionally the symptoms simulate the megalomanic phase of paresis; again the clinical picture may be distinctly depressive in character, accompanied by active hallucinosis and delusion formation. These various clinical states, however, are usually only episodic, while deterioration progresses. Marked dementia may have already become evident before these various episodes appear. Furthermore, there is no relationship between

the degree of choreic movements and the mental symptoms: either group may be much more or much less advanced than the other. Sometimes the choreic movements improve considerably during the course of the disease.

Diagnosis. — Where the mental symptoms antedate or predominate in the clinical picture, there may be some difficulty in differentiating paresis. In such cases one must depend upon the absence of pupillary disturbances or muscular paresis, the presence of only a hesitancy in speech with hastiness and tremor in writing, without defect in the content of speech and writing. In the mental field the emotional irritability is more disturbed, and there is proportionately less defect of memory and orientation. The history of Huntingdon's chorea in the antecedents should leave little doubt as to the true character of the disease.

The *pathological anatomy* of Huntingdon's chorea presents chronic leptomeningitis, with thickening of the pia and small cell infiltration, general cerebral atrophy with shrinking of the cortex, white matter, and basal ganglia. The vessels exhibit extensive thickening of the adventitia with increase in the perivascular spaces, and in places residuals of old hemorrhages. In four of the writer's cases, cell shrinkage was observed, and in one case also grave alteration. Trabantan cells were present in most sections, while glia nuclei were uniformly increased in the deeper layers of the cortex. In all, vascular alteration was present, with round cell infiltration, as well as the presence of free pigment about the vessels. In one case there was a slight degree of ependymitis, and in another, numerous areas of thrombotic softening were found scattered over the cortex.

Multiple Sclerosis. — When the disease process in *multiple sclerosis* involves the brain, there develops more or less mental deterioration. In 215 cases reported by Berger in 1904, dementia occurred in only 24 cases (more than 10 per cent). The type of mental disturbance is usually that of simple deterioration with failure of memory and judg-

ment, together with apathy, as seen in an unnatural complacency and anergy. Besides the emotional apathy, there is sometimes present a tendency to uncontrollable laughter, and other emotional outbursts of an episodic character. The mental symptoms, however, are rarely of such pronounced character as to bring the patient to insane hospitals. An atypical case of multiple sclerosis may be confounded with dementia paralytica, particularly if nystagmus, scanning speech, and intention tremor are tardy in appearance or absent. The burden of proof against dementia paralytica then rests upon the absence of pupillary disturbance, and of the characteristic paretic speech; while in the mental field there is absence of faulty time orientation and prominent defect of memory.

Cerebral Syphilis. — In *cerebral syphilis* there are two groups of cases: *simple syphilitic dementia*, and *syphilitic pseudoparesis*. Under this term are not included the mental disturbances occurring during the early manifestations, such as the occasional deliria similar in nature to infectious deliria, or the hysterical and neurasthenic syndromes, in all of which syphilis seems to play the role only of an exciting factor. The distinctively characteristic syphilitic psychoses develop only during the late period, when there is involvement of the cerebral vessels and the development of gummata, vascular occlusion, and malacia. The vessel alteration is typically syphilitic and gives rise to a profound nutritional disturbance in the cortex. It is to be differentiated from that occurring in paresis by the pathological fact that there is only very slight infiltration into the adventitia of the vessels, and mast cells are rare; but there is a marked proliferation of the intimal cells, with a tendency to form vascular foramina within the vessel itself. The new vessel formation is extensive and typical. The elastic fibres of the vessels tend to split into layers, while the vascular cells do not show pigmentation.

In *simple syphilitic dementia* there usually appears first, defective memory and judgment, and some absent-mindedness, as well as lack of insight into these defects. Coincident with the onset there usually occurs some sort of an apoplectiform seizure, which may be either of a mild or a severe grade. Emotionally there is a slight degree of elation. The patients are fond of boasting of their strength and ability, and plan extensively for the future. If there happens to be present some feeling of illness, they are confident of recovery. But more prominent still is the greatly increased emotional irritability, which often leads to strife and outbursts of passion. Delusions of influence and reference are sometimes present, also ideas of oppression and mistreatment, to which are ascribed sordid motives; but such delusional ideas are transient and rarely elaborated. Volitionally there is evident weakness of will, as shown in their tractability and fickleness. They tend to be thoughtless, disorderly in their work, neglect important for unimportant matters, and do all sorts of extravagant things. Finally, there is a striking susceptibility to alcohol.

The *course* of the disease is usually slow, although it may soon reach a stage of quiescence, with subsidence of the prominent symptoms. Recovery is rare, in spite of antisyphilitic treatment, because the cortex has become extensively involved. There are occasional exacerbations. Physically, the onset is usually with an apoplectiform attack; and as the result of this there may be residual hemiplegia or monoplegia, sometimes paresis of the eye muscles, some slight fault of articulation, and also complete or reflex iridoplegia.

This group of cases should also include that form of progressive deterioration appearing in youth which arises from congenital syphilis and is accompanied by forms of paralysis. The pathological distinction between these cases and juvenile paresis is that in the former there exists only the vascular lesions characteristic of syphilis. However, Meyer and Kaplan have described some cases in which there was a mixture of paretic and syphilitic lesions.

To this group also should be added the cases described by Barrett, Bechterew, and Jurgens, in which the lesion is one of disseminated syphilitic encephalitis.

In Barrett's case the deterioration was very rapid, leading to complete dementia and death within two months, while in the case of Bechterew the course of the disease extended through two years.

Amer. Jour, of Med. Sc, Vol. 129, p. 390.

'Handbuch der path. Anat. des Nervensystems. Flatan-JacobsohnMinor. Ref. Oppenheim, Syphilitische Erkrank des Gebirns. *Syphilitic pseudoparesis* includes those cases of cerebral syphilis which present pronounced mental symptoms, in addition to the evidences of focal brain lesions. The gradations between simple syphilitic dementia and pseudoparesis are so imperceptible in many cases that some authors do not attempt a differentiation, but describe both groups under cerebral syphilis. The onset of pseudoparesis, as in simple syphilitic dementia, may be with paralytic attacks. The attacks may be only syncopal, or aphasiform and of short duration, or there may be loss of consciousness with more or less severe paralysis. Such attacks may antedate many months the mental symptoms, or they may be tardy in appearing and sometimes they never develop. Of the mental symptoms, despondency is the first to appear, in which either hypochondriasis or apprehensiveness predominate. The patients feel stupid, the food does not agree with them, they are self-accusatory, fearful, and speak of infidelity. There is a change of character, and they become indifferent, forgetful, confused in thought; at other times they are irritable, excitable, and aggressive. Even delirious excitement may develop. Hallucinations are usually present and often very prominent, mostly of hearing, though sometimes of sight and smell. The megalomanic delusions so characteristic of paresis predominate and with this there is emotional elation and a tendency to facetiousness, although some patients are irritable, suspicious, and hostile. Many patients are productive both in speech and writing, exhibiting incoherence and even neologisms; others are inactive, sleepy, and reticent, and again others vary from 'one state to another. *Physically,* besides the residuals of syphilitic infection, and of the earlier apoplectiform attacks, such as hemiparesis, hemianopsia, and paraphasia, etc., there may be present optic atrophy, an increase, absence or weakening, and particularly inequality of the tendon reflexes, and complete or almost complete loss of the light reaction of one or both pupils. Speech and writing, however, show insignificant changes.

The *course* of the disease is slow, leading regularly to a considerable degree of dementia. Some patients continue orderly and are able to live at home; they possess the ability to read and amuse themselves, and follow up a simple daily routine, but are wholly incapable of profitable employment, lack insight into their condition, and are thoughtless of the future. They continue oriented, but memory for events of the psychosis and sometimes even for earlier life is faulty. The hallucinations and delusions tend to reappear; these are never modified but only forgotten.

In the severer cases the dementia is more profound; the patients are continuously confused, maintaining their various expansive and persecutory delusions, exhibiting restlessness, excitement, and aggressiveness, or they may be childishly good-natured and thoroughly tractable. Transitory conditions of profound stupidity and confusion arise. Paralytic attacks, either epileptiform or syncopal, with or without residuals, reappear with more or less regularity throughout the course and may terminate the disease. The course of the symptoms may not be as progressive, but after reaching a certain stage remain unchanged a long time, until an exacerbation or some intercurrent disease causes death.

The *pathology* of pseudoparesis exhibits the following syphilitic lesions: meningitis, foci of malacia, gummata, and particularly the syphilitic vascular lesions. Throughout the entire cortex there is a hyperplasia of glia cells, so much so that in places the *"gliarasen"* of Nissl is found, indicating a profound degeneration of nerve cells. The nerve fibres, however, are not much involved, and there is also very little development of glia fibres, and hence practically no reduction of the cortex. Regressive changes may be seen in many neuroglia cells. In the deeper layers of the cortex there is a large increase of small round glia nuclei. The large vessels are deeply stained (Nissl's stain) and the perivascular spaces are enlarged, although there is no infiltration of the adventitia similar to what one finds in dementia paralytica. The small vessels are greatly increased in number, dilated, and present many anastamoses, appearing everywhere to be overlaid with glia cells. According to Nissl, this proliferation does not take place by budding as in paresis, but by the formation of new vessel openings through the thickened endothelium among the numerous layers of the elastic coat. The muscular coat disappears. Finally, rod cells are very rarely found. These lesions extend throughout the cortex, but to a varying degree, in places being almost imperceptible. They are always more marked in the superficial layers of the cortex. Occasionally small old or fresh hemorrhagic foci are found.

The similarity of pseudoparesis to general paresis is so striking that the *differential diagnosis* is very difficult and depends mostly upon the presence and persistence of the residuals of the paralytic attacks. These often exist from the onset, which is not true in paresis. The characteristic paretic faults of speech and writing, with the aphasia and stumbling over syllables, the transposition and the repetition of syllables and letters, are absent, as well as the disturbances of the sensibility to pain. Memory is better than in paresis, and except in the very bad cases, orientation is preserved, *i.e.* names of persons are recalled and the patients remember striking incidents in their environment, and also take some pride in neatness and order. At the onset, when differentiation is most difficult, one observes that in paresis the memory defect is out of pro-

portion to the disorder in the rest of the mental life, and hallucinations are less prominent than in pseudoparesis. The *treatment* of pseudoparesis presents but little hope, although the few favorable cases following antisyphilitic treatment warrant a trial in all (see p. 319).

Tabetic Psychoses. — In most cases where mental symptoms develop during the course of tabes, the disease terminates as paresis, but there are a few cases which never become paretic. Very mild mental symptoms often appear during the early stages of tabes, *i.e.* some fault of memory, and an increased sense of fatigue, but more especially a change in disposition. Many patients become gloomy and hopeless, and have forebodings and fears, but others are cheerful, happy, and confident, sometimes reminding one of the feeling of well-being of the paretic.

The characteristic *tabetic psychosis,* however, is an acute hallucinosis with some excitement resembling the acute alcoholic hallucinosis. The onset of the hallucinosis is sudden, with hallucinations of hearing, accompanied by some anxiety and restlessness. Later hallucinations of the other senses appear. The hallucinations are of a threatening, disturbing type: such as the voices of relatives calling for help, threats against their lives, the odor of sulphur, or the sensation of electricity, to all of which the patients react. Orientation remains clear. The duration of the attack may be for a few weeks or several months, when the symptoms often disappear suddenly. There may be remissions.

The psychosis may resemble a short hallucinatory delirium, or it may simulate a chronic psychosis with hallucinations and paranoid delusions, both of persecution and grandeur. Again all of these different forms may represent different clinical stages of the same disease process, similar to the acute and chronic disease pictures which one sees in paresis, alcoholism, and dementia praecox. In some of the chronic cases there is a similarity to syphilitic pseudoparesis. Besides these forms of tabetic psychoses there may develop in tabes the manic-depressive syndrome, the cata-

tonic or the senile psychoses. The tabetic psychoses are differentiated from the forms of paresis by the fact that the disease process is not progressive. The grade of deterioration remains at a standstill, and furthermore, attention and memory is not disturbed to the degree that it is in paresis.

Arteriosclerotic Insanity.—Arteriosclerotic changes in the brain are very common in the senile period of life, yet it is doubtful if one is justified in considering them only as evidence of early senility, particularly in view of the fact that extensive arteriosclerosis may exist without accompanying mental impairment. One must conclude either that the vascular disease in arteriosclerotic insanity is not, in spite its great similarity, identical with that occurring in normal senility, or that in the former case the vascular change is an accompaniment of only secondary importance in a disease process which is highly destructive of nerve tissue. The varying extent of the vessel change, especially whether it involves the smaller or greater vessels, may account for the absence or presence of mental manifestations.

'Alzheimer, Allgem. Zeitschr. f. Psy. , LI, 809; *idem, LIU,* 863; *idem,* LIX, 695.

Binswanger, Berl. Klin. Wochenschr, 1894, 49.

Alzheimer, Histologische und Histopathologische Arbeiten liber die GroBshirurinde-Nissl, Jena, 1904.

This psychosis appears about the sixtieth year; yet some cases develop before fifty, but in the latter instance there is usually present a strong hereditary tendency to vascular disease. Alcoholism and syphilis may be regarded as etiological factors. When the disease occurs later in life, the arteriosclerosis may be associated with the characteristic senile changes of the nervous tissue which are dependent upon the vascular changes. Alzheimer speaks of these cases as "Senile Decay." This form of disease attacks especially the cortical vessels that pass in from the pia, leading to the formation of deep wedge-shaped foci with destruction of the nerve tissue and an increase of glia.

Pathological Anatomy.—There is regularly found, besides the evidences of general arteriosclerosis, cardiac involvement, either cardiac hypertrophy or dilation, and interstitial nephritis. The cerebral vessels are thickened and rigid, the dura and pia thickened, the latter being cloudy, and the entire brain is more or less atrophied. Several areas of hemorrhagic softening, either fresh or old, are usually found in the cortex, and the ventricles are much dilated. Microscopically, the numerous disease foci are found, especially along the path of the altered vessels. In these areas the nervous tissue has disappeared, being replaced by a luxuriant growth of neuroglia, which shows little or no tendency to regressive changes; The blood vessels, in addition to the usual arteriosclerotic changes, namely, a splitting and swelling of the elastica, thickening of the walls, and regressive changes in the muscularis and adventitia, also show a tendency to hyaline infiltration. In the lymph spaces there is increase of connective tissue, pigmentation, and granular cells. Comparing the normal with the arteriosclerotic cortex, as seen inFigures 1 and 2, Plate 10,

Plate 10 Fig. 1 — Arteriosclerotic cortex. Fig. 2 —Normal cortex.
it is apparent how extensive the degeneration of cells has been. The few remaining nerve cells present a high-grade alteration in the intercellular tissue. Deeply stained glia nuclei are scattered everywhere, mostly surrounded by a clear space, and gathered in groups, particularly about vessels. The vessels themselves, both large and small, present few nuclei, are hyaline and greatly thickened. Some vessels appear to have a double lumen, which is very frequently found in the arteriosclerotic cortex. The disease process is not evenly distributed throughout the entire cortex, as there are foci where only moderate changes are noted. Further, one cannot judge of the extent of the vascular change in the cortical vessels by the appearance of the larger vessels in the pia, as the latter may be much altered, while the former show little change. The nerve fibres, both in the cortex and in the white matter, show changes proportionate to the vascular disease. There usually are numerous cavities in the white matter, particularly along the line of the vessels. This condition, called *6tat cr1ble,* presents a very characteristic picture. Where this state is very pronounced and where the subcortical region is more involved than the cortex, it has been called, by Binswanger, chronic subcortical encephalitis. Clinically these cases are characterized by very many limited focal symptoms and a very pronounced dementia. The pyramidal tracts may show atrophy in the pons and medulla. Symptomatology. — The first symptoms of arteriosclerotic insanity consist of a diminution of energy, and forgetfulness. The patients tire easily, lack the characteristic freshness and energy for work. They not only hesitate to undertake anything new, but lack ability to do original work. Emotionally, they are easily depressed, disheartened, at times whining; again, they may be irritable, and subject to emotional outbursts. Emotional instability is apt to be present, as seen in rapid changes from one emotional state to another and in frequent weeping and laughing. Patients are forgetful and flighty, and mix up their work. There is always present a very definite feeling of illness that may even border on hypochondriasis. This may lead to suicidal attempts. Under the influence of alcohol or some emotional stress a moderate degree of dazedness may develop. Later in the course of the disease delusions of reference and particularly of infidelity are prone to appear.

The prominent physical symptoms are more or less pronounced attacks of dizziness, syncope, or even convulsive attacks, which may be accompanied by paraphasic disturbances, disturbances of sensation, paresis, and even paralysis. Residuals of these attacks usually persist. Pupillary reaction is retained, or at most is only slightly sluggish. The usual vascular and cardiac symptoms of arteriosclerosis are present, and there is albumen in the urine.

These symptoms may remain at a standstill for years, particularly if the patient's method of living is carefully regulated, but sooner or later apoplexy appears with its residuals. With each recurring attack there is further dementia, in which attention and memory suffer. Later there develops complete disorientation, and indifference, but at times there is childish irritability and at others happiness. Finally deterioration becomes so pronounced that they have to be cared for and fed like little children. Not all cases develop this degree of deterioration; indeed, there may be all grades of dementia. Aphasia, agraphia, apraxia, and asymbolism, also word and mind blindness, are frequent complications of these vascular lesions, which tend to make the mental deterioration appear even greater than it really is. There are old apoplectics of ten years' or more duration who present only an increased sense of mental fatigue, ill-humor, and some weakness of will, rendering them particularly susceptible to outside influences. In such cases the vascular lesions are supposed to be more circumscribed or to have come to a standstill.

There is a group of cases of arteriosclerotic insanity that deserve special attention; namely, those comprising the *severe progressive form.* These cases are characterized by a very rapid course leading to profound dementia and death. The disease usually begins with an apoplectiform attack, although there may have been prodromal headaches, some forgetfulness, and lack of energy. Following this there develops a condition of marked anxiety and apprehensiveness, sometimes with pronounced delusions of a persecutory nature, occasionally hallucinations and delusions of self-accusation. The patients are usually clouded and confused, so much so that they do not even understand what goes on about them or what is said to them. They are irritable, restless, aggressive, wandering about, attempt escape, trying to jump from the window, or commit suicide. Nocturnal restlessness is particularly marked. Nutrition and sleep suffer profoundly. There regularly develop for longer or shorter periods conditions of even greater bewilderment and more active restlessness. The patients become even more clouded, so that they perceive practically nothing and their attention cannot be fixed. Obstacles placed before them are not perceived or are handled in a wholly automatic manner. They will not avoid a test needle, although they wince from pain. Emotionally, they manifest lack of feeling, although occasionally there may be some anxiety or again some elation. Insight is absent. The patients present an almost incessant, motiveless activity, and they have no care of themselves. The speech is usually wholly incoherent, sort of babbling, and often unintelligible. Such mental states usually end in death. Yet the excitement may disappear, leaving the patient in a condition of dementia which then becomes gradually progressive. The patients are wholly listless, disoriented, and comprehend only the simplest questions. They have neither the energy to busy themselves nor the interest to mingle much in their environment. There is *great emotional weakness* and the patients laugh and cry very easily; even spasmodic laughing and crying may exist. In spite of their great deterioration, they may be able to solve simple mathematical problems, and not only recognize the members of their family, but derive some enjoyment from their visits. Physically, in addition to the residuals of the apoplectic attacks, in which paraphasic disturbances are apt to be prominent, there is also a peculiar impediment of speech which may sometimes lead to genuine scanning. The writing also presents marked changes. Individual letters are barely legible, even though ataxia is not evident. The patients lose their ability to write the single strokes into a complete word. In the words that can be read omissions are found. These faults of writing are present from the beginning and may be regarded as a sign of rapid fatigue. The pupillary reaction is always maintained, although sometimes it is sluggish. The entire duration of the disease is about four years, though there are cases of six to seven years' duration; and again, some cases run a course of only a few months. The prognosis in

any case is always influenced by the general physical condition, especially the condition of the heart, lungs, and kidneys, as well as the age of the patient.

The *diagnosis* of arteriosclerotic insanity may be difficult, particularly the differentiation from *paresis* occurring in late life. In the first place, it must be remembered that paresis is a diffuse lesion of the cortex, while in arteriosclerotic insanity there are many scattered foci. Therefore, we find in paresis that the general psychic alteration is more prominent than the physical signs. Paretics are usually clouded and exhibit loss of judgment before the physical symptoms appear, while in arteriosclerotic insanity the apoplectiform attacks are very often the startingpoint of the psychical disturbances. In arteriosclerotic insanity disturbances of perception are more striking than disturbances of memory, while in paresis both are equally impaired. Emotionally, the paretic shows greater elation or depression; while the arteriosclerotic patient is usually indifferent and apathetic, or he presents either hypochondriacal despondency or indefinite fear. The great elation of some paretics and the profusion of delusions is wholly lacking in the arteriosclerotic condition. Fabrication, although a prominent symptom in paresis, is seldom indulged in by the arteriosclerotic patient, and then it is of an altogether different character, being meagre and without the florid embellishments of the paretic fabrication. These patients also present in a marked degree lack of mental power; yet at times they suddenly surprise one with their knowledge, although at other times they appear much demented. There does not appear to be such a complete loss of mental power as in paresis, but an inability to control it, and corresponding to this there is a greatly increased sense of fatigue which is not present in paresis. Finally, in spite of the apparent great dementia, many of the arteriosclerotic patients remain oriented to the end, recognize their relatives and enjoy their visits, having good insight into their physical and mental helplessness. Fur-

ther, physically there is a marked contrast between the paretic and arteriosclerotic symptoms. In the arteriosclerotic state the physical symptoms are prominent; such as persistent, well-defined paralyses with spasms, contractures, aphasia, asymbolism, word blindness, mind blindness, hemianopsia, and astereognosis. The speech disturbance is more of the type that arises from paralysis, while in writing, simple omissions are more prominent than the ataxia and the transposition of syllables seen in paresis. Very often perseveration is present. The pupils remain normal. The presence of arteriosclerotic changes elsewhere in the body point to a similar condition in the brain, but the former is no sure criterion of the extent of the brain involvement. In the earliest stages of the disease, when the diagnosis may be most difficult, the predominance of the general physical symptoms over the mental symptoms, the latter of which are more apparent to the patient himself than to the friends, always favors a diagnosis of arteriosclerotic insanity.

Simple syphilitic dementia may be differentiated from arteriosclerotic insanity only with difficulty, particularly in the early stages. In the syphilitic psychosis, we perceive a slower development of the symptoms, and the disturbances of memory and perception are less pronounced, while the focal symptoms are more uniform, less manifold and variable than in the arteriosclerotic condition; again, the tendency to oculomotor disturbance, of optic disorder, and paralysis of the pupils is of importance as well as the knowledge of syphilitic disease elsewhere in the body. In differentiating pseudoparesis we find that the course is not as progressive as in arteriosclerotic insanity, while the hallucinations and delusions are not nearly as prominent and are often absent in arteriosclerotic insanity. The degree of deterioration does not become as great; memory is better, orientation is retained, and the patients continue conscious.

The *treatment* of arteriosclerotic insanity demands, first of all, rest, freedom from occupation, avoidance of excitement and all articles of diet that interfere with the vascular system; namely, alcohol, coffee, tea, and much tobacco. Forms of excessive exercise should also be avoided, as swimming, rowing, bicycle riding, etc. It is doubtful if the administration of potassium iodide or the employment of foods containing calcium have any beneficial effect. In the later stages of the disease the patients are apt to become bedridden, and require very careful nursing.

Cerebral Tumor. — In cerebral tumor all cases do not develop mental symptoms. Of 318 cases Gianelli discovered but 299 that developed a psychosis. If the cortex is not much involved or if the tumor is of slow growth, mental symptoms may not appear. On the other hand, they may develop where there is a small circumscribed growth, but in such cases there is always the possibility of chemical or other destructive agencies extending over a broader area. If the growth is of considerable size, mental symptoms are sure to appear. According to Schusters, tumors of the hypophysis in about two-thirds of the cases develop a psychosis, of the cerebellum in one-third of the cases, and of the stem in one-fourth of the cases.

In these cases the influence upon the cortex may arise from increase of the general pressure and interference with the blood supply, both venous and arterial. In tumors of the corpus callosum the destruction of the association fibres beween the two hemispheres has some effect upon the mentality. In general, then, the effect of tumors outside the cortex upon the mental processes depends upon their size. This theory re ceives some support from the fact that extensive tumors, involving even the cortex, may run their course without mental symptoms, if the tissue is gradually destroyed, and not put under pressure; while, on the other hand, even small tumors of the brain are often observed to produce pronounced mental symptoms because they exert either local or general pressure. Schuster observes in his experience that those tumors lying nearest the cortex produce far more mental symptoms than those lying at a distance. The latter cause only a simple progressive disappearance of the mental activity, indicating a cortical paralysis, while the former indicate signs of irritation.

The mental symptoms of brain tumor are naturally quite varied. Schuster in about fifty-six per cent of 775 cases of brain tumor accompanied by mental symptoms finds that these symptoms consist of a gradually progressive mental weakness. The patients become sleepy, inattentive, forgetful, unproductive in thought, indifferent, fatigue easily, and are without either their characteristic energy or facility for prolonged work. Mental application calls for an unusual effort. They exhibit a degree of drowsiness and stupidity which may even extend to coma. In addition to this, there develop the various symptoms indicative of tissue irritation and destruction, the character of which depends somewhat upon the situation and growth of the tumor, such as apoplectiform attacks, convulsions, aphasia, hemianopsia, etc. Where these symptoms are slight or altogether absent, the picture may appear very much like a case of paresis of the demented form. In such cases the differentiation depends upon the absence of reflex pupillary disturbance and the absence of speech disorder.

Other symptoms emphasized by Schuster are greatly increased irritability with transitory periods of excitement, less often periods of despondency with delusions of persecution and self-accusation. Tumors of the dorsal regions of the brain are apt to be accompanied by delirious states with pronounced hallucinosis, although mental symptoms accompanying tumors of this region are less frequent than in tumors of the frontal lobes.

Occasionally in brain tumors there exists a condition of elation, even with distractibility of attention, productiveness, flight of ideas, and some increased activity; but more frequently there exists a condition of childish happiness, with a tendency to joking and punning. This mental state Schuster finds more characteristic of tumors of the frontal lobes. Finally the hysterical syndrome may exist in brain tumor.

The *differential diagnosis* in this state as well as in all of those already mentioned depends almost wholly upon the presence and character of the physical symptoms, indicative of focal lesions. As regards *treatment,* one should resort to anti-syphilitic treatment in cases of suspected syphilitic gumma, and to surgical interference where the location of the tumor is suitable for such procedure. In recent years there is a gowing tendency to operate in all cases of cerebral tumor, if only for the temporary relief of distressing symptoms.

Brain Abscess.—*Brain abscess* may be unaccompanied by mental symptoms, particularly if it be of slow development. In recent traumatic abscesses stupor is a prominent symptom. The patients are completely disoriented, and do not comprehend what is said to them. They are restless, resistive, and sometimes in a dreamy, delirious state. Besides this, there may develop catalepsy, aphasia, epilepsy, slow pulse, Cheyne-Stokes breathing, and other signs of irritation.

Cerebral Apoplexy. — The mental symptoms of cerebral *hemorrhage, embolism,* and *thrombosis* usually depend in small measure only upon the focal disorder. Immediately following the apoplexy the patients are usually unconscious, completely disoriented, and perform all sorts of strange acts. Sometimes there develop transitory states of active excitement, with noisiness and display of resistance. These acute disturbances usually disappear in the course of a few days or weeks, leaving as residuals the symptoms of the original disease process, which almost always is an arteriosclerosis or syphilitic endarteritis. The patients may become wholly clear mentally, or may exhibit the various symptoms of arteriosclerotic or syphilitic insanity, already sufficiently described. In *embolism,* the mental symptoms may suddenly and entirely disappear. However, the persistence of aphasic or paraphasic disturbances may make it appear that the patient exhibits more marked mental weakness than really exists.

Cerebral Trauma. — Mental disturbances accompanying *head injury,* widely designated as traumatic insanity, comprise a considerable group of cases. It has been demonstrated that in cases of severe trauma there exist profound cellular changes in the cortex, and besides this, areas of contusion and punctate hemorrhages at a distance from the point of injury, particularly on the inferior surface of the brain, and at the tips of the frontal lobes, in the temporal and occipital lobes.

Traumatic insanity in the narrow sense comprises *traumatic delirium* and *traumatic dementia* (post traumatic constitution, Meyer). Cerebral trauma should also be regarded as a prominent etiological factor in epilepsy and in the traumatic neuroses. Insolation is regarded as a form of cerebral trauma.

Meyer, Am. Jour, of Ins., LX, 373; Guder, Die Geistesstorungen nach Kopfverletzungen, 1886; Koppen, Archiv f. Psy. , XXXIII, 568. *Traumatic delirium* (primary traumatic insanity) develops following the loss of consciousness incident to the head injury. The patients, instead of becoming clear, present befogged states with complete disorientation, difficulty of thought, and very little or no memory of the accident. Sometimes the amnesia includes a period just preceding the accident, and not infrequently there is amnesia for other isolated periods of the life of the patients. They perceive poorly, and have difficulty in seeing the connection of things. There is often a marked tendency to *fabrication.* Emotionally, they are irritable or indifferent. They are apt to be restless, at times aggressive, often whining and talking considerably, the content of the speech being rambling and incoherent. Delusions and hallucinations are rarely present. There is no clear insight into the disease, and the patients speak of themselves as being perfectly well. This state is sometimes accompanied by transitory aphasic states. The symptoms of traumatic delirium may last for many weeks, some cases persisting for several months, after which the patients usually recover, although sometimes the condi-

tion of traumatic dementia supervenes. In *traumatic dementia* there develops sooner or later after the immediate effects of the injury, and in some cases even where there never has been a loss of consciousness, a change of disposition. This alteration may even be so indefinite that all the friends can say is that he is a changed man. This change usually consists of an increased susceptibility to fatigue; *i.e.* unusual fatigue upon slight exertion; some forgetfulness, confusion of thought, inattention, unwonted timidity, occasional slight despondency, with a tendency to complain of many disagreeable sensations, as dizziness, ringing in the ears, head pressure, and a certain sense of heaviness and stupidity. Accompanying these complaints there is usually a keen sense of illness. The patient is irritable, irascible, and at times even exhibits some passion. Isolated convulsions sometimes develop, or even attacks of *petite mal,* or temporary dazed spells. Not only a tendency to alcoholism, but also a striking intolerance to the influence of alcohol and other drugs, often appears, as well as great intolerance to the sun's rays. The capacity for employment is impaired, in explanation of which the patient refers to various subjective sensations. Even games and conversations are avoided for the same reason.

The *course* of the disease is not distinctly progressive, but is sometimes characterized by distinct exacerbations. Many of these exacerbations can be traced to alcoholic indulgence or trivial emotional causes. Deterioration is most pronounced where the trauma is associated with alcoholism or arteriosclerosis, or where the injury has occurred during youth. Usually there are some nervous manifestations indicative of focal lesions of the brain, such as changing pupillary disorders, tremors, paresis of facial muscles, and exaggeration of the tendon reflexes. There are a few cases of traumatic dementia which for a time may appear like paresis, but are differentiated from this disease by the changing character of the pupillary disturbance and the characteristic speech disorder, and the relatively slow

progress of the disease. Undoubtedly some cases of paresis do develop from brain trauma as a starting-point. This, however, is a mooted point, yet there are many observations, including those of Meyer and Koppen, which indicate its validity. Some of the doubtful cases of traumatic dementia, simulating paresis, have presented on post-mortem examination an extensive arteriosclerosis of the brain.

The *treatment* of traumatic insanity rests in early cases with operative procedure, particularly where there is an indication of focal disorder. In traumatic dementia, surgical interference, even though there may be indications of focal irritation, is far less successful.

VIII. INVOLUTION PSYCHOSES

The forms of mental disease, described as involution psychoses seem to bear some relationship to the general physical changes accompanying involution. Undoubtedly, the forms of mental disease included here can occur in other periods of life, also there are many other psychoses unrelated to involution that may occur during the involution period; as for instance, the alcoholic and infection psychoses, manicdepressive insanity, etc. The mental disturbances of the early involutional period are of a somewhat different stamp than those characteristic of senility, though there are many symptoms common to both. Those occurring in the former period are called *melancholia* and *presenile delusional insanity,* and in the latter, *senile dementia. A.* MELANCHOLIA

Melancholia is restricted to certain conditions of mental depression occurring during the period of involution. It includes all of the morbidly anxious states not represented in other forms of insanity, and is characterized by *uniform despondency with fear, various delusions of self-accusation, of persecution, and of a hypochondriacal nature, with moderate clouding of consciousness, leading in the greater number of cases, after a prolonged course, to moderate mental deterioration.* v. Krafft-Ebing, Die Melancholic; Christian, Etude sur la Melancolie, 1876; Voisin, De la Mflancolie, 1881; Dumas, Les

Etats Intellectuals dans la Melancolie, 1895; Roubinowitsch et Toulouse, La Melancolie, 1897. Hoch, Rev. Ed. of Reference Handbook of Medicine, p. 117.

Etiology. — The disease is essentially one of the early senile period, as the majority of cases occur between the ages of fifty and sixty. It seldom develops under forty or over sixty. Sixty per cent. of the cases are women, in whom the disease tends to occur somewhat earlier, apparently bearing some relation to the climacterium. Defective heredity occurs in only a little over one-half of the cases, but it is a striking fact that the parents and brothers and sisters of melancholiacs frequently suffer from apoplexy, senile dementia, or alcoholism. External influences, such as mental shock, especially illness and loss of friends, acute and chronic diseases, and surgical operations, seem to play a rather important role as exciting causes of the disease.

Pathological Anatomy. — In many cases there is found extensive arteriosclerosis and its attendant results in the heart and kidneys. Sometimes there is evidence of beginning brain atrophy. Alzheimer found, in the deeper layers of the cortex, in addition to the changes in the nerve cells, an extensive fibril production of the neuroglia.

Symptomatology. — The onset of the disease is gradual, and is often preceded for months and even years by many indefinite prodromal symptoms; such as, persistent headache, vertigo, indefinite pains, general debility, insomnia, loss of appetite, constipation, palpitation of the heart, ringing in the ears, and increasing difficulty with work. The patients at first become sad, dejected, and apprehensive, and find no enjoyment in their work or home environment. They are overshadowed by doubts, fears, and self-accusations, and cannot be consoled. They feel ill, complain of being dull, confused, and forgetful, and find it difficult to do anything. During this period there are occasional days when they are free from fear and sorrow.

Delusions of *self-accusation* become prominent. Sometimes the patients ac-

cuse themselves only in a general way: they are wicked, are not worth anything, have made fools of themselves, have been impure, and are not worthy to live. But usually the self-accusations refer to definite experiences. Patients become retrospective, and refer to many misdeeds in going over the past life which are held as an adequate basis for their sorrow. Remote and often insignificant facts are recalled, such as the stealing of fruit in childhood, disobedience to parents and neglect of friends, which now cause them the greatest sorrow and anxiety. Their whole life has been made up of similar misdeeds. A patient was miserable because she had requested her sick sister to remain out of the kitchen; another, because at the death of her mother she had allowed herself to think of and mention the division of property. Many refer to former sexual indiscretions. Some patients reproach themselves for everything; they cannot do anything right. Everything in the environment is a source of special anxiety to themselves; the lamentations of a fellow-patient are directly the result of their own misdeeds. Others want for food if they eat. These references vary from day to day, or may be maintained with great firmness for a long time. Quite often the self-accusations refer to religious experiences. The patients are not as fervent in prayer as formerly; they no longer possess real religious feeling, or have sinned against the Holy Ghost, are possessed by the devil, etc. Occasionally their self-accusations center about actual misdeeds, which during health long since ceased to cause anxiety.

In addition to these self-accusations the patients sometimes harbor the conviction that they themselves must be killed or that one of their children is to be sacrificed. They, furthermore, are constantly finding "signs" and " meanings" which God has intended for them. There are often associated with these delusions of self-accusations many other depressive delusional ideas, chief among which are the fears of punishment. The patients believe themselves so wicked that God has forsaken them

and they are doomed to hell, they will be turned out of their home, brought to court, thrown into prison, or killed outright. People are waiting outside to carry them off, a death warrant is already signed. There is no need of taking food; they would rather starve and suffer for their misconduct, and even ask to be executed. Not infrequently they exaggerate their misdeeds and confess crimes which they have never committed, in order to secure severer punishment and to relieve their guilty consciences.

In other cases the delusions are of a more *hypochondriacal nature.* Patients insist that they are the most unfortunate individuals in the world; the stomach is gone, the lungs are filled up, the limbs shrunken, and all sensation lost. The brain and nerves are rotting away as the result of former sexual abuse. They fear that they are dying of consumption or cancer, and that they are going out of their minds and must end their days in an asylum. They maintain that the body has been poisoned, destroying all appetite, and now they must starve. They also express considerable fear for themselves and families; they will be deprived of their home, some great calamity will visit them, the children will die, or they themselves will be robbed and killed, will be driven from the church and damned by God. These depressive delusions so thoroughly influence their actions that they become seclusive, eat sparingly or not at all, refuse to spend money, and clothe themselves and their children scantily. They give up everything because they have only a short time to live.

Hallucinations of hearing and sight often accompany this condition, but they are usually indefinite and of short duration. The patients also refer to an inner voice which commands them to commit suicide, or constantly repeats to them that they are wicked and guilty. The *consciousness* is usually clear. The patients are well oriented, with the possible exception of some delusional ideas, in accordance with which they may claim that they are in a prison, or they may mistake strangers for acquaintances and insist that the letters which they receive are not real; but in spite of these ideas, it may be readily seen that apprehension itself is not much disordered. *Thought* is coherent and relevant, but the content is usually monotonous and centered about the depressive ideas, to which they constantly recur, recounting their various misdeeds and fears. Very often they show a tendency to repeat certain phrases, as " Let me go home," "Let me go home;" "I want to see my children," " I want to see my children." There is usually some *insight* into the change which they have undergone and they will complain that their head is not right, but they fail to recognize many symptoms of the disease as such.

There is a *smaller group of cases of melancholia of involution* occurring somewhat later in life, in which the various delusions of self-accusation, of fear, misfortune, and persecution are much more fantastic and senseless. In these cases the entire environment appears to the patients to be changed. Their home is transformed into a dungeon, into a house of ill repute, or a deserted prison from which there are no means of escape. Things about them seem unnatural and have a gloomy aspect; passing carriages are regarded as a funeral procession; the tolling of the church bell indicates that some one has died. A spoon lying on the table means that medicine has been taken by some one who is now at the point of death. Hammer and nails found on the floor signify that a scaffold is being secretly built for their execution. Chance remarks have a hidden meaning. Their food is the flesh and blood of their relatives. Everything is awfully changed for them; friends and relatives are not real; the sun and the moon look different; the end of the world has come; and they are now to be passed into a lion's den. The patients accuse themselves of horrible crimes, for which they are exiled or must die on the gallows; have murdered their husbands, devoured their children, or have brought sin upon the whole world. All wickedness is due to them; they have desecrated the communion bread, or have spat upon the image of Christ. They are totally unworthy, should be buried alive, no one should speak to them, hanging is too good, and they should be thrown into molten metal.

In some cases the so-called " *nlhilistic delusions" (d6lire de negation)* predominate, when the patients claim that nothing exists, there is no more food, no more houses, no more trees, no cities, no day or night, no sun or moon, no living being. They are alone in the universe, as there is no world. They themselves have no name, no wife, no children. They cannot eat, cannot speak, cannot die. Their body is all shrunken up, their bowels never move, and food has been accumulating in them for months. They no longer possess a heart or lungs; they cannot breathe or even walk.

Extremely absurd hypochondriacal ideas are apt to be expressed. The patients claim that they have no breath, the blood has stopped circulating, the veins have dried up, the eyes are rotting away, maggots are crawling under the skin, their brain is solid rock, their limbs are transformed to hoofs and the face to that of a wild animal. Occasionally sexual delusions of a silly character are present, the patients maintaining that they have been outraged at night, are now in a house of ill repute, or surrounded by men disguised as women. These depressive delusions are definite, coherent, and usually well-retained. There are a few cases, especially those with progressive mental deterioration, in which a few expansive delusions appear.

Hallucinations, especially of hearing, and also of sight are prominent. Voices and bells are heard, the devil commands them, strangers insult them, and they hear the evil thoughts of others. They see strange forms beside them at night, moving bodies and spirits. Occasionally they detect strange odors and tastes in food, and smell vapors at night. *Consciousness* in these cases is usually clouded and there is some disorientation for time, place, and persons. The *train of thought* is somewhat confused and monotonous, with a tendency to repeat compulsively such phrases as, " What did I do?" "What did I do?" "My God! my God!" Yet it is sometimes surprising to find how well patients answer questions and describe their symptoms. Sometimes the patients are partially conscious of the nature of their illness and complain that they have been made foolish and crazy by poison placed in their food or hypnotic influence. In other cases the patients are wholly unable to recognize the contradictions in their absurd statements: at one minute they will claim that they have been destroyed by poison, and at the next that they cannot die.

The *emotional attitude* is uniformly one of depression. The basis for this emotional depression seems to be *fear, a feeling of oppression, an inner anxiety.* Some patients claim that it is as if a heavy weight were upon the chest. They are timid, uneasy, and feel as though homesick. The fear is increased by association with those who are accustomed to arouse in them the deepest feelings, while strangers and new environment create little emotional reaction. Emotional outbreaks may be present at times, when the patients are greatly agitated, and may even present a dreamy disturbance of consciousness. These frequently follow visits of relatives or some unusual occurrence.

In *conduct,* the patients no longer feel the impulse to work; work is hard to finish. Yet they cannot remain quiet, they cannot remain in bed, and wander about the house in an aimless manner. They complain, lament, and pray; visit physicians and the clergy in order to receive sympathy, although they know that no one can help them. Many patients develop a feverish activity, they beg piteously for work, they work at night and struggle along until completely exhausted in order to take their minds off their sorrow and fear.

The countenances of the patients give clear evidence of their anxiety. Occasionally in very severe cases there may appear transiently a peculiar indefinite laughter, which by no means represents an elated emotional state, but is rather an expression of desperate irony. They feel compelled to talk about their condition. They always have something to communicate to the doctor, but one finds that it is always the same old story. It is a striking peculiarity that these patients become quiet when transferred to a new environment. They become natural in their manner, are approachable, and are able to conceal their anxiety. They claim that everything will be all right again if they could only return home and to work, but careful observation shows the real depth of their emotional excitement. After the disease has been in existence some time, the patients may be able to remain quiet and more or less indifferent for a much longer time. But as soon as one comes into close companionship with them, he will observe occasional evidences of emotional outbursts.

Commands are carried out without delay, unless they create some anxiety. The individual movements are usually free and unrestrained, although they are usually performed without any special strength or rapidity, especially in patients much reduced physically. There is no striking disorder in writing.

The patients eat irregularly and many even refuse food altogether, sometimes because they wish to die, at others because they are not worthy of food. Others suspect poison or excrement in their food. Similarly, patients refuse to take medicines and to bathe themselves. Some patients are untidy and even soil themselves.

The tendency to commit *suicide* is more pronounced and more to be guarded against in melancholia than in any other form of mental disease. The desire to end life may be the outcome of deliberation, or because they are repudiated by God. But usually the thoughts of death arise suddenly and are impulsive. Not infrequently they suddenly develop during convalescence. Often their attempts at suicide are not remembered. Sometimes the suicidal attempts are among the first symptoms of the disease. Every melancholiac should, therefore, be regarded as a dangerous patient, and the more so, the more conscious he is and the more capable of concealing his anxiety. Determined to commit

suicide, these patients resort to all sorts of devices to accomplish their purpose. Some attempt to drown themselves in the bathtub, others ram their heads against the wall; many hang or attempt to strangle themselves by tying something about their necks. In their agitation they seem to be quite insensible to pain. One of my patients reduced her scalp to pulp with a hammer, fracturing her skull in several places. Other patients swallow glass, nails, ink, or in fact anything that they can secure.

In case the anxiety is accompanied by greater excitement, the patients cannot remain quiet, but pace back and forth, wringing their hands, pulling at their hair, moaning and lamenting until so hoarse that they can barely speak aloud. In their great anguish they persistently pick at their nose, face, or fingers until smeared with blood, pull out their hair, tear their clothing, and pound themselves. Kraepelin questions whether this extreme picture really belongs to melancholia or should be classified in a group as yet undifferentiated. These cases, anatomically, usually present severe and extensive lesions in the cortex in which there is destruction of very many nerve cells.

Physical Symptoms. — *Insomnia* is an early and prominent symptom. The sleep is scanty, much disturbed by dreams, and unrefreshing. Occasionally there are observed the early signs of the senile changes; such as attacks of dizziness, sluggish pupillary reaction, paresis of the facial muscles, and tremor of the tongue and hands. The patients also complain of uncomfortable sensations about the heart; a sort of tension, a pressure, or an " anxious feeling," which is regularly worse at night. The muscular power is diminished and there is some general physical weakness. The nutrition suffers and the weight falls. Appetite is poor or completely lacking, the bowels are very sluggish, the tongue coated, and the breath foul. The mucous surfaces are anaemic. The temperature frequently remains below normal. Circulatory disturbances are often present; as, cyanosis, coldness and edema of the limbs. The pulse may be small and ir-

regular or slow, and the arteries may give evidence of beginning sclerosis. Other changes, indicative of senility, are sluggish reaction of pupils, grayness of the hair, cessation of the menses, dryness and harshness of the skin.

Course. — There is a gradual development, a prolonged duration, and a still more gradual convalescence. In cases of recovery the whole course lasts at least twelve months to two years. Short remissions, during which there is only a partial disappearance of the symptoms, are characteristic of the entire course. There is often present a daily improvement toward evening, and an exacerbation of the symptoms during the morning. Exacerbations often arise as the result of annoyance, fatigue, and excitation, such as that induced by visits. A gradual improvement of the sleep and nutrition, especially an increase in weight, may be regarded as a favorable sign. The remissions become longer and more marked, and the anxiety gives way to irritability and fretfulness; the patients then begin to display interest in work and reading. Even when convalescence is well established, it is not unusual for them to have " bad days," during which they are troubled and fearful.

Diagnosis. — The distinguishing characteristics of melancholia of involution are a slow development, uniform course, long duration, gradual improvement, and doubtful prognosis. These characteristics only partially suffice for the differentiation of melancholia from the depressive phase of *manic-depressive insanity*. In addition, the disquietude of the melancholiac is contrasted with the more dejected and hopeless attitude of the manic-depressive patient. This difference is especially well marked in the early stages of the disease, when the melancholiac shows more clearly anxiety and restlessness and the manic-depressive patient a dismal despondency and sadness. In melancholia the emotional attitude is much more uniform. Although the melancholiac may show some variation in the intensity of his feelings, the anxiety is always present, and it is not possible, as it sometimes is in manic-depressive insanity, by consoling or joking with them, to make them cheerful and smiling. Furthermore, in the psychomotor field we do not observe the retardation, which is usually so pronounced in manic-depressive insanity. The patients have no difficulty in expressing themselves orally or by writing; they are unhampered in their movements and actions. If they happen to be silent and refuse to speak, it is evident that this arises from their desperation or their delusions. They are usually communicative and talkative enough whenever they can secure consolation.

The differentiation is by no means as easy in some of the *mixed phrases of manic-depressive insanity,* in which the despondency is associated with some excitement and not with retardation. In such cases the distinction depends upon the fact that the emotional state in the mixed phases is usually less anxious than irritable, is accompanied by grumbling and at times faint-heartedness, that restless patients can be easily influenced by conversation to become quiet and even cheerful, and finally, that the excitement is not an expression of the feelings, but an independent disturbance which stands in no relation to the intensity of the feelings.

The *depression of catatonia* developing during involution is distinguished from melancholy by the presence and persistence of hallucinations and the inaccessibility of the patients. The melancholiac is resistive and inaccessible only in connection with his anxiety or his delusions. He is usually influenced by conversation, and participates in the conversation when visited by friends, while the catatonic shows emotional indifference, negativism, and constrained and manneristic conduct. The uniform lamentation and wringing of the hands in melancholia contrasts with the senseless stereotypy of the catatonic.

Symptoms characteristic of *senile dementia* sometimes develop in melancholia, rendering the prognosis less favorable. Such symptoms are, chiefly, the interference with the impressibility of memory, the tendency to fabrications, loss of orientation, emotional in-

difference, silly obstinacy, and nocturnal restlessness. The fantastic and nihilistic character of delusions is not an unfavorable sign, but senile physical changes are; namely, decrepitude, atrophic changes in the skin, bones, and muscles, and the evidences of arteriosclerosis in the heart and vessels.

Melancholia has no connection with the arteriosclerotic brain lesions. The depressed states occurring in *arteriosclerotic insanity* are distinctly hypochondriacal and accompanied by evidences of dementia and of severe brain lesions.

Considerable trouble may be experienced in differentiating the depressed form of *dementia paralytica.* In melancholia one finds a subacute onset following definite prodromal symptoms, greater or less clouding of consciousness, a more consistent emotional attitude, and absence of evidences of mental deterioration early in the disease, while in dementia paralytica there is a gradual onset with early evidence of mental deterioration, defective time orientation, poor judgment and memory, silly and contradictory delusions. Furthermore, the emotional attitude does not always correspond with the ideas expressed, and consciousness is more deeply clouded.

Prognosis. — The prognosis is not favorable, considering that only one-third of the cases fully recover. Twentythree per cent. of the cases improve so as to be able to return home and live comfortably, sometimes aiding in the maintenance of the family, twenty-six per cent. become demented, and nineteen per cent. die within two or three years. The patients, being apathetic and anergetic, and taking little exercise and insufficient food, become more and more emaciated, and finally succumb to cardiac weakness or some infectious or chronic disease. The prognosis is less favorable in cases occurring after fifty-five years of age.

In those cases that improve, but do not recover, the depression and the delusions gradually disappear, and the consciousness becomes perfectly clear, but the patients fail to develop full in-

terest in the surroundings and to adapt themselves to any kind of work. They are dull, sluggish, and indifferent, and tend to be low spirited and tearful. In those that become more demented the delusions fade very gradually, but the patients fail to gain insight and show poverty of thought. They are forgetful, apathetic, and entirely unable to apply themselves. They stand around stupidly or lament in a monotonous fashion. Others develop the typical picture of senile dementia. Residuals of former delusions, as well as a few hallucinations and some expansive ideas, remain.

Treatment. — The chief essential is the establishment of a "rest cure," which, first of all, demands the removal of the patients from all deleterious influences, including the nearest relatives, the home environment, and the customary occupation. Hence it is usually necessary to send the patient to a sanitarium or hospital. This is particularly urgent if suicidal tendencies develop.

It is necessary in most cases that the patients be *confined in bed* with short intermissions, with sufficient and constant attendance. If the patient can be confined in bed out of doors in a secluded, partially sheltered, and sunny place, it will be found decidedly beneficial. It aids in alleviating insomnia and affords a more interesting and attractive environment. In very light cases a suitable change may be found in removal to a different boarding-place or into the associations of a happy family. It is decidedly not advisable to attempt such distractions as might be afforded by long journeys, sight-seeing, and constant company. The rest in bed should not be too prolonged; later it is best that it be gradually replaced by short drives or walks, combined with daily change of scenery.

Of next importance is *nutrition.* The food should be nutritious, given in small quantities and at frequent intervals. Monotony in diet should always be avoided by consulting the tastes of the patient. Careful regulation of the intestines, combined, if necessary, with rectal injections, usually improves the appetite. Extreme anxiety and restlessness often necessitate artificial feeding by stomach or nasal tube in order to maintain nutrition. When this is contraindicated by cardiac weakness, it is necessary to resort to saline infusions.

Insomnia, which is both troublesome and often difficult to overcome, is best combated at first by prolonged warm baths in the early evening, warm packs, or gentle massage provided it does not increase the agitation. Hot malted milk before retiring may aid in inducing sleep. These measures, well carried out, often render hypnotics unnecessary, the use of which is always inadvisable because of the prolonged course of the disease. Of the hypnotics, alcohol is the most useful. Paraldehyde, one-half to one fluid dram, trional in ten to fifteen grain doses, veronal seven and one-half grains, and somnos are the most useful. The distressing condition of *anxious restlessness* may be combated with opium. It is best given in rapidly increasing doses beginning with five drops and reaching thirty to fifty drops of the tincture of opium three times daily, which is gradually reduced as soon as the restlessness begins to subside. This drug sometimes not only fails, but serves to aggravate the symptoms, when it must be withdrawn gradually. Improvement from this source, if it is to occur, appears within a few days. *Suicidal tendencies* necessitate painstaking, careful, and constant watching, as melancholiacs are the most difficult to thwart in their attempts at suicide. This care must be as strenuously observed until recovery is well established.

The *psychical influence* which may be constantly exerted over the patients by those in attendance is of the greatest value in alleviating distress, modifying the delusions, and relieving the anxiety. For this reason the manner should be gentle, friendly, and assuring, and some attempts should always be made to lead the thoughts of the patients away from their depressive ideas. As the patients improve there should be a systematic effort to gradually engage them in some light employment, as sewing, reading, writing, etc. Visits from relatives are always deleterious and in the height of the disease must be forbidden Finally, it is of the utmost importance that the patients be kept under observation and treatment until thoroughly recovered. A safe index of this may be found in their insight into the disease and the return of normal sleep and nutrition.

B. PRESENILE DELUSIONAL INSANITY
There is a small group of cases appearing during involution which are unlike either melancholia or senile dementia, showing many of the characteristics of dementia preecox. It has been tentatively differentiated and characterized by the *gradual development of marked impairment of judgment, accompanied by numerous unsystematized delusions of suspicion and greatly increased emotional irritability.*

Etiology. — The psychosis is rare, occurring only twelve times in ten years' experience. The majority of the cases are women, in whom the disease appears between fifty-five to sixty-five years of age; while in men it occurs about the fiftieth year. There seems to be marked hereditary predisposition to the disease.

Symptomatology. — The onset of the disease is gradual, with a change of disposition. The patients at first become quiet, seclusive, discontented, moody, suspicious, and irritable. Then delusions gradually develop which at first are vague and transitory, but later become more permanent and definite. Among the first to appear are the *hypochondriacal delusions.* The patients complain of the most varied and changeable nervous sensations and pains, spasmodic twitchings, vertigo, troubled dreams, debility, malaise, roaring in the ear, etc., which remind one of hysterical complaints. These ideas later usually become somewhat senseless, and the patients complain that the spine is dried up, the brain shrunken, all strength has departed, etc.

Meanwhile, fantastic *delusions of suspicion appear.* The patients claim that their clothing has been exchanged or stolen; that articles of furniture have been removed and others of less value substituted; thieves are about. They suspect poison in the food; accuse the physician of trying to get rid of them, of being obscene, of removing the womb, or making them ill for the purpose of studying their case. The husband believes that the wife is secretly dosing him.

Delusions of infidelity are usually very numerous and prominent. The husband is accused of eying women on the street, of flirting with every one he meets, of caressing the servant, and receiving letters from the schoolmates of his daughter. He arranges to meet women whenever he leaves home, and has intercourse with every one possible. The husband is suspicious of his wife because she leaves him at night, or is surprised when he returns home unexpectedly.

It is characteristic of all these delusions that they are exceedingly unstable. They appear at one moment, are abandoned in the next, and again recur in another form. As regards *insight,* many patients admit that they might have been mistaken and that they are sick, but they fail to really appreciate the senselessness of their ideas. Half an hour later you may find them in the greatest distress, because they have been poisoned, or because some one has hidden under the bed; they are going to die, etc. A soothing word usually suffices to quiet them and dispel their fear.

Hallucinations accompany the delusions in only a few cases. The patients are sometimes threatened, or hear strangers boast of intercourse with their wives. The cries of their ill-treated children reach them. At night they may see dark forms stealing out of the room, or feel some one lying beside their wives. It is a noteworthy fact that the patients do not make a genuine attempt to intercept these guilty parties. If a search is instituted and they fail to find any one, they express anger only because connubial fidelity was violated with such shamelessness and slyness in their-own presence. *Consciousness* is unclouded and orientation unimpaired. *Thought* is coherent, but *judgment* shows a marked weakness, noted in the retention of the most fantastic delusions, while the consciousness of the patient is perfectly clear. The patients cannot see the senselessness of the delusions, and while they may claim that they are open to conviction, they can never be convinced. Their *memory* for remote events is unimpaired. However, in the narration of their delusions, they add all sorts of embellishments and misrepresentations.

The *emotional attitude* at first is one of depression and fear; occasionally it leads to suicidal attempts. Later there usually appear some excitement and irritability. The patients then talk a good deal, make verbose complaints, stir up boisterous scenes, fly into violent passion, and are abusive, but they are usually quieted without difficulty. They sometimes laugh and cry without cause.

The *conduct* is characterized by all sorts of senseless actions. In accord with their delusions many patients run about from one physician to another, and solicit much advice without attempting to follow any of it. Some stop eating, seclude themselves, destroy everything within reach, and become violent. Jealousy leads to strict surveillance of the husband or wife. The servant is sent out in search of them; torn letters in the waste basket are placed together in order to obtain proof of guilt, and the supposed seducers may be publicly accused.

With the advance of the disease the delusions become more senseless; the patients claim that the wife and children are being tortured, the son nailed to the floor, or suspended on a fence; the wife wanders nightly from place to place, and every one is talking about it. Female patients believe that their husbands have intercourse with their own children, and even with other men, disguised as women. They are aware of this only through sensations in their own bodies, whenever they are deceived. The precious Lord proclaims everything, talks to them, and lies beside them at night like a shadow. Persons and the environment are changed; their bodies are disfigured and influenced. For this reason, many patients remain in seclusion, veil themselves, and at times refuse to speak and then suddenly become very friendly and communicative. These delusions frequently change, and may temporarily fade away, although some general signs of them are constantly recurring. In spite of progressing mental deterioration, the patients do not become incoherent. Diagnosis. — Some regard these cases as *paranoia,* but they certainly differ from paranoia, in that the delusions are not systematized. The persecutors remain indefinite or change frequently, the suspected consorts are not regarded as enemies, but are often thought to have been seduced. Moreover, the patients do not find in their delusions any broad basis for action, and except for their occasional violent outbreaks, do not treat the supposed persecutor as especially hostile; they associate with their faithless wives, in fact even force themselves into their company, and surprise one by becoming friendly toward those persons whom they have just previously suspected and accused. They often prefer to be confined in the hospital in spite of complaining of all sorts of persecution, because they enjoy the protection afforded them there. Finally, the delusions do not continue stable, but change frequently, and sometimes even in a short time. The conditions of excitement seem to depend less upon deliberation than emotional vacillations.

Some consider these cases of *dementia prcecox,* which may occur at this age, although not frequently. These patients do not present catatonic symptoms. The peculiar resistiveness and excitement occasionally manifested are not compulsive or spontaneous, but depend upon delusions or moods. The patients do not become apathetic rapidly, but, on the contrary, continue irritable and interested, while disturbances of judgment greatly predominate over those of the emotions and actions.

Prognosis. — The outcome is never characterized by profound dementia or confusion of speech, but by a moderate deterioration, with isolated, changeable, and incoherent delusions. Recoveries or marked improvements are not likely to occur.

Treatment. — The treatment is wholly symptomatic. Most patients are troublesome and need hospital treatment, but some, under favorable conditions, are able to remain at home.

C. SENILE DEMENTIA

Senile Dementia is *characterized by a gradually progressive mental deterioration, occurring during the period of involution and accompanied by a series of lesions in the central nervous system.* It comprises several groups of cases, including *simple senile deterioration* of lighter and severer grades, *presbyophrenia, senile delirium,* and *senile delusional insanity.*

Etiology. — The disease may appear at any time during involution, but is encountered most frequently between sixty and seventy-five years of age. Individuals with a faulty constitutional endowment, worn with hardships, and especially those addicted to excesses, may succumb before sixty. Men who have been more exposed to overwork and excesses develop the disease earlier than women. Defective heredity occurs in about fifty per cent. of cases, but is confined mostly to senile deterioration in parents and in brothers and sisters. Very frequently the disease develops immediately following an injury, particularly head injury, emotional shocks, also acute febrile diseases, especially influenza and bronchitis.

Fuerstner, Archiv f. Psychiatrie, XX, 2; Noetzli, Uber Dementia Senilis, Diss. Zuerich, 1895; Alzheimer, Monatsschrift f. Psychiatrie u. Neurologie, 1898, 101; Scholoess, Wiener Klinik, XXV, 9 u. 10, 1899; Colella, Annali di Neurologia, 1899, 6; Zingerle, Jahrb. f. Psychiatrie, XVIII, 256. Pickett, The Jour, of Nervous and Mental Disease, 1904, p. 81.

Pathological Anatomy. — All advanced cases of senile dementia present, both macroscopically and microscopically, atrophy of the nerve substance. The *brain weight* is from two hundred to five hundred grams below normal. There may be compensatory thickening of the cranium, and increase of the cerebrospinal fluid (hydrocephalus ex-vacuo). The *dura* is usually adherent to the calvarium. The Pacchionian granulations are increased in size. Pachymeningitis interna haemorrhagica is often present, and sometimes to an extreme degree. The *pia* is somewhat thickened uniformly over the entire cortex, may contain many corpora amylacea, and is almost always edematous. The *convolutions* are narrow and shrunken, and the gaping fissures contain blebs filled with serous fluid. Minute hemorrhages are sometimes found in the cortex, corona radialis, and basal ganglia. The *ventricles* are much dilated and ependymal walls thickened, and occasionally granular. The choroid plexuses usually present various stages of cystic degeneration. The cerebral vessels exhibit arteriosclerosis, in which there are often evidences of hyaline changes, but it is more characteristic of the vessels in senile dementia to show a rich pigmentation of the endothelial and adventitial cells. The fact that the blood vessels, in simple senile deterioration, are only moderately involved, favors the view that the vascular changes in senile dementia cannot be regarded as the particular cause of the disease. Further proof of this is found in the fact that there are many individuals with extensive vascular lesions of the brain who do not exhibit signs of senile dementia. Nevertheless, more or less extensive. vascular lesions commonly accompany senile dementia. There occasionally occur combined forms of senile and arteriosclerotic insanity, called by Alzheimer *"senile decay"* (see p. 334).

Microscopically, the nerve cells present different grades of the chronic cell change in addition to much pigmentation. Complicating the chronic cell change there may occur any of those acute cell changes described in paresis (see p. 282). Both the tangential and radical fibre tracts in the corona present more or less atrophy. The neuroglia cells are more numerous and show an increase in the number of nuclei, the cell bodies often forming distinct clumps *(raseri)* with a thick network of fine glia fibrils. Many of the neuroglia cells show evidences of extensive degenerative processes; such as, vacuolization, marked pigmentation, and atrophy of the nucleus. The *spinal cord* presents an atrophy in its ganglion cells

and fibre tracts. Calcareous placques are sometimes found in the pia. The entire pathological picture, however, varies, as well as the clinical picture, but as yet it is impossible to establish any definite relationship between the different pathological and clinical pictures.

The other organs of the body present senile atrophy and arteriosclerotic changes. The condition of the heart, with chronic endocarditis and fibroid changes in the myocardium, is of importance, as it interferes with cerebral circulation.

Symptomatology. — The *apprehension* of external impressions is slow and difficult. The patients fail to note details and to understand the connection of things that are complicated. They, therefore, become easily disoriented, cannot see the point in a discussion, and overlook important matters. They are drowsy, disinclined to think, somewhat dazed, and easily lose the thread of a conversation. *Thought* becomes stagnant and the patients are unable to change their viewpoints or to gain new ones. The old trains of thought, being inaccessible to new ideas, do not get beyond the beaten paths. Ideas, once aroused, are constantly recurring, without any regard for the circumstances. The mental elaboration of external impressions, the consideration of cause and effect, and the critical examination of ideas is always inadequate and uncertain. This explains the patients' total inability to comprehend the views and conditions of others, as well as the inflexibility of their opinions and their susceptibility to delusional ideas. Their *delusional ideas* consist mostly of excessive fear of illness, senseless distrust, or childish egoism. Other prominent delusions are those of reference and robbery. They commonly believe that many things are done to annoy them and that their property has been taken from them. A *lack of genuine insight* into their infirmity, necessitating the appointment of a trustee or conservator, creates still other ideas of persecution. *Hallucinations* and especially *illusions* are common.

The *failure of memory* is always a

prominent symptom, especially memory for recent events. Present and passing events within a short time seem to be completely effaced from memory. Patients forget where they were yesterday, or where they have placed things, do not realize that they are relating the same story that they told yesterday or perhaps a few hours ago, cannot recall the names of recent acquaintances, and even forget the names of old friends. On the other hand, memory for events of early life is well retained and furnishes the chief topics for conversation. The gaps of recent memory are very often made good by extensive *fabrications.* Finally, as the result of the progressive impairment of memory, to which nothing new is ever added, there develops an increasing impoverishment of the store of ideas, with an extraordinary dearth and uniformity of the content of thought.

In *emotional attitude,* indifference and lack of sympathy are the prominent characteristics. The patients become apathetic; they fail to enter into the sorrows and joys of those about them, and do not grieve at the loss of friends. Self-interest, with the gratification of personal whims, precedes everything. They are no longer interested in their family or home. This may advance to genuine avarice, the feeling of greed overwhelming even filial affection. The fundamental emotional tone is sometimes that of surly dissatisfaction, and at others a childish happiness and an exalted self-confidence. There may be irritability for short periods. The patients are inconsiderate, arbitrary, dogmatic, and offended at any opposition. The emotional states are both superficial and transitory; extreme and tearful sympathy or silly happiness may be aroused on the slightest pretext and just as rapidly disappear. The *sexual feelings* are frequently increased, impelling the patients to enter into improper sexual relations, especially with children; to use obscene language, to dress in an attractive manner, plan marriages, and in extreme conditions to expose themselves. The *conduct* of the patients varies greatly. Many remain quiet, orderly, and contented, and, in spite of increasing dementia, cause no trouble and can be kept at home. Other patients gradually develop an increasing restlessness: they grumble, quarrel, curse, abuse those about them at every opportunity, and often threaten and become aggressive. Many patients begin to idulge in excesses, to masturbate, to wander away from home, to make foolish purchases and plans, to hoard all sorts of plunder, and ultimately get themselves into many difficulties. But *nocturnal restlessness* is most characteristic. It consists in getting out of and dishevelling the bed, wandering about the house with a light, and rummaging chests and closets without evident purpose. During the day these patients are weary and drowsy and frequently fall to sleep during conversation and meals. Patients are unable to care for themselves properly and are dirty about their clothing.

Physical Symptoms. — In addition to the insomnia, there is usually a pronounced deterioration in the general physique and some anorexia. The patients usually look older than they really are, the musculature is reduced, and the strength below par. A fine tremor is characteristic of the senile, and can be distinguished from the tremor of the paretic and the alcoholic by the numerous irregularities in the separate strokes. Furthermore, there are a series of physical symptoms corresponding to the cortical lesions; namely, headache, vertigo, convulsive seizures with transitory or permanent aphasic symptoms, hemianaesthesias, hemianopsia, ptosis, hemiparesis of the muscles of the eye, tongue, or extremities. The pupils are sometimes small, or unequal, and react sluggishly or not at all. The reflexes are usually increased, seldom diminished. The speech is often indistinct. Neuritic disturbances are frequent. Finally, evidences of arteriosclerosis are frequently observed.

In the severer grade of senile dementia there develops *great clouding of consciousness and complete disorientation.* These patients apprehend what is said to them and respond briefly in a sensible manner, but they are wholly unable to grasp what is taking place about them. They have no idea of where they are, address their associates by the names of friends long since dead, and even fail to recognize their relatives. They have very little memory for what occurs in their daily lives, and gradually lose even their remote knowledge. They cannot tell how old they are, or how many children they have. They say they are twenty-five years of age, have had twenty-five children, the oldest of which is twenty-five years, that they still menstruate, and are now pregnant. They undress at midday, thinking it night, and call the physician by their husbands' names. They are easily distracted and cannot hold long to one thought. The store of ideas is greatly impoverished and the same remarks are repeated over and over again. They occasionally indulge in a peculiar senseless rhyming and a half-singing repetition of words and syllables.

Numerous changing fantastic *delusions* are present, both depressive and expansive, and often also hypochondriacal and nihilistic. They cannot speak, eat, or sleep; nothing has passed then bowels in weeks, and the liver has rotted away. They have leaned against a radiator and burned a hole in the lungs which has caused the heart to cease beating. Their abdomens have been cut open and organs removed, or they will be buried alive. On the other hand, they may claim that they possess much property, hold an important position, or are in communication with God. The delusions are apt to be embellished with numerous *fabrications. Hallucinations* of sight and hearing are frequently present.

The *emotional attitude* varies. The patients are sometimes apprehensive and dejected, sometimes irritable, and at others, elated and happy, while rapid changes from one mood to another are common. In *actions* they display more or less restless activity, which is especially marked at night. They regularly tear and throw about then-bedding, creep about the room, picking into the corners, destroying and smearing their clothing, or they laugh, sing, and run about in a silly manner. They are very untidy, and wholly incapable of caring for themselves. Insomnia is pronounced, and very little nourishment is taken.

In the group of cases of senile dementia called presbyophrenia, the patients, *in spite of a marked disturbance of the impressibility of memory, retain fairly well their mental alertness, the coherence of thought, and to a certain extent, also, good judgment.* Women predominate in this group, and chiefly robust individuals are affected. Usually the disease develops gradually, sometimes following more or less definite prodromal symptoms which have been in existence for some weeks. It may appear as an episode during the course of simple senile deterioration.

The patients are capable of entering into a long conversation, and of comprehending in great measure the occurrences in their environment, but they utterly fail in obtaining any conception of their own condition or of their relation to the environment. They *forget* almost immediately what they have been doing or what they have heard. Only an occasional impression is retained, and especially those accompanied by some feeling. Place and, particularly, time *orientation* is disturbed. Patients cannot tell where they are or those about them. They greet strangers as acquaintances; regretting that they cannot just recall the name, but they are confident that they have seen them before. They know neither the day nor the week. They make all sorts of contradictory statements as to their age, speak as if their parents were still living, and refer to their own infant children. The *store of knowledge* also is faulty. Their ability to reckon may be fairly well retained, as well as knowledge of the small affairs of daily life, like the price of articles of food, cooking receipts, etc., but all beyond that is lost. They cannot recall historical and geographical facts, the name of the President, and, indeed, sometimes even the names and ages of their own children, but yet they may be able to recall a few remote facts, as their own maiden name and the playmates of their childhood.

The patients do not appreciate these marked defects. When quizzed, they will explain their inability to answer such questions by the fact that they were never interested in such things, that women are not supposed to bother about such matters, etc. They usually make good the lapses in their recent memories by simple *fabrications;* such as, that they were busy in the morning, had been out to call on their parents, other relatives were there, and they all drank some coffee. Now they have come here to help with some work, but are soon going to return to their place of employment, where they are earning good wages. These patients rarely express *delusions* or have *hallucinations.*

Their *judgment* is fairly well retained as far as it involves their early knowledge and facts which are at their disposal. For instance, such senseless expressions as that " the snow is black," or "that ball is square" cause them to smile, and they become indignant if told that they steal or perjure themselves. On the other hand, the patients fail to recognize the most absurd contradictions as regards the temporal relation of events, even when their attention is called to them. They will say that their parents are no older than they, that their daughter is only three years younger, though she was born more than ten years ago. In their conversation the patients are often energetic and loquacious, although they frequently digress.

The *emotional attitude* of the patients is usually that of happiness with an occasional brief show of peevishness or irritability. They exhibit an interest and readily familiarize themselves with their environment and can appreciate a joke. In conduct they are, in general, orderly, and busy themselves in one way or another. Occasionally there is some nocturnal restlessness. Symptoms of severe brain lesions, particularly paralysis and apoplectic attacks, are rarely encountered.

This picture of presbyophrenia may persist unchanged for a number of years. Again it may pass over into a state of simple stupid dementia.

Senile Delirium. — This form is *characterized by a more acute onset and a short course urith great clouding of consciousness, active hallucinations, and delirious conduct.* It often appears as an episode in the course of senile deterioration; indeed, signs of beginning senile dementia usually precede the outbreak. Exciting causes are prominent; such as acute illnesses, mental shock, or injuries.

The patients rapidly develop many *hallucinations* of sight and hearing. They hear voices, threats, singing, see the devil, or crowds of men pressing upon them with knives. They are anxious and restless, claiming that they are in the world below, surrounded by mighty powers, are bewitched and poisoned, the house is being flooded and huge boulders rolled about the room. Disorientation is complete. The speech is irrelevant, incoherent, and flighty, and is often limited to unintelligible, disjointed words, or to a repetition of senseless syllables. There is usually great pressure of speech. The activity is greatly increased; they rattle doors and windows, shout for help, refuse food, resist, tear up the bedding, and crawl about the floor, etc. Insomnia is extreme.

The *course* of the delirium presents many fluctuations and sudden remissions, with more or less complete return to clear consciousness. The delirium may reappear after a short interval, or it may pass over into a state of anxiety with peevishness, which may persist, or in time entirely disappear. In unfavorable cases the delirium becomes extreme, leading to collapse and death from exhaustion, injuries, or acute febrile diseases.

Finally, there is a characteristic group of cases in senile dementia which has been called senile delusional insanity. These cases develop gradually. The patients become reticent, irritable, and suspicious. It soon becomes apparent that they are dominated by *delusions;* that they believe that they are being robbed, are being ridiculed and insulted by their neighbors, and are hindered in their work; that poison is being placed in their food. These delusions are apparently scanty, somewhat incoherent, and are rarely elaborated, though they may remain unchanged a long time. *Hallucinations* are often present, especially in deaf patients. The patients remain completely *oriented.* However, persons in the environment, who are involved in their delusions, may be mistaken for others. The *emotional attitude* usually becomes indifferent, though occasionally the patients are irritable and egotistical. In *conduct* they are orderly and tractable; they busy themselves and only occasionally are excited.

Diagnosis. — The physiological changes common to *normal senility,* such as the defect in the impressibility of memory, an impoverishment of the store of ideas, an emotional indifference, a paralysis of activity, and the development of stubborn unruliness, renders very difficult the differentiation of the milder forms of senile dementia. To a certain extent this distinction is wholly arbitrary. The appearance of delusions and of excitement should leave no doubt as to the presence of a psychosis. The depressive states in senile dementia may be differentiated from *melancholia* by the dearth and the incoherence of the delusions and the defective memory and emotional dulness.

The differentiation of senile dementia from *arteriosclerotic insanity* is difficult. It has already been indicated that focal symptoms of themselves are not particularly characteristic of senile dementia, and point only to the fact that there is an accompanying vascular disease. Therefore, the more prominent such symptoms are, the greater the role of arteriosclerotic changes. Inversely, a rapid and general decay of the mental activity, particularly a severe disorder of memory, indicates senile dementia. The same observation holds true in *syphilitic insanity,* in which the dementia never becomes very pronounced until after a long duration, while hallucinations and delusions are more prominent.

The senile delirium, except for the underlying basis of deterioration, does not differ from the delirium encountered in other psychoses.

Treatment. — The treatment is wholly symptomatic. The condition of faulty *nutrition* needs careful watching in order to secure the ingestion of a sufficient amount of easily digested food. The *insomnia* of the senile is most intractable. In combating it, one should first employ the simplest remedies; as, warm nourishment at the time the patient awakes after the sleep of the early night, prolonged warm baths, and sufficiently warm bed clothing, together with, if necessary, hot-water bottles. Warm packs should be employed most cautiously. Of the hypnotic remedies, alcohol is most useful. Paraldehyde, chloralamide, and somnos are at times also efficient. Occasionally small and repeated doses of nitroglycerin give excellent results. These patients, if kept at home, must be watched closely at night, and placed in rooms without lights and with guarded windows in order to prevent injuries to self and danger from fire to others. If the insomnia and restlessness become extreme, the prolonged warm bath (see p. 140) may be used. Failing in this, one should improvise a padded room or a bed with high padded sides. In the cases accompanied by great anxiety, opium (see p. 362) is indicated and often brings the desired relief.

IX. MANIC-DEPRESSIVE INSANITY

Manic-depressive insanity is *characterized by the recurrence of groups of mental symptoms throughout the life of the individual, not leading to mental deterioration. These groups of symptoms are sufficiently well defined to be termed the manic, the depressive, and the mixed phases of the disease. The chief symptoms usually appearing in the manic phase are: psychomotor excitement with pressure of activity, flight of ideas, distractibility, and happy though unstable emotional attitude. In the depressive phase we expect to find psychomotor retardation, absence of spontaneous activity, dearth of ideas, and depressed emotional attitude; while the symptoms of the mixed phase consist of various combinations of the symptoms characteristic of both the manic and depressive phases.*

Etiology. — Manic-depressive insanity is one of the most prominent forms of mental disease, and comprises from twelve to twenty per cent. of admissions to insane hospitals. Of the etiological factors, defective heredity is the most important, occurring in from seventy to eighty per cent. of cases. The relatives have often suffered from the same form of disease. The defective constitutional basis is often apparent in individuals previous to the onset of the psychosis; some are peculiar, some are abnormally bright, others are of an excitable disposition and subject to frequent and apparently causeless changes of mood, and still others are excessively shy and reserved; while a few are imbecile from birth. Physical stigmata may also be present. Women predominate in the disease and represent about two-thirds of the patients. The disease almost always appears independently of external causes. In a few cases the appearance of the first attack is coincident with the first menstruation. The first and subsequent attacks may occur during succeeding periods of childbearing, but it is also a conspicuous fact that the attacks do not cease at the climacterium. In twothirds of the cases the first attack appears before twenty-five years of age, and in less than ten per cent. after the fortieth year, in both of which periods women greatly predominate. The first attack may occur as early as ten years of age, and as late as seventy years.

Kirn, Die periodischen Psychosen, 1878; Mendel, Die Manie, eine Monographie, 1881; Emmerich, Schmidt's Jahrbucher, CXC, 2; Pick, Circulares Irresein, Eulenburgs Realencyclopaedie, 2. Auflage; Hoche, Ueber die leichteren Formen des periodischen Irreseins, 1897; Hecke, Zeitschrift ftlr praktische Aertze, 1898, 1; Pilcz, Die periodischen Geistesstorungen, 1901; Thalbitzer, Den manic-depressive Psykose, Stemmingssindsygdom, 1902; Hoch, Ref. Hand. Med. Soc., Vol. V, 120.

The *nature* of manic-depressive insanity is still obscure. Several hypotheses have been formulated, but none are adequate. There are no demonstrable *anatomical, pathological lesions* characteristic of this disease.

Symptomatology. — *Apprehension* of external impressions in the manic states, with the exception of hypomania, is more or less disturbed. This disturbance is due largely to the great *distractibUity* of attention. The patients lose the ability to select and elaborate their impressions, because each striking sensory stimulus forces itself upon them so strongly that it absorbs their entire attention. Their attention may be held for a moment by holding objects before them, but it is quickly distracted by something else. Hence, the environment is never fully apprehended, and the picture remains disconnected and incomplete, although there is no serious disorder of the perceptive process. In the depressive forms apprehension is more manifestly and extensively disturbed; especially is this true in stupor. Even in the lighter depressive states the patients are unable to elaborate and comprehend well their impressions.

Consciousness is regularly disturbed in the severer forms of the disease. At the height of the manic excitement the hazy impressions lead to disorientation. Patients do not correctly understand where they are, mistake persons, and greet the physicians and nurses by the names of relatives or neighbors. This mistaking of persons sometimes arises from slight similarities of dress or facial expression, but at other times it seems to be due altogether to the capriciousness of the patients. In the less severe manic forms consciousness is very slightly disturbed. On the other hand, in the depressive states of the disease consciousness is more clouded, particularly in the stuporous conditions. *Hallucinations* are rare, except in the delirious form of the manic phase, and in the more marked stuporous depressive conditions, but even here they are neither a prominent nor persistent feature. Furthermore, the hallucinations do not have the same sensory distinctness common to the sense deceptions of dementia praecox. On the other hand, numerous and varied *false sensations* often accompany the pronounced hypochondriacal fears of the depressive patients. These are experienced all over the body. Patients claim that they feel the food as it courses through the veins, that they feel their organs being consumed, that nerves are dissolving, and that little white worms are crawling under the skin, etc. This increased sensitiveness to the internal processes of the body stands out in contrast to the loss of central sensitiveness to external impressions in the manic states, as seen in the remarkable insensibility of the manic patients to extremes of heat and cold, to hunger, and to pain. *Memory* does not suffer much injury from the disease itself, although patients often temporarily lose control over their store of ideas. Especially in the depressive states the patients are often unable to recall even simple facts. It takes them a very long time to solve a simple problem or to relate some experience. During the disease process the *impressibility of memory* is impaired. It has been shown by special tests that manic patients make more errors than normal individuals in recalling to memory their perceptions. There is sometimes a tendency to fabrications and to depict grotesque experiences. Memory for events of the attack is usually somewhat indistinct, particularly where there has been pronounced excitement or profound stupor. *Delusions* are often present in manic-depressive insanity. In the manic phases they are changeable and frequently appear in the form of playful boasts and exaggerations. Where the consciousness is somewhat clouded, the patients tend to elaborate more permanent expansive and persecutory delusions, the latter being directed particularly against the family; also delusions of jealousy and poisoning. In the depressive states hypochondriacal ideas are most prominent, and are often associated with delusions of persecution and of self-accusation. The depressive delusions sometimes beome markedly fantastic, similar to those expressed by paretics. Patients usually express some *insight;* they appreciate having undergone a change, but they are quite apt to attribute it to misfortune or abuse of some sort, rather than to mental illness. *Disturbances of thought* are prominent symptoms. In the manic states a definite line of thought cannot be followed out; ideas pass abruptly from one subject to

another, and the line of discourse is lost in a mass of detail. A short question may be answered correctly, but with the addition of a host of details and side remarks that have only a distant relation to the subject — *circumstantiality.* It is impossible for the patients to relate any event coherently without frequent inquiries and suggestions on the part of the listener to recall him from his digressions. There is a lack of voluntary guidance of the train of thought; hence there are abrupt changes in the succession of ideas influenced by objects that happen to come into the field of vision, or by sounds caught up from the surroundings. On the whole, there is a multitude of ideas which are not well connected. There is no controlling goal idea. The association of ideas follows along accustomed tracks, especially those that play an important part in daily expressions; such as bits of slang and common phrases. The resulting incoherence of thought gives rise to the so-called *flight of ideas.* Observation of external objects may seem to be very accurate and complete, but in reality it is superficial. A striking object attracts the attention, is apprehended, and starts a train of thought, but before this has proceeded far something else obtrudes upon the sensorium, and another is started. In spite of appearances, genuine thought is delayed. Instead of an acceleration of the train of ideas, there is only flightiness and an instability. There is an abundance of words, not of ideas. Sometimes in the depressive forms there is a slight degree of flight of ideas. As a counterpart to flight of ideas, we have *retardation of thought,* which regularly accompanies the depressive phases of the disease, and also some of the manic-stuporous states and the forms of manic excitement allied to them. Patients seem unable to marshal their ideas, and are often painfully aware of this. The individual ideas seem to develop slowly and only after very strong stimuli. Hence, external impressions do not quickly and easily arouse a group of associations, but the train of thought has to progress slowly and requires an especial effort of the will. On the other hand,

an idea once developed is not pushed aside by the appearance of new ideas, but it fades slowly and often sticks with great persistency, especially if it arises in connection with some feeling. Thus there result great difficulty and slowness of thought, monosyllabic answers to simple questions, and a dearth of ideas. This is apt to be regarded as evidence of dementia, until close observation demonstrates that there is no real deterioration.

The *emotional attitude* in the manic forms shows more or less elation and happiness. There is a feeling of well-being with a tendency to joke and to make facetious remarks. Expressions of emotion are unrestrained. Irritability is prominent, giving rise at times to outbursts of anger from trivial causes, but rapid changes in the emotional attitude are still more characteristic: in the midst of joy patients become tearful, and complain of abuse and misfortune; again, in spite of profound misery, they may burst out into boisterous laughter. These varying states appear and disappear with the greatest rapidity. Depression of spirits sometimes appears for a few hours at a time during manic states. In the depressive states of the disease the emotional attitude is regularly that of gloominess, despair, doubt, and anxiety. Patients complain particularly of the loss of interest in things; "everything is the same to them," " they are desolate and empty," " they are dead, because they have no feeling," "music does not sound natural," and "the crying of the children no longer creates sympathy." They feel as if they no longer belong to this world. One sometimes encounters moments when patients exhibit feeble attempts at laughter and even brief gayety. There are some cases of simple retardation in which there is no especial emotional tone. In the transition states and mixed phases there is stupor with silent mirth, or restless mischievousness with anxiety.

The disturbances found in the *psychomotor sphere* are prominent symptoms. In the manic states the increased facility for the conveyance of stimuli into action gives rise to *pressure of ac-*

tivity. Every sort of impulse leads to an action, completely inhibiting all normal volitional impulses, or even if a volitional action is begun, it is overwhelmed before half accomplished. Furthermore, almost imperceptible impulses excite the greatest variety of movements, which are executed with unusual energy. In the mildest manic states there appears a characteristic busyness and an excessive display of energy over trifles. If the disease is more severe, the actions become disconnected, and new impulses intrude before any one object can be accomplished. In the severest excitement, the actions change as rapidly as the ideas. The actions, however, depend upon and bear a definite relation to the ideas and emotions. The intensity of the motor excitement is due to an increased irritability and depends largely upon external stimuli, the removal of which reduces the activity. Unrestrained activity tends to increase the excitement. The ready release of the motor impulses perhaps accounts for the unusual *absence of fatigue.* In these conditions excitement may persist for weeks or even months without any signs of exhaustion.

The psychomotor pressure of activity is prominent also in the field of *speech,* and aids in the production of flight of ideas. The easily aroused motor-speech dispositions have a stronger influence in directing the train of thought than the ideas arising from purely intellective processes. Instead of a logical sequence of ideas, we find that motor coordinations determine their succession; thus, we encounter those associations common in the everyday life; such as, set phrases, slang, and rhymes, and finally a predominance of pure sound associations, when are heard such productions as, "Sam, jam, bang, slam, hell, shell, bells," etc. Silence is impossible. The patients prattle away and shout at the top of their voices, scream, declaim with many gestures and in a pompous manner, perhaps ending in unrestrained laughter, or they sing, now softly, now slowly. The following is a sample of the manic production: —

"I was looking at you, the sweet voice, that does not want sweet Boap. You always work Harvard, for the hardware store. Here is the right hand, the hand that they shot off yesterday. The love of God don't win gray hairs. I don't care if I am nineteen, my father taught me to love. Neatness of feet don't win feet, but feet win the neatness of men. Run don't run west, but west runs east. I like west strawberries best. Rebels don't shoot devils at night. For three years I got over seven dollars a month and some old rags. Take your time and be not disobedient, be grateful when judgment day comes. God's laws are all right, but Royal Baking Powder is compressed yeast. Women should never chew gum. Women should never smoke. Women should mind their own business. Fish-hooks are between the American flag, red, white, and blue, Fourth of July. You must pay for your own fiddler, Prudence. I am no tobacco chewer, I am no street walker, I am vaccinated, but McKinley does not win. My father is a Democrat. He had no work for three years."

Such incoherence is not the outcome of an excessive repletion of ideas, but results from an inability to give direction to the train of ideas. A normal individual, at times, might give expression to a similar production if he could utter a sequence of ideas as they came into his mind. In the disease picture this ideomotor excitability regularly leads to the expression of every idea that presents itself.

The letter-writing of manic patients shows with equal clearness the same disturbance. Single phrases and sentences may be well started, but are soon resolved into a senseless enumeration of catch phrases, bits of slang, and rhyme. The script is coarse and bold, while underlining, overwriting, and punctuation marks predominate.

The psychomotor field in the depressive form presents a *retardation of activity,* due to the slowness of conversion of sensory and ideational stimuli into impulses. In the mildest degree this retardation appears as a deficiency in the power of resolution. Actions may not only be performed slowly, but even after being started may fail of completion. The simplest movements, such as walking and talking, are performed very slowly and without energy. Unless extreme, the retardation may be overcome by an emotional excitement, such as impending danger or some unusual stimulus. In the severest forms the retardation leads to a complete abolition of all voluntary movements, producing a condition of stupor, when the patients are unable to leave the bed or attend to their physical needs.

Retardation may vary considerably in the extent to which it influences the different spheres of voluntary activity. The patients may perhaps be able to dress themselves and to employ themselves without difficulty, but they shrink from any act that demands resolution. Some patients are so taciturn and monosyllabic that it is impossible to engage them in conversation, and although they are able to count or read aloud as rapidly as ever, they will sit for hours with a letter in front of them, unable to finish writing it. Again there are patients who read rapidly, but cannot write a line; and there are others who write long letters, but become speechless as soon as you address them. The symptoms enumerated above portray the disease picture as a whole. As already indicated, these symptoms tend to arrange themselves into two large groups, representing the manic and the depressive phases of the disease, and a third smaller group, the mixed phase. Occasionally, individual cases fail to present sufficiently clear pictures to permit their definite assignment to any one of these phases, which condition, together with the occurrence of numerous transition stages from one phase to another, emphasizes the fact that it is impossible to draw a distinct border line between the prominent phases of the disease.

Manic States

The manic states comprise hypomania, mania, and delirious mania.

Hypomania represents the mildest form of the manic states, and has been variously designated "mania mitis," or " mitissima," and " folie raisonnante."

Consciousness, apprehension, and

memory are undisturbed. The activity of the mind and of the attention is often increased; indeed, the patients may appear brighter and clearer minded than usual, because of their ability to grasp faint resemblances, but in reality they cannot make use of any valid comparisons. In the realm of ideation they show a *moderate flight of ideas,* which is more especially noticed in letters. They shift abruptly from one subject to another, and are quite unable to bring a thought to a logical conclusion. They are very talkative, the content of conversation being centered about commonplace affairs, their experiences and difficulties. They revel in minute details, and often distort the facts with exaggerations and frequent misrepresentations. In the severer grades there is a striking lack of coherence in the train of thought. The patients are unable to arrange logically a series of ideas without abrupt transitions from one subject to another. In their writings and rhymes they often develop a flight of ideas. Upon effort they may be able, for short periods, to gain the mastery over their incoherent thoughts, as well as over their excessive activity. There may occur, for short periods, more marked excitement and dazedness.

Memory for recent events is not always correct. Patients in their conversation are easily carried away with exaggerations and distortions, which arise in part from their keener perception and in part from accessory interpretations, which never really come clearly into consciousness. Although there are no genuine *delusions,* yet there is a greatly exaggerated self-esteem. Patients boast of their own deeds and show a proportionate lack of appreciation for those of others. Hence, they lack insight into their condition. While they may admit a previous attack, they cannot regard their present state as anything but normal. They justify their actions in a most persistent way, and never lack plausible excuses. Moreover, they believe themselves misjudged or falsely confined, as they never were more healthy or capable of work. Usually, in their estimation, the relatives and friends, or those who have been instrumental in their confinement, are the ones in need of treatment.

As to the *emotional attitude* the patients are usually elated, happy, cheerful, and often exuberant. They derive great pleasure from their associations and undertakings. Some patients develop a pronounced humorous vein and a tendency to see the funny side of things, to make facetious remarks, to invent nicknames, and to make sport of themselves and others. They are jovial and friendly, but distinctly selfish, while their own desires and wishes prevail. On the other hand, increased irritability may develop, when the patients become discontented, intolerant, and quarrelsome with their environment. They are apt to become inconsiderate, saucy, and rude, whenever any one opposes them. Insignificant occasions may lead to violent fits of anger and even aggressiveness. They are completely under the control of sudden impressions and emotions, which quickly acquire an irresistible power over them. Their general conduct bears the stamp of impulsiveness and rashness; hence, on account of the slight disturbance of intellect, their conduct is often regarded as unscrupulous.

The most striking symptom of all is the *increased psychomotor activity.* The patients feel compelled to be doing something all the time. They must take part in whatever goes on about them. Since the sense of fatigue is diminished, they do not feel the need for rest, so they busy themselves until late at night and are up again early in the morning, bustling about on all sorts of business. They take long walks, devote much time to pleasure, begin a diary, write many letters, undertake long journeys to renew old acquaintances, and do many other things which they never would have thought of before. They suddenly change their occupation, attempt journalism, write verse, purchase property, give away many presents, build castles in the air, and start in numerous undertakings that are beyond both their capital and physical strength. Their actual capacity for work, however, is much diminished. They lack perseverance, become negligent, and apply themselves only to that which is agreeable.

In general demeanor it is obvious that the patients are self-conscious and attempt to attract attention. They dress in a conspicuous manner, and adorn themselves with flowers and cosmetics. Their handwriting is characteristically large and coarse, with a display of many exclamation and interrogation marks and much underlining. In the presence of others they always press forward, seek to assert themselves, talk a great deal, gesticulate, and boast. They are apt to be discourteous and offensive in manner. In spite of deep mourning they indulge in boisterous pleasures. In the presence of women they relate questionable tales. They make free with strangers and persons of high rank, as if they were old friends. Their tendency to indulge in all sorts of extravagances is particularly prominent. They often begin to drink and smoke, remain out late at night, keep questionable company, frequent saloons, and eat excessively of rich foods. Women are particularly apt to show increased sexual desires, and to dress in a striking manner, to attend dances, to read trashy novels, and to fall in love. Not infrequently, betrothals and pregnancies result during such attacks. Patients show extraordinary craftiness in this peculiar and senseless behavior. All attempts on the part of relatives to control them are vain, often irritate the patient, and give rise to passionate outbursts and even aggressiveness.

The disease picture as seen in the individual cases varies considerably. The milder the disease process, the greater the opportunity for the individual's characteristics to enter into the symptom picture. Personal peculiarities are particularly apt to show themselves in the emotional field. While many patients remain amiable, tractable, and approachable, and are troublesome only because of their restlessness, others are extremely disagreeable on account of their imperiousness, irritability, and reckless pressure of activity.

Physical Symptoms. — The number of hours of sleep is cut short by late retiring and early rising, but the actual sleep is profound. The appetite is regularly improved, and the weight may increase. The skin appears healthy, and the movements are strong and elastic.

The *course* in this form is usually uniform. Improvement is very gradual, and often accompanied by remissions. The duration is seldom less than several months, and sometimes lasts over a year. The disease may, however, last for only a few days. This condition often follows mania.

Mania (Tobsucht). — The border line between hypomania and the less severe forms of manic excitement is not always sharply denned. The onset of mania is almost always sudden, following a short period of headache or malaise, although a few days of simple depression may precede the onset. The patients rapidly develop *great psychomotor restlessness, with a pronounced flight of ideas, clouding of consciousness, disorientation, and great impulsiveness. Consciousness* is more or less clouded. This is seen in partial or complete disorientation. Patients know the time and where they are, but they perceive only in a superficial way the events of the environment. They mistake those about them for old acquaintances. Sometimes they designate them as historical personages, as congressmen, public officials, or well-known millionnaires. Apprehension is greatly interfered with by the *extraordinary distractibility:* sounds from the surroundings are caught up and woven into their speech; an object held by the physician, or parts of his clothing, attract the attention and quickly lead the thought in another direction, which is just as abruptly left before the thought is half expressed, aiding in the production of a flight of ideas. Patients understand what is said to them, and are able to give short, correct, and pertinent answers to questions. In this way facts concerning their past lives and occupation can be obtained by piecemeal. Very often a patient shows some *insight* into his disordered condition, admitting that he is crazy and cannot control himself.

In *emotional attitude* the patients are mostly happy and exuberant. Irritability, on the other hand, is very marked. Trifling affairs, such as interference or contradictions, may lead to outbursts of passion with profane abuse, assaults, or destruction of the clothing or other objects. The rapid changes of the emotions are still more characteristic. In the midst of joy they begin to lament and weep at the thought of home, or because of abuse by their nurse. Abrupt changes to a condition of passion and rage are not infrequent.

In the *psychomotor field* there is great activity and excitement. Patients cannot sit or lie still; they run back and forth, dance about, turn handsprings, sing, shout, and prattle incessantly, make all sorts of gestures, tear off clothing, pull down the hair, clap the hands, smear the person and room with grotesque designs, and ornament themselves in the most fantastic manner with clothing which has been torn into strips, as shown in Plate 11. Everything that they can lay their hands upon, from watch to shoes, is taken to pieces. Bits of straw and pieces of stone, glass, and food are hoarded to plaster up a crevice in the wall or to pack a keyhole. In the absence of tobacco all sorts of material are used, — leaves and bits of bread and even dried feces. They are especially apt to cram the nostrils and ears with foreign material, and to carry bits of glass, nails, stones, and nutshells in the mouth. One of my patients secreted a four-inch nail and an extracted tooth in his mouth for months. They are quarrelsome and domineering, or mischievous and playful. Because of great irritability, the most trivial affairs may lead to extreme violence and abuse. Female patients are more apt to show this tendency than male. Sexual excitement is manifest in shameless masturbations, exposure, and demands for intercourse, by indecent attitudes and insinuating remarks.

Some of these cases of mania may show for a longer or shorter period complete dazedness. The patients then apprehend their environment only in a fragmentary manner and are wholly disorientated. There is also great incoherence of speech, often combined with pronounced hallucinations and delusions. The *haUucinations* are usually transitory. Sometimes faces are seen on the wall, shining objects appear on the ceiling, and flash-lights are seen as signals in the sky. Noises are heard, floors creak, locomotives whistle, bells ring, and poisonous vapors are set free in their rooms at night. Sometimes they complain of feeling electric shocks. *Delusions* are mostly expansive, seldom depressive. They are changeable and embellished by numerous fabrications. Patients claim that they are royal personages or generals, that they have supernatural strength, can produce planets, and are related to God, etc. Many of these ideas are recognized by the patients as pure fabrications, are expressed with a laugh, and forgotten the next moment.

Physical Symptoms.—The sleep is usually much disturbed, and the patients may go weeks with almost no sleep. Nutrition suffers in spite of increased appetite, but food is taken hurriedly and irregularly. There often occur attacks of syncope, and sometimes even convulsive attacks of a hysteroid character. The heart's activity is usually increased and the pulse slowed, while the blood pressure is diminished. The urine is found to show a striking diminution of the phosphates, while calcium and magnesium are increased. The quantity of urine also is often increased. Pilcz has shown that both in the manic and depressive phases there is excreted an abnormal amount of acetone, diacetic acid, indocan, and albumoses, which, however, bear no definite relation to the intensity of the symptoms.

Course. — The height of the disease is usually reached in the course of a week or two, and in some cases within a few days. The intensity of the symptoms is fairly uniform, with only slight fluctuations. Occasionally there may appear a sorrowful and depressed emotional condition, with disappearance of the motor activity, or even a transient stupor, indicating a transitory depressive state. Genuine improvement is very gradual; furthermore, for some time after the return of comparative clearness, the patients are apt, under strain, to show a flight of ideas and some increased activity. Even after apparent complete recovery, trying conditions, reverses and misfortunes, and more often intoxication can cause a recurrence of the symptoms. The duration varies considerably, from a few weeks and even days to many months, and sometimes two or three years. The usual duration is many months. Some cases extend over several years. The cases with many delusions and those with exacerbations of excitement last longer.

Delirious Mania. — This, the extreme of the manic states, is characterized by *pronounced dreamy clouding of consciousness, intense psychomotor activity, great incoherence of speech, a marked flight of ideas, numerous hallucinations, and dreamlike delusions.*

These cases are very rare, and there is a question if they really belong to manic-depressive insanity. The onset is sudden, following a few days of indisposition, uneasiness, and insomnia. The patients suddenly develop the greatest possible restlessness with many hallucinations, which are present in all of the sensory fields: they see beautiful sights, strange faces, and scenes of torture; hear distant music, ringing bells, cannonading, and the roar of wild animals. Their food has a peculiar odor and taste, and small objects crawl on the skin. They see fire and hear the crackling timbers. Everything is changed. At the same time manifold, confused, and dreamlike *delusions* appear, both of an expansive and of a depressive nature: they are the " chosen ones," have been elected Presidents, have wonderful power, can create and destroy nations, possess millions; they have lost all friends, are to be murdered, must enter hell, have been taken to an immense height, and are now to be cast into the sea, etc.

From the first the *consciousness* is greatly clouded, and disorientation is almost complete. The patients are thoroughly confused as to time, place, and persons; they mistake their environment, and even their friends.

Their *speech* is incoherent, abounding in sound associations, rhymes, and numerous repetitions of single syllables and phrases, in which one can always detect many fragmentary references to objects in their environment. *Attention* usually cannot be attracted except momentarily, when a fragment of the desired response can be detected in the incoherent speech. Striking objects, such as a penny dropped on the floor, will divert the attention and the train of thought for a moment.

As to the *emotional attitude,* the patients show various changes between extreme happiness and profound distress, ecstatic joy and timidity, exuberance and apathy. Irritability is very marked.

In the *psychomotor field* the patients exhibit, from the beginning, signs of the most extreme excitement. They run about shouting and singing, disrobing, destroying everything within reach, and they become recklessly violent and smear themselves. Occasionally they impulsively attempt suicide. At one moment they are praying, at the next cursing with the vilest language, or singing an obscene song; at one time they are insulting in speech and action, and a minute later are profuse in apologies and distastefully affectionate. They chatter away, scream and stamp their feet, pound the window or door, race about at the greatest speed, mount the furniture and declaim in a loud voice with profuse and exaggerated gestures.

Physical Symptoms. — The state of nutrition suffers profoundly because of the small amount of food taken and the excessive expenditure of energy. Occasionally there is a general muscular tremor. Sleep is greatly disturbed, and at the height of the disease is entirely lacking; the pulse is accelerated and the reflexes are exaggerated. Sometimes the conjunctivas are injected, and the vessels of the head and face distended. Occasionally there is profuse perspiration.

Course. — The height of the attack is quickly reached, usually within a few days or weeks, and the symptoms begin to abate at the third or fourth week. Brief intervals of composure often occur for a few minutes or a few hours, during which the consciousness remains clouded. The improvement may be rapid, *i.e.* over night, but usually is gradual. For some time the patients, although clear, usually retain residuals of their hallucinations, delusions, and peculiarities of conduct, and are especially inclined to be irritable and distrustful. But even these signs entirely disappear in the course of a few weeks. There is rarely any memory for the events of the acute stage of the psychosis. The disease may terminate fatally as the result of exhaustion, injuries, fat embolism of the lungs, or intercurrent infections.

It very often happens that following a manic attack the patients exhibit a low-spirited condition with more or less general weakness, which sometimes is regarded as a sort of reaction, but which really represents a transition into a characteristic depressed phase. These patients tire very easily, and are unable to apply themselves to either physical or mental work, are despondent, worry about the future, are reticent, sluggish, and indecisive. These symptoms gradually disappear with the increase of weight. In some instances, where the condition is more severe, there may remain a permanent lack of judgment and insight, some emotional irritability, and also restlessness.

Depressive States

The depressive states comprise *simple retardation* and the *delusional form.*

The mildest form of the depressive states is characterized by the presence of *simple retardation unaccompanied by any hallucinations or delusions,* and is, therefore, termed simple retardation.

The onset is generally gradual, except in a few cases which follow acute illness or mental shock. There appears gradually a sort of mental sluggishness: mental processes become retarded, thought is difficult, and patients find difficulty in coming to a decision, in forming sentences, and in finding words with which to express themselves. It is hard for them to follow the thought in reading or ordinary conversation. The process of *association of ideas* is remarkably retarded; the patients do not talk, because they have nothing to say; there is a dearth of ideas and a poverty of thought. Familiar facts are no longer at their command, and it is hard to remember the most commonplace things.

In spite of this great slowness of apprehension and thought, consciousness and *orientation* are well retained. Patients appear dull and sluggish, and explain that they really feel tired and exhausted. They sit about as if benumbed, with folded hands and bowed head, exhibiting no initiative and rarely uttering a word voluntarily. What is said is uttered in low, inexpressive tones. Customary actions, such as walking, dressing, and eating, are performed very slowly, as if under constraint. When started for a walk, they halt at the doorway or at the first turning-point, undecided which way to go. Their usual duties loom before them as huge tasks, because they lack strength to overcome the retardation, and anything new appears unsurmountable. Sometimes they become bedridden. Because of this extreme retardation, the patients rarely commit suicide, although they often express the desire to die. Attempts at suicide are more to be feared when the retardation has disappeared, and while the despondency still persists.

In the *emotional attitude* there is a uniform depression. The patient sees only the dark side of life. The past and the future are alike, full of unhappiness and misfortune. Life has lost its charm; they are unsuited to their environment, are a failure in their profession, have lost religious faith, and live from day to day in gloomy submission to their fate. Everything is spoiled for them; they take no pleasure in life and do not care to live longer. They are ill-humored, gloomy, shy, sometimes pettish or anxious, and sometimes irritable and sullen. They fear business reverses and begin to economize, even denying themselves and their families the necessaries of life.

Sometimes numerous *compulsive ideas* appear. Patients feel compelled, against their will, to ponder over certain things, and to busy themselves with depicting unpleasant scenes. Others worry themselves over the thoughts of how they might be martyred or torn limb from limb. Even compulsions to act

arise, such as to commit injury or to set fire.

Insight is frequently present, the patients appreciating that a change has come over them. This very often is characteristically expressed as a *feeling of inadequacy*. The patients say: " I am not sick, I am only lacking a will of my own." "I can't pull myself together." "I have no energy, I can't get hold of myself." "I feel all gone and I can't make up my mind to do anything." Sometimes the recurring sadness is ascribed to external influences, such as, unpleasant experiences, changes in the environment, etc.

The condition of retardation may, at some time during the course of the psychosis, become so pronounced as to produce a condition of *stupor.* Patients then lie abed perfectly dumb, unable to comprehend their surroundings, or to understand even simple questions. There is no particular emotional change to be noted, except occasionally when a look of anxiety or perplexity flits across the countenance. Voluntarily, the patients almost never speak. If able to answer questions, their responses are exceedingly slow. They sit helplessly before their meals, allowing themselves to be fed by spoon, and holding firmly whatever may be pressed into their hands. These patients are unable to care for themselves, but are not filthy. This condition of stupor tends to disappear rapidly, and leaves no memory of the events of the period.

Simple retardation runs a rather uniform *course,* with few variations. The improvement is gradual, and the duration varies from a few months to over a year.

A second group of depressive cases has been termed the delusional form, which is characterized by *the presence of varied depreciatory delusions, especially of self-accusation and of a hypochondriacal nature, in addition to the evidences of retardation.*

The *onset* of this form is usually subacute, following a period of indisposition, and occasionally even a short period of exhilaration and buoyancy of spirits; a few cases appear after an acute illness or mental shock.

The patients become profoundly despondent, and indulge in all sorts of *self-accusations.* They feel that they have been great sinners, have neglected their duties and made many enemies, have never done anything right, and their whole life has been one long series of mistakes. They accuse themselves of bringing misfortune on others or of causing some great calamity. They claim that they are devoid of feeling and sympathy for others. They feel that they are being watched, fear arrest and imprisonment, they must die, are to be poisoned or shot. Others hold them in derision, laugh, and jeer at them. Their families are incriminated by their misdeeds, and are suffering imprisonment. They have lost everything, and will be driven into the street with their families, to wander about in utter misery.

Hypochondriacal delusions are prominent and are usually associated with numerous false bodily sensations: their health is ruined as the result of masturbation; they are succumbing to some malignant disease, and their organs are wasting away; cloudy urine signifies profound disease of the kidneys; they can never recover, and their body and face are altered. Female patients complain of being pregnant, and often accuse themselves of immorality and masturbation.

These various delusions often become absurd and fantastic. A common delusion is that everything about them is altered: their home is not their own; their friends and relatives have disappeared forever; they do not belong to this world; they themselves are changed, are but a skeleton without life, they cannot live and cannot die. Though struck on the head or pierced in the heart, they would still live on. *Their* heart has ceased to beat; their stomach and intestines are entirely gone; there are no feces; they are full to the throat with decomposing food; their skin is all dried up; their bones are softening, etc.

Hallucinations are occasionally associated with this condition, when groans and moans are heard, disagreeable odors permeate the room, terrible apparitions appear at night, and fearful scenes are depicted.

The *consciousness* is for the most part unclouded, and the patients are usually oriented, and comprehend correctly what transpires in their environment, although occasionally they develop some delusional ideas in reference to the home or institution and the persons around them. They understand questions and answer coherently, but the content of thought and *speech* shows a constant tendency to revert to their depressive delusions. Thought is retarded, as shown in their attempts to write letters or to solve a problem.

Insight into the condition is very often present, yet while admitting recovery from previous similar attacks, they declare that their present condition is so much worse that they can never recover. Some of these patients go to an institution of their own accord. The *emotional attitude* is uniformly one of depression. The patients are dejected, gloomy, and perplexed, and lament for hours in monotonous tones. They say little to those about them, but sit staring into space and paying very little attention to their environment. It, however, becomes evident during the visits of friends and relatives that they are not only not apathetic, but capable of showing considerable feeling. *Psychomotor retardation* of thought and action is evident in their dearth of ideas, their silence, and slow and hesitating replies to questions, their sluggish and languid movements, their lack of independent activity and inability to apply themselves to mental work. Some patients at times exhibit anxious restlessness, pacing up and down the room, swaying the body or rocking uneasily in a chair, picking at the clothing or rubbing some part of the body. Suicidal attempts are not infrequent. *Stuporous states* may also develop in this delusional type of depressive cases. The patients then develop a condition of befogged consciousness, in which almost no external impressions are apprehended and consciousness is dominated by numerous variegated and incoherent delusions and hallucinations. Everything appears changed in the most fan-

tastic manner; the whole world is being consumed by fire or congealed into ice. They themselves are removed from everybody, have been taken up into a cloud and carried off to the farthest point of the universe, and left there alone. They are to be shoved off into space, where they will keep falling forever, or they are crowded into a narrow grave from which they can never escape. The walls of the room are closing in upon them, and passing troops have arrived to attend their execution. Crowds jeer at them; they are made to wear a crown of thorns, or are turned loose to run naked in the street. Everything about them has a most mysterious aspect; they are in the midst of historical personages, and are made to do penance for the whole world. They have been transformed in a most horrible manner, are of a different sex, are swollen to the size of a cask, have two heads, the body of a serpent, and the feet of an elephant. While in this dreamy state their *retardation* is shown by their inability to speak, to feed themselves, or to care for themselves in any way. They do not show active feelings, but lie stupidly in bed, are inaccessible and indifferent. An occasional anxious expression, the resistance to passive movements, peculiar postures, and unexpected, impulsive attempts at suicide betray their anxiety and fear. Sometimes a few words or sentences are uttered very slowly and in low tones. These stuporous states disappear gradually, but even after consciousness has become clear, a few hallucinations and delusions usually persist for some time.

There are a few cases which present coherent delusions of persecution accompanied by many hallucinations with clear consciousness. The hallucinations play a rather important part and persist for a long time, reminding one very much of acute alcoholic hallucinosis, save for the psychomotor retardation.

Physical Symptoms. — The patients complain of numbness in the head, ringing in the ears, dizziness, palpitation, chilliness in the neck, heaviness in the limbs, and of a feeling as if there was a weight upon the chest. The appetite is

poor, the tongue coated, and the bowels constipated. There is usually a strong aversion to food, and it often requires considerable urging to administer sufficient nourishment. The sleep is much broken and disturbed by anxious dreams. The facial expression and the general attitude are sleepy and languid, the speech low, the eyes lustreless, the skin sallow and without its accustomed firmness. The body weight always sinks. Respiration and cardiac activity are weakened and slower, and blood pressure is increased, while the pulse is slow. The quantity of urine is diminished as well as the excretion of urea, phosphoric acid, and magnesia. The height of the disturbance is reached in a few weeks and runs a shorter *course* than the manic states.

Mixed States'

In these states *there occur simultaneously varying combinations of some of the fundamental symptoms characteristic of both the manic and depressive phases of the disease.*

The mixed states are most clearly seen during the transition periods when patients pass from a manic to a depressive phase or *vice versa*. At these times all the symptoms of one phase do not disappear simultaneously, so that symptoms of the depressive phase develop before all of the symptoms of the manic disappear. For instance, the characteristic manic flight of ideas may have given way to typical retardation of thought, while there still remains emotional elation and pressure of activity. A few days farther along in this transition period, we find that there still is some elation, but retardation of activity has also developed. Later still, and the elation has given way to depression, and we have the typical picture of the depressive phase. In another case during this transition period, the emotional elation may be the first symptom to subside and pass into despondency, while there still remain pressure of activity and flight of ideas. In a few days the flight of ideas also has gone over into retardation of thought, while there is still some pressure of activity. Farther along, we find the pressure of activity replaced by retardation and the typical depressive picture. All together there have thus far been recognized six chief types of mixed states.

(1) Irascible mania, in which a depressed emotional state replaces the usual elation. These are the cases of pronounced manic excitement in which the patients exhibit a more or less constant irritability; they heap abuse upon the environment, and become passionately angry and even aggressive upon the slightest provocation. If the excitement is not quite so pronounced, there is produced the picture of the *grumbling mania,* in which the patients show a feeling of somewhat increased self-confidence, but without elation. They are dissatisfied, intolerant, perhaps a little anxious, have some fault to find with everything, always feel that they are mistreated, are served poor food, and have to sleep on a wretched bed. They have a facility for offending and vexing others, and for instigating trouble for every one about them. Each day they have a new complaint, and become irritable if they are not heeded. The fundamental manic symptoms are seen in the moderate flight of ideas, the great instability, and restlessness. Weygandt, Ueber die Mischzustaende des manisch-depressiven Irreseins. Habilitationsschrift, 1899. (2) Depressive excitement comprises those depressive cases in which the restlessness is out of all proportion to the intensity of their emotional despondency. These patients talk incessantly, but always about the same thing; they torment themselves and their environment by the same old complaints; they are forever expressing the same delusional ideas, mostly of a hypochondriacal nature and usually in the same phraseology. They complain that they have been mistreated, have been poisoned, can never recover, and are going to die, but at the same time they are not especially anxious or sad, and they are able to apply themselves without fatigue. They may even, for short periods, make humorous or sarcastic remarks, and show some irritability and aggressiveness. (3) Unproductive mania is the manic state with dearth of ideas. This form is often encountered. The patients are very slow and inaccurate in perceiving. One often has to repeat a question several times before they understand it. They don't pay attention, give many false and evasive answers. They give one the impression that they are weak-minded, but later they prove themselves to be quite intellectual. This condition of unproductive mania fluctuates considerably; at one time the patients may temporarily give ready answers, while at another it is impossible to get anything out of them.

The emotional attitude is one of elation, happiness, and exuberance; they laugh readily and without sufficient cause and make fun over every little thing. Then speech is incoherent and the content limited. They speak slowly and do not have much to say; indeed, if left to themselves, they remain speechless for long periods. It is characteristic of the thinking difficulty to be more intense at the beginning of an interview, but as the conversation is prolonged, the patients gradually develop considerable pressue of speech. There is always present an increased emotional irritability. The pressure of activity is usually confined to grimacing, occasional dancing around, changing the clothing, and fussing with the hair, but the patients never show the restless busyness so characteristic of mania. Many of these patients ordinarily conduct themselves so well and quietly that a superficial examination fails to reveal any excitement. Nevertheless, they are in an elated frame of mind, at times showing irritability; they are tractable or rude, and often break out in boisterous laughter. Other patients are inactive and sit around, but upon the slightest provocation they laugh uproariously, or, for no apparent reason, become saucy. They are incapable of any orderly employment, but are rather given to all sorts of mischievous tricks, stealing and hoarding a lot of things, tearing up papers and clothing and tying knots in them, plugging up keyholes, and pasting paper designs all over the walls. Sometimes they suddenly burst out in great anger. Also, they may show transient periods of genuine mania with flight of ideas and pronounced pressure of activity.

(4) Manic stupor is the depressive state in which emotional elation takes the place of the usual despondency. The patients are quite unapproachable; they do not bother themselves about their environment, will not answer questions, laugh without apparent cause, he quietly in bed, sometimes all rolled up in the clothing, or dress them up in a fantastic manner, but all of this is done without evidence of restlessness or emotional agitation. Sometimes a few changeable delusions are expressed. They are usually well oriented. Occasionally catalepsy is present. In the midst of this stupor the patients suddenly develop great activity, rush about, disrobe, tear their clothing, destroy furniture, smear their food, sing and talk loudly and freely, often making bright and striking remarks, and then after a few hours as quickly return to the previous state. At other times one finds them quiet, perfectly clear and intelligent in conversation, but this is only for short periods. Many patients pace about in measured steps, never speak except to make an occasional witty remark, or rub up against the doctor in an erotic manner, and laugh. These patients often have a good memory for what occurs, but they are wholly unable to explain their peculiar conduct. In some cases the facial expression is fixed and staring, in others it is more cheerful, happy, and amorous.

Manic stupor often develops for a short time in a pronounced manic state, but it more frequently represents a transition state between a depressive stupor and a manic state.

(5) Depression with a Flight of Ideas. — These depressive cases are easily aroused when they can show a facility of thought. They read a good deal, show interest in and comprehend their environment, and, indeed, even evince some curiosity, in spite of the fact that they are retarded in their general attitude, are almost mute, and are despondent. These patients tell us as soon as they begin to talk again that they could not control their thoughts, that a whole host of things would come into their minds

which they had never thought of before. It seems, therefore, that there really exists a flight of ideas which, however, is not apparent to others because of the retardation of the movements of articulation. Some of these patients cannot express themselves orally, but can write, and often astonish one with their numerous productions, containing delusional ideas of persecution and fear. (6) Finally there is the depressive state with flight of ideas and emotional elation. These patients are happy, sometimes somewhat irritable, are distractible, prone to witty remarks, and are easily aroused during conversation to a flight of ideas and at times even sound associations, but in general their demeanor is quiet. They he quietly in bed, and now and then interpolate a remark or laugh loudly. Nevertheless there seems to exist an inner tension, because the patients can suddenly become very violent.

The mixed states occur most frequently in the transition periods from manic to depressive states and *vice versa*. Indeed, it is only by the history of their development and their transition into the well-known phases of the disease that we are able to recognize them as mixed phases and as a type of manic-depressive insanity. This observation is of especial importance in those cases in which mixed states almost wholly replace the typical manic and depressive phases. In such cases the recognition of the disease, particularly in the first attack, is extremely difficult, if not impossible.

Course. — The course of manic-depressive insanity is marked by a recurrence of attacks separated by lucid intervals. With but very few exceptions, attacks recur throughout the life of the individual, appearing with greater frequency between the ages of eighteen to thirty and forty to fifty. In five per cent. of cases the attacks from the first pass directly from one phase into another, sometimes with such regularity that the name " alternating insanity " has been applied to them, or if short intervals of lucidity have intervened, "circular insanity." If only one or two attacks occur during the life of an individual, the separate attacks are in no way essentially different from those recurring frequently. It seldom happens that all are of the same type; at some time or other a depressive attack is sure to appear. On the other hand, one patient during life may suffer from all possible forms, from hypomania to profound stupor.

The first attack in sixty per cent. of the cases is depressive. This is especially true in women, and when the disease develops early in life. The first depressive attack usually runs a mild course, and in about fifty per cent. of the cases is followed immediately by a lucid interval. In the other fifty per cent. of the cases it is immediately followed by a manic attack, which in turn is followed by a lucid interval. A first manic attack is almost always followed by a lucid interval, seldom by a depressive attack. If the first attack is manic, the majority of the succeeding attacks are manic. Similarly, several depressive attacks may recur before a manic attack appears; in other words, the occurrence of several attacks of one type to the exclusion of other types indicates that the greater number of attacks throughout life will be of the same character. Later in the course of the disease there may be a regular alternation between manic and depressive attacks. After a long duration of the disease there is more apt to be a regular alternation from one type to the other, if the early attacks have been mostly of one type. The mixed forms usually do not appear until after two or more manic or depressive attacks.

The *duration* of the individual attack may vary from a few days to five years, but the usual duration is from six to twelve months. The depressive attacks average longer. The first attacks rarely last longer than a few months. In the circular type of the disease it has been observed that hypomania usually alternates with simple retardation, while severe manic states are followed by deep stupor, and again, when delusions and hallucinations occur in the manic states, they are usually also present in the depressive states.

The *lucid intervals* vary considerably in length, from a few days or weeks to many years, and stand in no definite relation to the duration of the attacks. They are apt, however, to be longer at the beginning and shorter as the attacks recur, until finally they may disappear altogether, the attacks then passing directly from one into another. At the beginning of the disease the intervals are usually of at least one or more years' duration. Sometimes the intervals are of such a definite duration that the patients know just when to expect the attacks. The intervals tend to become shorter during the climacterium and to lengthen out again later. Sometimes, especially in young females, the disease begins with a series of several short attacks with brief intervals, which are then followed by a prolonged interval of several years. In the small group of cases in which from the beginning the attacks succeed each other without lucid intervals, the type of the attack is usually light, mostly hypomania and simple retardation. Sometimes, even after a long series of such recurring attacks, there may appear a long lucid interval.

During the intervals the patients are perfectly lucid, except in a few cases where the attacks are long, frequent, and severe. They are able to reenter the family, to employ themselves profitably, and to return to their profession. The few who do not thoroughly recover are also usually able to return home, but are apt to show some restraint, lack of independence, a tendency to be morose, an unusual susceptibility to fatigue, some sleepiness, and a diminished capacity for work, or they may be irritable, quarrelsome, markedly egotistical, or unstable and easily excitable. During the interval some of the patients fail to show a thorough appreciation of their disease. They will admit that they have been " excited and nervous," but attribute it to some family trouble or confinement.

It very often happens that during the intervals the patients may suddenly develop short periods of moderate exhilaration, flightiness, irritability, and unusual activity, or on the other hand, they may be unnaturally apprehensive, suspicious, despondent, inactive, and indifferent. These symptoms disappear abruptly, and without the history of other attacks might not be recognized as disease symptoms.

The *transition* from a manic to a depressive phase, and *vice versa,* is usually gradual, though it may be sudden, often occurring during the night. In this transition the stages of alteration are usually quite perceptible. At first the countenance of the depressed patient becomes more illuminated and the eyes appear brighter and the skin firmer and more elastic. The patient is more affable, shows more interest in the surroundings, and expresses a desire for freedom. His activity, at first increasing slowly, now becomes prominent; he is busy all the time, is happy, never felt better in his life, and everything pleases. From this time the manic state becomes quite evident. The manic patient at first gradually loses weight, the pressure of activity abates, he is calmer and more in earnest, his many schemes recede to the background and then entirely disappear. Soon his movements become languid, he himself is seclusive, talks less, only occasionally mentioning his ill-feelings and misfortunes. His countenance loses its freshness, and at last we have a typical depressive state.

Diagnosis. — There is usually little difficulty in recognizing the psychosis, where there has been a previous attack; yet the occurrence of more than one attack is by no means pathognomic of manic-depressive insanity, as it may happen in dementia praecox, especially in the catatonic form, in paresis, melancholia, and in amentia.

It is difficult to distinguish between the mildest forms of manic-depressive insanity and certain *morbid personal peculiarities* which manifest themselves chiefly as a more or less regular vacillation of the emotional state. The manicdepressive periods of ill-humor on the one hand, and of impetuous exhilaration on the other, are sometimes mistaken as simple whims and ascribed to all sorts of deleterious influences, or they are apt to be designated as *hysteria, neurasthenia,* and *hypochondriasis,* since it is only in the depressive states that the patients are considered ill. These same patients themselves, however, often have insight into their periods of excitement and dread their approach. Usually the true nature of the disease is disclosed by the transition from one phase to another, and by the periodic recurrence of different phases. The simple lack of decision— the inability of the depressive patients to come to a conclusion — is so characteristic that it alone often suffices in making the diagnosis. These borderline cases are numerous, and are often encountered in sanitaria.

In the mild forms of the manic states, when one sees the patient in the first attack and is without a history of the patient's life, it is often difficult to distinguish the patients from some normal individuals. The distinction depends chiefly upon the fact that the increased busyness and activity is not uniform, but shows variations. In the forms of *constitutional mania* there are also noticeable aggravations of the condition and regular transitions into opposite moods. Such patients, because of their frequent conflicts with their environment and the law, are usually considered swindlers and vagabonds, or are regarded as morally insane. In addition to the vacillations, the clinical picture also shows an attitude of overconfidence, an irritability, a lack of plan in their excessive busyness, an excessive emotional irritability, and a lack of criminal tendencies.

The differentiation of the disease from the *exhaustion psychoses* and from the excited stages of the catatonic and hebephrenic forms of dementia praecox will be found fully detailed in the differential diagnosis of those diseases.

The manic forms are differentiated from *hysterical excitement* by the presence of the flight of ideas, pressure of activity, the exuberant emotional state, and the great distractibility. The hysterical excitement comes in the form of brief separate attacks with definite outbursts of temper. Hysterical excitement usually subsides quickly and completely after a very short duration.

It is more difficult to distinguish simple retardation from the initial period of *depression* in *dementia præcox.* In the manic-depressive patients the psychomotor retardation, with slowness of movement, low tone of voice, difficulty of thought with sparsity of ideas, slowness of application of attention, and slight clouding of consciousness, stands out in contrast to the absence of retardation, freedom of movements and thought, and to the clearness of consciousness in dementia praecox. Rapid appearance of senseless delusions and numerous hallucinations without clouding of consciousness speak for dementia praecox.

The differentiation of the depressive states from *dementia paralytica* and *melancholia* have been discussed under these psychoses.

Acquired neurasthenia is sufficiently differentiated from the depressed forms under that disease.

The unproductive mania is often mistaken for *imbecility urith excitement,* but can be distinguished by the evidences of flight of ideas and the manic demeanor of the patients with only moderate restlessness.

Manic stupor sometimes must be differentiated from *catatonia.* If, in manic stupor, the patients struggle, the cause for it lies in the irritable, fretful disposition which almost always leads to abuse and violence. Again, the patients pay more attention to their environment, and are influenced in their actions by circumstances, in contradistinction to the stupid or wilful indifference of the catatonic. Furthermore, the manic-stuporous patient displays a poverty of thought and not a stereotyped and senseless speech production. The movements of the catatonic are apt to be planless, impulsive, and with a uniform pressure of movement, while in stuporous mania they are purposeful, playful, and adapted to the environment.

Prognosis. — The prognosis of the disease is unfavorable in view of the certainty of recurrence of the attacks throughout the life of the individual. It is favorable for recovery from the individual attacks, except in five per cent. of cases, which from the onset pass directly from one attack into another. While, with this exception, there are almost certain to be other attacks and recoveries, the frequency of their recurrence and the duration of the lucid intervals is wholly uncertain. At present we have no means of judging just what the future course will be. In general it may be said, however, that it is safe to predict frequent recurrence of attacks with short intervals where the psychosis manifests itself early and without external cause. On the other hand, if the first attack occurs late and following some external cause, such as childbirth, there probably will be but few attacks. If pronounced mixed states predominate, the disease will probably be more severe. If the onset is previous to the period of involution, one should expect a recurrence during the climacterium.

Mental deterioration occurs in only a few cases, where the attacks appear during the period of development and are long, frequent, and severe. Even these patients in the intervals are conscious, well oriented, and retain a very good memory. They simply show some indifference, irritability, an increased susceptibility to alcohol, and slight deficiency in judgment. There are a few cases that have very long manic attacks, lasting even ten years and more, which have been designated *chronic mania.* This condition is not one of dementia, but one in which there are incomplete remissions. If observed carefully, these cases usually present not only manic states of varying intensity, but also evidences of depressive and mixed states. Furthermore, it is usually found that even in the lucid intervals the patients have always been somewhat unstable, freakish, irritable, or have been schemers and incapable of any consistent and productive employment. These cases are better termed *constitutional mania.*

There is a corresponding series of transitions from the depressive states. There are manic cases which in the intervals are shy, low spirited, and slow to make up their minds. This defective constitution is more characteristic in those individuals who suffer from periodic depressive states. Finally there are cases in which the separate attacks of periodical ill-humor present themselves without sharp differentiation, and are simple aggravations of a *constitutional depression.* Arteriosclerosis, or marked senile changes, developing during the course of manic-depressive insanity, usually lead to states of dementia which obliterate the original mental picture.

Treatment. — The disease, being deeply rooted in the personality of the individual, offers little chance to eradicate the underlying causes. Individuals who seem to be predisposed to the disease certainly derive benefit from leading a careful life under favorable conditions and abstaining absolutely from the use of alcohol. Such persons should not marry.

Individuals suffering from frequently and regularly recurring attacks can sometimes ward off an approaching attack by the use of large doses of the bromides, even up to three hundred and sixty grains a day for a few days before the anticipated attack. Atropia, hypodermically, or belladonna in the form of the extract in full doses, is highly recommended for the same purpose. In those cases in which the attacks tend to develop during pregnancy or puerperium, artificial abortion has occasionally been performed for the purpose of either warding off the attack or cutting it short. Kraepelin himself has not derived much benefit from this procedure, but finds that, in spite of abortion, the disease recurs and runs its regular course. In all such cases measures should be adopted for the prevention of pregnancy. Individuals who have already suffered from an attack of the disease should be compelled to lead a quiet life, free from irritating influences. The susceptibility to alcohol is increased, hence its use should be most scrupulously avoided.

In the treatment of the patient during the manic attacks, the first essential is the removal of all forms of external excitation. Except in the mild cases, it is unsatisfactory to attempt to care for the patient at home, and even the milder forms run a more moderate course under the influence of a quiet and well-regulated hospital or sanitarium environment than at home. Unrestrained activity tends to increase the excitement; therefore the pressure of activity should be limited as much as possible. One of the best means of accomplishing this is confinement in bed. Bed treatment is especially indicated in anemic and debilitated cases.

In *severe excitement* prolonged warm baths (see p. 140), used in connection with the bed treatment, give the most satisfactory results. The patients should alternate from the bath to the bed; *i. e.* when the excitement subsides in the bath, he can be returned to the bed until it reappears. It may be necessary in order to first introduce the patient to the bath to give a preliminary dose of hyoscin hydrobromate (j to grain). The prolonged warm bath properly applied will often relieve the greatest excitement, and usually renders medicinal treatment unnecessary. If the bath is not available, the use of hyoscin hydrobromate hypodermically, or by mouth, is the best remedy for subduing the intense psychomotor activity. Scopolamin hydrobromate *(hf* to *.£$* grain) or paraldehyde may be substituted for the hyoscin. As the excitement permanently subsides, confinement in bed can be gradually relaxed and the patient given an opportunity to exercise in the open. In very extreme excitement with impending collapse the administration of whiskey or brandy or camphor is necessary, and in the case of coexisting cardiac weakness, digitalis or caffein should be added. The general management of the patient is usually a very important adjuvant in controlling the excitement. This requires the greatest amount of tact and patience on the part of the nurse; gentle friendliness at suitable moments sometimes renders what appears to be a most dangerous patient quite tractable. The nurse must exercise self-control, be free from all prejudice, avoid the use of discipline, and above all be frank and truthful.

The *nutrition* of the patients demands special attention. An abundance of nutritious and easily digested food should be given the patients at regular intervals. They should not be allowed to gulp their food, and hence it usually requires the constant attendance of the nurse at meal-time. Because of the great restlessness, it often requires considerable patience to get an excited patient to take sufficient nourishment. In severe cases the patients should be weighed frequently in order to ascertain if the body weight is falling off, and, where necessary, artificial feeding by stomach or nasal tube can be employed.

It is very often a difficult matter to determine just when manic patients have recovered sufficiently to be discharged from treatment. Because of their great importunity and impatience to be set free, there is a tendency to discharge them while some symptoms still remain. One of the dangers in premature release is the tendency to alcoholic indulgence, which regularly leads to a recurrence of the symptoms. The safest guide in deciding this question may be found in the body weight, which should have returned to normal.

In the *depressed states* the patients should at once be given the benefit of the rest treatment with confinement in bed and ample feeding. Except in debilitated and anemic cases, the patient should be permitted to leave the bed for a short period during the day to take exercise in the open. If this is not feasible, massage should be administered. The rest treatment taken in the open on a shielded but sunny porch should always be tried in preference to indoor confinement. If there is great agitation, opium in increasing doses (see p. 362) is often given with benefit.

The *insomnia* should be controlled, if possible, by the aid of the various physical measures, such as, hot baths at night, hot liquid nourishment upon retiring, gentle massage, etc. Failing with these, one may employ on alternate days and for short periods trional 15 grains, veronal *1* grains, or paraldehyde 1 to 2 drachms. During prolonged periods of administration, these hypnotics should be varied.

The *nutrition* also demands careful attention, for which purpose the patient should be frequently weighed. The food should be carefully selected and easily digestible. Abstinence from food often requires artificial feeding by nasal or stomach tube. The relief of constipation, which often exists, usually improves the appetite.

The patient must be relieved from all forms of excitation, and visits from relatives, long conversations, letter-writing, etc., should be avoided. Rational conversation and encouragement is helpful, except at the height of the disease, when it sometimes seems to be aggravating. In the lighter cases hypnotic suggestion has been used to great advantage in relieving the insomnia, despondency, and disagreeable somatic sensations. The greatest care must be exercised to prevent suicidal attempts, which are often to be most guarded against at times when the patients, though still convalescing, believe themselves recovered, and also in the transition periods between attacks.

X. PARANOIA

Paranoia is *a chronic progressive psychosis occurring mostly in early adult life, characterized by the gradual development of a stable progressive system of delusions, without marked mental deterioration, clouding of consciousness, or disorder of thought, will, or conduct.*

Etiology. — The disease is uncommon, constituting only one to four per cent. of the cases admitted to insane hospitals. Men are more often afflicted than women. The disease begins between the ages of twenty-five and forty. It develops on a defective constitutional basis, either congenital or acquired, defective heredity existing in a very large percentage of the cases. Peculiar traits and eccentricities may be recognized early in life, the patients being moody, dreamy, or seclusive. Some show perverted sexual instincts, or a marked aptitude for study or mental activity in special, limited fields. Some have been abnormally bright; others have always been flighty, entering into many projects which they were unable to pursue successfully; many show stigmata of degeneration. Exciting causes occasionally form the starting-point of the psychosis, such as an acute illness, excessive mental stress, shock, business reverses, deprivation, and disappointment.

Snell, Allgem. Zeitschr. f. Psy., XXII, 368; Griesinger, Archiv. f. Psy., I, 148; Sander, *ibid.*, 387; Westphal, Allgem. Zeitschr. f. Psy., XXXIV, 252; Mercklin, Studien liber prim (ire Verrilckheit, 1879; Amadie e Tonnini, Archivio italiano per le malattie nervose, 1884, 1, 2; Werner, Die Paranoia, 1891; Schttle, Allgem. Zeitschr. f. Psy., L, 1 u. 2; Cramer, *ibid.*, LI, 2; Sandberg, *ibid.,* LII, 619.

There is as yet no demonstrable, pathological, anatomical basis peculiar to paranoia.

Symptomatology. — The development of the psychosis is very gradual, extending sometimes over years, and is usually so insidious that the disease is in existence long before it is recognized. During this period it may have been noticed that the patient had changed in disposition, having become somewhat irritable, grumbling, suspicious, and easily discontented, and that he had made indefinite physical complaints, especially of malaise and insomnia.

The first symptom to be noticed is that the daily mental or manual labor becomes distasteful, and little affairs at home or in the shop cause displeasure and arouse suspicion. The wife seems less attentive, the children less loving, shopmates less friendly, and the overseer more stern. The accidental absence of the morning greeting, or imaginary slight on the part of a close friend, sets the patient to thinking that it cannot all be accidental. He becomes distrustful, is constantly seeking other evidences of unfriendliness, and careful watching soon satisfies him that he is neglected, both at home and at work. He begins to make complaints, accuses his friends of slights, and members of his fraternity of plots. He leaves his employment, holds aloof from his companions and friends, and often becomes rude and discourteous. Some patients are able to ignore for a time the apparent indifference of friends, but others become much disturbed and suspect a malicious purpose. They are morbidly sensitive, considering that such trifles as harmless jokes, smiles, or accidental nods of the head have special reference to themselves. Items in the paper indicate some intrigue, bill posters contain hints, some daily passer always lights his cigar or coughs when near them; men similarly dressed always meet them near the same corner, or are shadowing their footsteps. Any doubts as to an evident purpose in all this are sooner or later dispelled by remarks accidentally overheard. In this way false interpretations gradually assume greater prominence, and the resultant *persecutory delusions* are constantly increased and aggravated. Those who conscientiously approach and question friends or supposed intriguers are further alarmed and justified by the indifference displayed and the little satisfaction obtained; some ignore them, others answer evasively. Trivial matters which formerly passed unheeded are now falsely and absurdly interpreted and enter into the structure of their delusions. A spot on the coat, a calloused finger, a decayed tooth, or a headache are all regarded as positive proof of treachery and an effort to get them out of the way by a slow process of poisoning. The appearance of natural baldness is readily explained by the application of electricity during sleep.

Sooner or later, in connection with these delusions of persecution, which are firmly held and well moulded by a coherent train of reasoning, there may also appear *expansive delusions*. These may be coincident with the persecutory ideas at the onset of the disease, but more frequently are the outcome of the delusions of persecution. The increasing attention which the patients attract and the persistent persecution lead them to cast about for the reason. While some find this in property which they really possess, others believe that it lies in their personal charms, while still others conclude that they have been born for a special mission, or are of noble descent. A thrifty Irish woman, who had accumulated considerable property by dint of hardest labor, finds a sufficient cause for her persecution in attempts of her enemies to secure her hard-earned accumulations. A factory employee already approaching the limits of the climacteric finds the reasons for her persecution in her attractive appearance, and the desire of eminent men to seduce her. Where the expansive delusions are more directly evolved from the delusions of persecution, the patient asks himself why he is so molested and tormented, why so many, not only individuals, but nations, seem directly interested in him, and why he is constantly accompanied by a secret patrol. Gradually it dawns upon him that he is a kidnapped son of a millionnaire or of a crowned head, that he is of Napoleonic descent and lawful heir to the throne, while his extensive landed properties are unlawfully used by the government. This explanation first appears in the tendency to find evidences of persecution in many or all the events of their environment, and becomes prominent when the patients discover its purpose. Then all these supposed facts assume a place in the chain of evidence which confirms their conclusions.

These delusions may only assume the form of an exaggerated *feeling of self-importance*. The patient considers himself especially renowned in his profession, — a fine lawyer, an excellent teacher, an interesting talker, an ideal gentleman, a social favorite, or an individual worthy of great political distinction. Finally, a change of personality may result, and the patient announces himself as titled, or a direct descendant of Christ. The patients become aware of this in various ways, one once receiving a salutation from the President, another recognizing a striking similarity between himself and the equestrian statue of a famous general. Others are assured of their high station by the deference paid them by every one: people bow to them, their names are in the paper, the orchestra begins to play as they enter the theatre, the prima donna directs her song at them, and the birds chirp when they are near. The appearance of the sun from under a cloud, casting its rays upon them, indicates that they are under the special guidance of God.

All delusions, both persecutory and expansive, are held with great persistency, *and built out into a coherent system, which is an essential characteristic of the disease.*

In the systematization of the delusions another prominent feature is the frequent appearance of *retrospective falsification of memory*. While this symptom is mostly characteristic of paranoia, it may also be present in the paranoid forms of dementia praecox and in melancholia. Here the patients, in reviewing their past life, find evidences of persecution, or detect occurrences which at the time should have indicated their superiority. The loss of a situation many years ago, derisive remarks by fellow-workmen, or an injury, now become clear evidences of their persecution by enemies. One patient recalled that when thirteen years of age a priest took from her a book, claiming that it was unfit for her to read. This incident she now regards as the beginning of years of persecution by the priesthood, who would seduce her and then hold her up as an example before the world. Another patient led his class in marching, and later was chosen captain of the boys' brigade: these incidents at that time should have made him aware of the fact that he was to have been a famous general. Another remembered overhearing his parents whisper in an adjacent room, becoming mute at his entrance, and later a disguised woman, who was really his mother, visiting at the house, all of which pointed to a noble birth and his displacement by a younger brother. Many similar incidents scattered throughout life are pointed out as striking evidences which aid in fortifying their system of delusions.

An erotic element often appears in the delusions, which in some cases has been pronounced enough to lead to the recognition of an *erotic paranoia*. Likewise, the religious coloring is sometimes strong enough to establish a *religious paranoia*.

In the erotic cases the patient usually believes himself the object of admiration by some lady who is attracted to him and solicits his attention. She makes him aware of this by daily appearing at her window as he passes, or by casting sly glances as she drives by. Other evidence is gathered by anonymous love poems in daily papers. Numerous fantastic methods of communicating his love to her are devised, to which she responds by wearing certain articles of clothing, or arranging her hair differently. Their mutual admiration is publicly regarded as an open secret. He hears it indirectly referred to everywhere, and friends would have him infer, from casual remarks, that they are well pleased. Sometimes this fanciful, romantic, and even platonic love is maintained for years without action; at others the patient makes an effort to approach his supposed fiancee. Her rebuffs may at first be regarded as necessary for the accomplishment of her desires. Later she may appear to him in the guise of one of his companions.

Hallucinations are always present at some time, but do not play a very important part in the psychosis, and rarely persist through the whole course of the disease. Hallucinations of hearing are apt to be the most prominent. At first very indefinite noises annoy them. Later they hear their names mentioned, or derisive laughter from a crowd; nicknames are called out, some one curses below the window, and bits of conversation from adjoining rooms excite them. The remarks are more often of a depreciatory nature. Hallucinations of sight are rare, but those of general sensibility are quite frequent,— the hair is plucked at night, the skin irritated by poisonous powder, the flesh pierced by bullets, or the countenance transformed by the nightly application of an iron mask.

There is never genuine *insight* into the disease. The patient, on the other hand, may complain of all sorts of physical ailments, such as nervousness, indigestion, pains in the head and back, for which he seeks medical attendance, but he cannot be made to realize the fallacy of his delusional ideas. The *memory* is well retained, and *judgment,* except as biassed by the delusions, is unimpaired.

The *emotional attitude* of the patients stands in direct relation to the character of the delusions. They are irritated by their persecutors, are shy and excitable, and at first usually despondent; some, however, tolerate the persecution and regard it as essential to their spiritual welfare. All sooner or later become arrogant, proud, and dogmatic.

In *conduct* the patients appear quite normal for a considerable time. Some of them, long before the real nature of their disease becomes evident, attract attention by their eccentricities, peculiarities in dress, oddities in manner, excessive religious zeal, or an attitude of self-importance. Later they become seclusive, move about in their employment from city to city, leave one shop to enter another, where they soon detect the presence of their former persecutors, and are again compelled to leave. In this way an iron moulder travelled from San Francisco to Boston in order to avoid the persecutions of his trade-union. A change affords only temporary relief to the anxiety, as suspicious circumstances are soon noticed which leave no doubt that news about them has been passed on from their last situation until finally their existence becomes known the world over. They become unstable in their behavior and mode of living, are unable to conduct a successful business, and fail to support their families. In reaction to the delusions they attempt to call public attention to their persecution by writing newspaper articles and issuing pamphlets. Very often they apply to the police for protection. Frequently they assume the offensive, and take the matter of vengeance into their own hands. Not infrequently the first striking evidence of the disease is a murderous assault upon some one. The paranoiac is for this reason the most dangerous of all insane. One patient assaulted the mayor of the city for keeping him from his fiancee; another drew a pistol upon a man with whom he was having an altercation over business matters, in the belief that he was the secret agent of the French government sent to kill him.

In accordance with expansive ideas the patient may address the President as his father, or demand access to a millionnairess whose parents are keeping them apart. If confined in an institution, they may for a time ingeniously conceal their delusions until they find evidences of continued persecution in their new surroundings, when the fellowpatients appear to them only as accomplices placed there to aid in their discomfort. Sometimes their confinement is regarded as an effort of their persecutors to make them insane. Some patients submit gracefully to their detention, considering it but another cross to bear before their final rescue and the proclamation that they are rightful rulers. A few patients even consider that they are being treated with the utmost consideration and the greatest attention, provided with the best quarters, and granted every possible privilege by those who recognize the great injustice done them.

The course of the disease is protracted. The onset is always gradual, and usually the disease has been in progress for some time, even a few years, before recognition. When once established, the course is slowly progressive, with a gradual evolution of delusions which are constantly being further systematized and made to encompass new environment. Several psychiatrists claim that the course of the disease presents definite periods according to the stages of evolution of the delusions. At first there is the prolonged period of insidious onset, by Regis called the period of subjective analysis, followed by the persecutory period with the development of delusions of persecution with hallucinations, and finally the ambitious period accompanied by a change of personality. The patients usually are quite orderly, present an unclouded consciousness, and for many years are capable of considerable labor, both mental and manual. After a duration of many years there appears a moderate degree of mental weakness. Patients become unable to apply themselves, take less notice of their environment and less care of themselves. In some cases the disease may seem to be at a standstill for years, while in others partial remissions occur when the patients for a time are able to rejoin their families, but are rarely in a condition to resume their accustomed occupations.

The diagnosis depends upon the slow onset, the characteristic, coherent, and systematized delusions of persecution with retrospective falsifications of memory, often associated with a change of personality, unclouded consciousness, coherent thought, and absence of mental deterioration for many years.

The *paranoid forms of dementia pracox* have already been differentiated from paranoia under the former disease.

A few cases of *dementia paralytica* and *melancholia* may simulate paranoia. Dementia paralytica is to be distinguished by its rapid development, the early appearance of emotional weakness, and physical signs. The conduct of a paranoiac is entirely dependent upon the content of the delusions; he cannot be reasoned with, is persistent in the prosecution of his ideas, and is rarely submissive to confinement; while the paretic opposes his retention weakly or intermittently and with some stubbornness.

The *melancholiac* presents a more rapid onset (three to nine months), a marked disturbance of the emotional attitude, fear, self-accusations, occasional clouding of consciousness, an absence of system in the formation of delusions, and evidences of mental deterioration within the course of two years.

The prognosis of the disease is very poor, as no case of genuine paranoia ever recovers.

The treatment of the disease is naturally limited to the removal of irritating influences and to confinement in an institution where systematic routine, with out-of-door life and ample exercise, may ameliorate or ward off the condition of mental weakness.

There are a few cases of paranoia which have been designated by Hitzig as querulent insanity (Querulantenwahn) which deserve a brief description here. The psychosis is of gradual onset, and usually arises as the result of some legal injustice, — a defeat in court, an unjust award of damages, loss of property, or an unfair adjustment of claims, in which the patient has been the sufferer. He refuses to settle, carries the case from one court to another, and finally develops an insatiable desire to fight to the bitter end. He reaches a point where he is unable to view the standpoint of any one else with any sense of justice, and his personal belief and desire completely obscure his better judgment. The statutes appear inadequate, and even the fundamental principles of the law fail of comprehension. He sets aside all business in order to cany on the struggle, solicits sympathizers, and denounces those who do not side with him. Hearsay and bits of knowledge gathered at random are cited as evidence in his behalf, and money is squandered in the pursuit of justice to the most extreme limits. He cannot abide by the ultimate decision after all the usual means of justice have been exhausted. Failing to appreciate the needlessness of further struggle, he writes to magistrates, legislators, consuls, ambassadors, and finally to the President or foreign rulers. Answers to these letters only create greater embitterment. His letters are long and carefully written, usually upon a particular kind of paper, and sometimes written with colored ink.

Hitzig, Ueber den Querulantenwahn, 1895; Koppen, Archiv f. Pay., XXVIII, 221; Pfister, Allgem. Zeitschr. f. Psy., LIX, 589.

The patient is irritable and often becomes greatly excited in conversation, although at the same time priding himself upon his ability to exercise self-control!

Consciousness remains unclouded. Memory is well preserved; in fact, it is often surprising to see with what accuracy he is able to quote from law books, to repeat parts of speeches, and to enumerate various dates. Thought continues coherent, but there is a great tendency to monotonous repetitions of the delusions. One seldom misses them in even a short conversation.

There is no insight into the condition. On the other hand, the patient is often encouraged in his belief by the fact that there are always many men, and not a few physicians, who will testify to his sanity.

The few cases of querulency are apt, after a prolonged course, to present greater deterioration than other varieties of paranoia; the content of speech becomes more and more limited and somewhat incoherent, the irritability increases, the patient becoms peevish, indifferent, and sometimes even stupid.

XL EPILEPTIC INSANITY

Epileptic insanity is a psychosis based upon epilepsy which is characterized by a *variable degree of mental impairment and by the recurrence of certain transitory mental states, designated epileptic ill-humor and epileptic befogged states.* The befogged states include *pre-and post-epileptic excitement and stupor, anxious and conscious deliria, and possibly also dipsomania.*

Etiology. — *Defective heredity* is the most frequent *predisposing* cause of epilepsy, appearing in eighty-seven per cent. of cases, while in over twenty-five per cent. epilepsy exists in the parents. Spratling found in 1070 cases hereditary taint in fifty-six per cent., sixteen per cent. of which displayed parental epilepsy. He also found nearly similar ratios in parental alcoholism and tuberculosis. Fere" notes among progenitors and relatives of epileptics the extreme frequency of migraine, headaches, infantile convulsions, mental disturbances, and deterioration. All authorities agree that parental alcoholism is a prolific source of epilepsy in the offspring. Wildermuth considers its influence almost as powerful as that of mental disorders, including epilepsy. Other factors in the progenitors which predispose to epilepsy are insanity, syphilis, rheumatism, diabetes, and possibly chorea. Evidences of congenital defect are frequently found in malformation or asymmetry of skull, microcephaly, hydrocephalus, the socalled " epileptic physiognomy " (broad forehead, broad and flattened nose, prognathism, thick lips, and staring eyes with wide pupils), feeble-mindedness, precocity, moral delinquency, and sexual perversion.

Spratling, Epilepsy and its Treatment, 1904. Fere", Lea Epilepsies, 1890.

Among the *exciting* or immediate causes of epilepsy we find cerebral palsies, dentition, emotional shocks (fright, excitement, anxiety, grief), many acute infections, meningitis, thermic fever, overwork, gastro-intestinal disorders, disease of heart and kidneys, tobacco, lead, and other poisons, carious teeth, foreign bodies in the ear, and even sexual intercourse.

Head injuries, such as blows, falls, brain lesions (especially hemorrhages), are frequently assigned as the cause of epilepsy, and in a certain number of cases a direct relation between them can be traced. Wildermuth gives their frequency as three and eight-tenths per cent., and Heeres as four and two-tenths per cent. Spratling says that "trauma is more frequently the cause of epilepsy in men than in women (eight and five-tenths per cent. men: three and five-tenths per cent. women)." The numerous scars often found on the head are more frequently the results than the causes of the malady.

Alcoholic excesses are by far the most important causes of epilepsy beginning after the twentieth year. About ten per cent. of chronic alcoholics are thus afflicted. All epileptics present a marked intolerance to alcohol, and its use by them, even in small quantities, hastens the onset and intensifies the symptoms of mental disorder. Many imbeciles and idiots and a few seniles (thirty-four hundredths per cent.) develop epilepsy. Epilepsy is essentially a disease of youth, convulsions appearing in thirty-four per cent. of cases in infancy. Spratling found in ten hundred and seventy cases twentysix and five-tenths per cent. develop under the age of five years; nineteen per cent. from five to nine years; twentyfour and four-tenths per cent. from ten to fourteen years; and thirteen and six-tenths per cent. from fifteen to nineteen years, — a total of fifty-six and five-tenths per cent. under twenty years. Gowers found in fourteen hundred and fifty cases that in seventy-four and eight-tenths per cent. the onset occurred before the twentieth year.

Pathology. — As not all epileptics are insane, it is evident that the pathology of epileptic insanity must be based upon that of the seizures plus hereditary taint, constitutional defect, and other factors whose nature and influence are not yet thoroughly known. There is a wide variation in views as to the nature of epilepsy, but it is now generally regarded as a cortical disease which is general and profound. Gross *lesions* are of secondary importance and mostly act as contributing factors. Among the most important gross changes revealed by autopsy are alterations in the texture and shape of the skull, old lesions of infantile cerebral hemiplegia (four to ten per cent.), sclerosis of the cornu ammonis, porencephaly, encephalic scars, neoplasms, etc. Wildermuth asserts that thirteen and three-tenths per cent. of his cases were due to polioencephalitis, and five and eight-tenths per cent. to other gross lesions. In the remaining eighty-three and nine-tenths per cent. of his cases — called "genuine" or idiopathic epilepsy — various anatomical changes were found in the brain, which probably bore some relation to the clinical symptoms. The microscopic changes thus far found are cortical gliosis and numerous cortical cell changes, such as chromatolysis; while in late epilepsy we find arteriosclerosis and occasionally syphilitic lesions. It is possible and very probable that many of the lesions found in the brain are the results of epilepsy and not the causes.

The *periodicity* of the seizures may possibly be explained by the apparent tendency in the nervous system to a periodical reaction to any continued irritation. If the researches of Krainsky, Cabitto, Agostini, and others can be corroborated, it would seem probable that idiopathic epilepsy is due to a toxic condition arising from faulty metabolism, and that the immediate cause of the convulsions is the accumulation of deleterious substances in the blood or a faulty chemotaxis of the cortical cells. This theory receives further weight from the fact that the convulsions are frequently accompanied by symptoms which point to intoxication, as drowsiness, headache, nausea, etc.; and also from the fact that epileptiform attacks occur in many conditions of chronic intoxication, especially from alcohol, lead, and uremia. "From the nature of the cortical cell changes we have a right to expect that the inciting agents will be very active nuclear poisons."

It is now believed that the blood, sweat, urine, and gastric contents are hypertoxic for some time before, during, and after the seizures, and hypotoxic in the intervallary periods, but no definite conclusion as to the sources of this alteration in toxicity has been reached. Epilepsy due to circumscribed lesions, traumatic or otherwise, of the brain, can hardly be ascribed to toxicity alone. Even if we should base the known cerebral changes upon a chronic intoxication, we would still need to explain the periodicity of the attacks, the accumulation of toxins, and also the hereditary relationship of epilepsy to other mental and nervous diseases. On the whole, it seems probable that the ultimate and characteristic cause of the symptom-complex epilepsy is to be found in *morbid conditions of the nervous tissues, especially the cortical cells, most likely due to chemical changes*. Spratling, Epilepsy and its Treatment.

Symptomatology. — Epilepsy unquestionably produces some mental deterioration in every case, but in about fifty per cent. this is slight, chiefly affecting the memory. The most striking feature of the epileptic weakmindedness is the slow evolution of psychic processes, external stimuli arousing only a meagre response in consciousness. In the majority of cases of epileptic insanity the degree of deterioration once established may remain without marked progress for years or even life. In a few cases, however, a condition of profound deterioration may be reached.

Hallucinations are exceedingly infrequent except in the befogged states and anxious and conscious deliria. When present in the interparoxysmal periods, they generally have a religious character. *Illusions* are quite frequent for a short period before and after attacks of grand mal. *Consciousness* is usually clear and orientation normal in the intervallary periods, except during the befogged states. Apprehension of the daily routine is fairly keen, but attention is always somewhat impaired or easily fatigued. *Memory* is always impaired, sometimes to a great extent. While prominent events and the ordinary daily routine may be recalled, the recollection of the general course of life, whether remote or recent, is more or less hazy. In contrast to the memory defects found in other deterioration psychoses, patients are able to express clearly and coherently their remaining narrow circles of thought.

The *train of thought* shows a marked atrophy of the store of ideas with scanty assimilation of new impressions. In conversation and writing there is a strong tendency to detail and circumstantiality. Their narratives are obscured by a multitude of data and irrelevant or unessential accessories which greatly impede the progress toward and development of the goal ideas. The connection is not lost, however, and the goal is ultimately reached. The religious content of thought is another striking symptom, many patients spending a large part of their time in reading the Bible or in praying aloud. Patients adhere to familiar paths, and their vocabulary consists largely of set phrases, platitudes, Bible texts, proverbs, etc. The narrowness of thought naturally leads to a *greater prominence of the ego*. This is especially noticeable in the conversation of epileptics, in which they indulge in praise of self and family, and pay much attention to personal matters.

The *imagination* is practically inactive, if not entirely abolished, and epileptics show no ability to reconstruct or recombine the materials furnished by old experiences or new perceptions. They occasionally, however, write verse which shows an unruly and riotous fancy, as in the following:— "E is the eel who soars to the sky; F is the finch who is fond of pie." *Judgment* invariably becomes impaired as mental deterioration progresses, but *delusions* are not common except in some of the transitory epileptic mental states, when they are accompanied by hallucinations. Many epileptics become hypochondriacal. The true relation of ideas is obscured or even lost, and "common sense," tact, and discretion are seldom displayed. Patients never adequately

recognize the incongruity between their plans and their limited ability. One man with marked mental and physical defects, whose schooling had been meagre, gravely proposed to study theology; and another who could hardly name the simplest flowers desired to become a florist. As a rule, however, epileptics have some *insight* into their condition, realizing that they have convulsions, poor memory, and difficulty of thought.

Among the most marked symptoms are those occurring in the *emotional field*, even when mental deterioration is not advanced. There is almost always an increased irritability manifested by their peevishness, obstinacy, unruliness, also by frequent outbreaks of emotional excitement as well as sudden alternations from elation to depression, and the reverse. This is particularly apt to occur in the proximity of the convulsions and is easily aroused by alcohol. Some patients complain of an " internal anguish," or fear. They are easily angered, are threatening, quarrelsome, violent, and dangerous. Usually the finer feelings become blunted, and there often exists a uniform state of apathy. On the other hand there are a few patients who for years always display a placid, amiable disposition, free from evidences of irritability.

Morbid and sudden *impulses* are frequent and characteristic symptoms of epileptic insanity. These are largely due to increased irritability or lack of self-control. Patients will attack any one who disturbs them, and often in a blind rage suddenly inflict severe and dangerous injuries, even on innocent and inoffensive bystanders, without any provocation. These impulses are by no means confined to the pre-or post-paroxysmal stages, as many suppose, but may arise at long intervals between the seizures. The wild state of blind rage, where patients run amuck, striking and assaulting indiscriminately every one in their range, — the characteristic *epileptic furor*, — is a nerve storm which may justly be considered as an " equivalent." These sudden impulses to violence and even homicide render epileptics especially dangerous. Suicidal impulses are

very infrequent, and their accomplishment still more so.

The *conduct*, apart from the stubbornness and morbid impulses above described, is usually good. Epileptics as a rule are neat, orderly, and observe the usual conventionalities unless deterioration is quite marked. Some patients display marked sexual excitement, and some are inveterate masturbators. All epileptics show a diminished *capacity for work*, especially where the higher grades of mental and physical training are requisite. They may engage with fansuccess in simple routine occupations where little or no initiative is required, but unless carefully directed and supervised, are apt to slight their work or leave it unfinished.

Physical Symptoms. — The most important physical symptoms in epileptic insanity are the *convulsions*, which may assume the type of grand or petit mal. In the former there may be an aura, followed by a cry, a fall, and tonic followed by clonic convulsions, usually localized at first, but rapidly extending over the entire body. During the convulsions, which may last from two to ten minutes, consciousness is totally abolished, but returns gradually within a period of a few minutes up to several hours. In status epilepticus there may be from twenty to even several hundred attacks of grand mal, without a return to consciousness in the intervals. In petit mal there is a very brief loss of consciousness (usually only one or two seconds), either without any convulsive movements or with very slight ones which often elude observation.

The *reflexes* are abolished during the convulsions, and in some cases are not restored for one or more hours. In 1088 observations on male epileptics, Keniston' found that the normal plantar reflex (flexion of toes, etc.) was present in both feet immediately after clonus had ceased in forty-five, and one hour later in two hundred twenty-six, cases; the Babinski phenomenon (extension of toes with dorsiflexion of ankle) occurred in one hundred three cases directly after the seizure, and in one hundred twelve cases one hour later. An extensor response was found in right or left foot in ninetynine and fifty-three cases, respectively, and a flexor response in right or left foot in ninety-nine and two hundred eleven cases, respectively, while a mixed response, that is, extension in foot and flexion in the other, occurred in eighty-two cases directly after a seizure and in one hundred forty-seven cases one hour later. The plantar reflex was abolished in six hundred sixty cases immediately after the convulsions, and in three hundred thirty-nine cases one hour later. The kneejerks were active in three hundred ninety-six cases, moderate in one hundred thirty-seven, and absent in five hundred thirty-nine cases.

Keniston, Journ. of Amer. Med. Assoc., March 21, 1903.

The *speech* of epileptics is often altered and very characteristic. It is abrupt, with intervals after each phrase, often drawling, jerky, or strongly accented. During excitement it may be so rapid as to be indistinguishable, were it not for the fact that a few phrases are repeated over and over again. Tuberculosis and organic and functional diseases of the heart are quite frequent, and the pulse rate is often increased. Epileptics rarely complain of headache, and often show an insensibility to pain amounting to analgesia, while their frequent wounds usually heal rapidly. Richter found anaesthetic areas in forty per cent. of his cases, general analgesia in twelve and two-tenths per cent., and hemihypffisthesia in ten and two-tenths per cent. Paresthesias are very common. *Sleep* is often irregular and muscular strength diminished. *Appetite* is usually good, and most epileptics are greedy and gluttonous. As residuals of seizures we find scars of all kinds, especially on the head, broken noses, extensive burns, and absence of front teeth; and as causal residuals we see evidences of alcoholic abuses, sequellae of early brain diseases, syphilitu or arteriosclerotic alterations, and cranial scars. We occasionally find after seizures small cutaneous hemorrhages, particularly in the conjunctiva.

In addition to the above general mental and physical symptoms which constitute the epileptic dementia, there occur with more or less regularity *certain transitory epileptic mental states, which occur periodically and independently of external causes.*

The most important of these states is the periodical illhumor, which according to Aschaffenburg occurs in 78 per cent. of epileptics and is characterized by a *marked emotional tension without much involvement of consciousness.*

The separate attacks bear an extraordinary resemblance to each other. The same complaints, the same delusions, and the same impulses recur. The phraseology of the patients is definite, the behavior characteristic, and the expression similar. These attacks vary in intensity, and often come on in the morning. Sometimes the intervals are so regular that the time of recurrence can be foretold with tolerable accuracy. Patients usually awake peevish, irritable, fault-finding, threatening, and quarrelsome; often commit sudden and unprovoked assaults on the nearest person; break glass or destroy bedding and furniture, and use profane or obscene language. Very often the emotional condition is one of *anxiety,* when the patients complain of feeling homesick, and low spirited, and of being troubled with sad thoughts, have presentiments, and express delusions of self-accusation. Occasionally hallucinations also appear. At the same time the patients may complain of feelings of numbness, pressure in the head, ringing in the ears, and difficulty of thought. They are unable to work, wander about, sometimes remain in bed, and frequently attempt suicide. Less often the patients develop a state of *expansiveness* or *ecstasy.* They then run about with glaring eyes and happy countenances. They shout, throw things about, and get into all kinds of trouble, tease their mates, pray loudly, and express expansive religious ideas. Occasionally there is a flight of ideas. Furthermore there is great emotional irritability with a tendency to aggressiveness. Some patients rapidly develop a condition of marked excitement. Sometimes the patients develop a delusional state with emotional irritability and anxiety and also occasionally accompanied by hallucinations, which condition might be termed a *paranoid condition.*

While the ill-humor usually occurs after a seizure, it may precede it, in which case the convulsion generally clears the mental atmosphere. The attacks rarely last more than a few hours, but may persist for a week or more. Abatement is gradual, and is often followed by a feeling of complacency or well-being. In some cases the hallucinations and delusions may persist with little change for weeks or months, simulating closely certain conditions found in dementia praecox, but finally the hallucinations and delusions entirely disappear.

Befogged states represent the second large group of transitory epileptic states, and are characterized by a more or less *profound clouding of consciousness.* These states include *pre-and post-epileptic insanity, psychic epilepsy, epileptic stupor, anxious delirium, conscious delirium, some cases of somnambulism, and possibly dipsomania.* The befogged state? are sometimes preceded by the transitory states of ill-humor just described. Alcohol may predispose to them, even when taken in very moderate quantities.

Pre-epileptic Insanity.— Here all sorts of morbid sensory impressions may arise, — flashes of light, impairment of vision, indefinite or strange sounds, peculiar odors, and paresthesias, — which are not to be confounded with the individual aura, when such exists. There may be fixed ideas, falsified identifications, monotonous repetitions of words or phrases, involuntary or grotesque movements, and imperative impulses, as to strike, destroy furniture, or kill. In a short time — sometimes a few minutes or even seconds — consciousness becomes clouded, and the convulsion begins. In a few cases the latter passes over into a pronounced dreaminess lasting for hours or days. *Post-epileptic Insanity.—* It is more common and is characterized by deep dazedness after the seizure, lasting for hours or even days. Patients do not understand questions, speak confusedly (paraphasia), are completely disoriented, wander aimlessly about, collect all obtainable objects, and even drink their urine. While active sensory disturbances are undoubtedly present, no account can be obtained from the patients, who have complete amnesia of all that has happened. As a rule, they recover their normal mental and emotional attitude very gradually. *Psychic Epilepsy.*—Mental and emotional disturbances very similar to the above may appear in the intervallary periods, entirely independent of the convulsions, and are then called " equivalents," or psychic epilepsy. These conditions are by no means rare, and are frequently observed in hospitals. They are more liable to occur in patients who have seizures at long intervals. The essential feature of psychic epilepsy is the disturbance of consciousness. Patients are confused, move and act in a mechanical or automatic manner, and often present evidences of illusions, hallucinations, and delusions. They wander aimlessly about, and do not appear to recognize any one, but will sometimes reply incoherently to questions. Occasionally they assume fixed or peculiar positions, or gaze steadily at one point. In some instances they display a heightened excitement, and again a gloomy stupor, during which they may masturbate, expose their person, or attempt sexual assaults. Patients have been known to set fire to their bedding or furniture for such trivial purposes as boiling coffee, etc. The numerous criminal acts, such as theft, arson, assaults, and even homicide, committed during these periods demonstrate the extreme importance of the recognition of psychic equivalents in their medicolegal aspect. The history of previous attacks of grand or petit mal, even if very infrequent, the senselessness of the actions, with utter absence of motive or attempt at concealment, and either complete amnesia or only a very hazy recollection of what has happened, should make the diagnosis clear. These attacks usually last only a short time, — seconds or minutes,— but occasionally continue for an hour or more.

Under the head of psychic epilepsy should be included some cases of *somnambulism,* occurring in epileptics. Patients notice only those objects which are directly in front of them. The eyes may be closed, half-opened, or staring. Movements usually display evidences of automatism, but there may be traces of deliberation and purpose, as in avoiding obstacles. Sometimes higher psychic fields are involved, and patients may carry on long conversations, compose poems, or transact business. Next morning they do not remember what they have done, but may complain of lassitude, stiffness, or soreness.

Epileptic Stupor.—Here the clouding of consciousness is intense and prolonged. Patients may eat, speak, or perform certain mechanical movements, but always as if dreaming and without clear understanding. Sometimes the eyes are closed, or the face dazed or staring. The same attitude is maintained for hours or even days, and the expression justifies the inference that confused terrorizing delusions dominate the emotional sphere, although occasionally the demeanor indicates happiness or religious ecstasy. Patients show absolute indifference to their environment, never answer questions, remain in bed, and soil themselves. They sometimes show active resistance if disturbed, may make sudden impulsive attacks, and instinctive suicidal attempts are not infrequent. The reflexes are abolished, sensibility is blunted, and in single cases temporary catalepsy is seen. Nourishment is often refused, either wholly or partially. Epileptic stupor usually lasts from one to two weeks, but in severe cases the course is longer. Recollection of the events is mostly lost. Improvement is generally gradual, but in a few cases the confusion may disappear in one day. Where attacks are repeated and prolonged, patients may remain for a long time dull and inattentive. *Anxious Delirium.* — This form is more frequent than stupor and may occur independently of seizures. The mental disturbance is profound. The attack develops suddenly, and may be preceded by very brief periods of ill-humor, characteristic sensa-

tions, and numbness, or by fixed and regularly recurring hallucinations, as red objects, flames, etc. Apprehension is dulled, surroundings are changed, and orientation is lost. The hallucinations and delusions are usually terrifying: patients must be punished, must die, are surrounded by devils, animals, or throngs of people who come out of the walls or floor. They wade in blood, their parents are perishing, the house is blown into the air, or everything is sinking. Sometimes God or Christ appears and carries them in splendid chariots to heaven, but these transports are only transitory, and the predominant tone of their emotions is one of fear and dread. Patients are impelled to brutal and incredible outrages, as cutting up their parents or children, shooting, stabbing, etc. They run away to escape the horrors which confront them. With flushed faces, either silent or howling and shrieking, they rage furiously, with prodigious strength, destroying everything within reach. The duration of anxious delirium varies from a few hours to two weeks. Sometimes consciousness clears up suddenly after a long sleep, but usually gradually, so that transitory hallucinations, delusions, and normal ideas are mixed together in a characteristic manner. There is no recollection of events occurring during the height of the delirium. *Conscious Delirium.* — This is a rare form, which either follows a seizure or appears as a psychic equivalent. Patients appear from their conduct to be conscious, but in reality consciousness is greatly clouded, while numerous illusions and hallucinations may inspire false ideas of danger. Expansive ideas are not uncommon. Answers to simple questions are coherent and relevant, but the whole demeanor, if closely observed, discloses some confusion and disorientation. The disposition is irritable, usually anxious, but sometimes elated, and delusional ideas often lead to impulsive acts. Legrand du Saulle reports the case of a merchant who, on suddenly recovering from an attack, found himself on the way to Bombay. Others have committed, with seemingly unclouded consciousness, senseless and even criminal acts (thefts, arson, rebellion, desertion, indecent assaults) without any insight into their significance. Attacks of conscious delirium may last for days, weeks, or even months, and there may be a series of attacks separated by short intervals. *Dipsomania* in many respects resembles epilepsy, as it presents an apparently paroxysmal and periodical impulse to senseless alcoholic excesses. Among the prodromal symptoms are noted uneasiness, anxiety, fear, despondency, weariness of life, increased irritability, a feeling of heaviness in the head, anorexia, insomnia, and occasionally sexual excitement. Very rapidly after these manifestations there appears an impulsive and irresistible desire to obtain relief, which is found in a " mad rush " for liquor. Some patients develop a typical epileptic befogged state, in which they become abusive, aggressive, noisy, and undertake foolish journeys. One man had attacks once in two years, when in the space of two days he would drink several pints of whiskey, ultimately becoming completely unconscious, and often, on coming to his senses, finding himself in strange places. After several of these attacks, he arranged that friends should take him to a hospital on the first appearance of the prodromes.

Some dipsomaniacs present no typical epileptic disturbances, but in their attacks fall suddenly into a condition resembling inebriety, in which they continue without interruption — day and night — to drink large quantities of beer, wine, gin, or spirits, until they have spent their last cent, and even sold their clothing to obtain means for gratification of their morbid appetite. During these attacks intoxication is seldom complete, but consciousness is clouded, and patients retain only a hazy recollection of a few events of their debauch, but often manifest deep contrition and an abhorrence of alcohol. Convalescence is gradual, and sometimes accompanied by nausea, anorexia, gastric catarrh, unsteadiness, and tremors, while a few cases present symptoms of collapse, accompanied by delirium and hallucinations.

The attacks of dipsomania may recur without any external cause, and in the intervals, which may last for weeks, months, or even years in a few instances, patients have no craving for alcohol, and either totally abstain or drink very moderately. There are many transitions or variations from the characteristic picture of dipsomania. Some patients manifest a disposition similar to that of epileptics, and a few perhaps present during life only one instance of an epileptic befogged state accompanying an attack of inebriety.

Diagnosis. — The diagnosis of epileptic insanity is generally easy as soon as we can establish the existence of the characteristic convulsions. It should, however, be differentiated from hysteria, dementia paralytica, and the catatonic form of dementia praecox.

In *hysterical insanity* consciousness is less deeply disturbed in the seizures, and we almost never see sudden involuntary falls, serious injuries, or biting of the tongue. The seizures are also specially induced by external influences, as mental emotions, physicians' visits, etc. , and may be curtailed or suddenly aborted by very lively excitement or strenuous treatment. The development is more diversified than that of the epileptic seizure, which is always uniform. In hysteria tonic and clonic muscular contractions of the entire body, convulsions of the diaphragm, opisthotonus, jactitation, rolling on the ground, somersaults, lively movements of expression (dramatic and passionate attitudes), alternate even in the same attack, and consciousness is never abolished. Dilatation and immobility of the pupils, usually considered an important characteristic of epilepsy, have recently been found in hysteria also. We find in hysteria extravagant caprices, rapid changes of disposition, and dependence on external influences, while in epilepsy there is a rough irascibility, a limited waywardness, an independent periodicity, and a prominent ill-humor. Mental weakness is more frequent and pronounced in epilepsy.

In epilepsy coming on in middle life, we must consider the possibility of *de-mentia paralytica,* which sometimes begins with epileptiform seizures. Here the consideration of the other symptoms, such as impaired pupillary reflex and inequality, characteristic speech disturbances, ataxia, incoordination, etc., will soon clear up the diagnosis. When, however, the epileptiform attacks occur at long intervals, and are accompanied by one or more of the above symptoms, we should be prepared for the possibly gradually developing symptoms of dementia paralytica.

The epileptic befogged state has been mistaken for the initial stage of the catatonic form of *dementia prcecox.* In the latter we find negativism, passive resistance, senseless answers, rapid and correct execution of commands, eccentricities, and stereotypy, with absurd acts, and less disturbance of apprehension and orientation. In epilepsy there is anxious resistance with indifference to orders, and uniformity of conduct, while there are frequent assaults, atrocities, and attempts to escape. Special weight attaches to the previous history and the proof of separate attacks of vertigo or syncope, periodical ill-humor, and probable night attacks, as evidenced by occasional enuresis, injuries to the tongue, and severe lassitude or headache in the morning.

The diagnosis of the *befogged states,* when only one convulsion has been observed during life, or perhaps not even one, but only a brief syncope, presents some difficulties; but we must remember that while the convulsion is a very important symptom of epileptic insanity, it may be absent or replaced by an "equivalent." Hence the periodicity of the attacks, clouding of consciousness, morbid impulses, crimes committed without motive or attempt at concealment, amnesia, and rapid course will facilitate the diagnosis.

Prognosis. — This depends essentially on the cause of the epilepsy and the time of onset. When dependent on gross brain lesions, recovery is out of the question, and the mental weakness often progresses to complete deterioration. When following head injuries, some recoveries have occurred, and in many cases decided and long-continued improvement has resulted.

Genuine epilepsy may disappear spontaneously, but recurrence is common if life is prolonged, and in the interval there is usually some mental dulness with transient ill-humor. Improvement rarely occurs in cases where the befogged states, especially stupor, have occurred, if they have bees at all frequent. In some cases of anxious delirium death occurs from exhaustion. Conscious delirium is not dangerous to life, but, like anxious delirium, if recurring at short intervals, tends to hasten the progress of deterioration.

In epilepsy arising late in life the outlook is very unfavorable. On the other hand, in alcoholic epilepsy treatment is often successful in effecting a cure, or at least grea: improvement. On the whole, while in some cases patients may improve sufficiently to go home, especially where the disturbance is largely in the emotional sphere, the prognosis of epileptic insanity is unfavorable, and patients should be subjected to prolonged observation and treatment before one assumes the risk of discharging them. This is nll the more desirable as attacks of furor may occur without any seizures, and thus the patient becomes a danger to the community. As far as life is concerned, we must remember that serious and even fatal injuries may result from accidents occurring during the convulsions or from the development of status epilepticus. Worcester found that sixty per cent. of epileptics die as the result of their seizures.

Treatment. — As far as the medical treatment of epileptic insanity is concerned, little can be done except to attend to bodily needs and combat any unfavorable symptoms which may arise. On the other hand, moral treatment, by which is meant suitable occupation and diversion, out-door life, helpful suggestions, educational efforts to retard the progress of deterioration and conserve what mental equipment is left, is of the highest value and an absolute necessity. Every one who possesses a remnant of physical or mental power should be *obliged to do something.* Occupation

should be light, safe, avoiding high or dangerous places, varied, and with ample intervals of rest. Diversions should be simple and wholesome, and all reading should be carefully selected, consisting largely of history, biography, light essays, standard novels, and religious subjects which would help toward right living and avoid all exciting or controversial points which might intensify the religiosity to which almost all epileptics are prone.

The treatment of epilepsy itself should be based on wellknown principles. Nutrition should be fostered by careful attention to the alimentary system. The diet should be regulated, and may consist of fruits; cereals in moderation and thoroughly cooked; eggs, breads, milk, cocoa, chocolate, and a minimum of tea and coffee; simple puddings, such as rice, farina, and custard; fish and a moderate amount of meat, at noon only. The supper should be very light and taken at least two hours before retiring. All meals should be regular, and patients should be carefully supervised to insure thorough mastication and prevent " bolting " food. The reduction of salt in food has been advocated, not only to diminish the irritability arising therefrom, but to enable us to materially decrease the amounts of bromids prescribed. It is said that this method diminishes by one-half the chance of bromism. Toulouse and Richet have introduced the *hypochlorization* method, which consists in using sodium bromid in place of ordinary salt, ten grains of the former being equal to twenty grains of the latter.

The kidneys require attention, and the secretion of urine Bhould be stimulated by a free use of water. The skin should be kept in good condition, and occasional *hot* baths employed to induce perspiration. If eye strain or other ocular symptoms are present, they should be remedied. The teeth and mouth must be kept in a healthy state.

It is very important to insist on complete and permanent abstinence from alcohol in all cases, and not merely in alcoholic epilepsy and dipsomania. Every epileptic is more or less intolerant of

its effects, very severe mental and emotional disturbances often result from its use, and nothing is to be gained from it in any case.

While innumerable remedies have been used to control or abort the seizures, their utility is somewhat doubtful, since the convulsions are practically safety valves, which allow the elimination of toxins. Unless the cause can be removed, it is perhaps better to allow the insane epileptic to have his fits, as they often clear the mental atmosphere. Nevertheless, in the present state of medical and lay opinion, it is advisable in every case, at the beginning, to administer the bromids, either singly or in various combinations, with proper precautions, until after due trial we can decide from the general condition of each patient — mentally, emotionally, and physically — whether or no it is best to continue their use. They should be given at the start in very small doses (6 to 8 grains) three times daily, after meals, in plenty of water, gradually increasing the amount until the point of saturation is reached, which is indicated by the disappearance of the throat reflex. Then the dose, which varies with the individual, should be reduced more or less gradually until we establish a norm which can be continued for a lone time, even years, with occasional short interruptions. In some cases the epileptic disturbances disappear, not even returning when the medicine is suspended, and we may perhaps regard the case as cured. It must be borne in mind, however, that in a certain number of cases the seizures cease spontaneously without any treatment, not to recur for years, if ever. Hence we must not attach too much importance to the curative power of the bromids.

Should bromism occur, as evidenced by acne, digestive disturbances, bronchial disorders, cardiac weakness, increase of the reflexes, anaesthesias, impairment of memory, stupor, etc., the bromids should at once be discontinued and an eliminative and supporting treatment instituted, — free and regular evacuations of bowels and bladder, promotion of normal skin action, and the use of digitalis and strychnin in small and decreasing doses, supplemented by absolute rest in bed and a simple, easily digested diet.

Among the other countless remedies employed to control the seizures may be mentioned argenti nitras, brom-ethyl, atropia, oxid of zinc, borax, adonis vernalis, and the Flechsig treatment by a regular course of opium in increasing doses, followed by bromids, with rectal lavage, and strict confinement to bed. While all these have given satisfactory results in some cases, none are so generally useful as the bromids.

When *status epilepticus,* which is comparatively infrequent among the insane, occurs, compression of the carotids should be tried if the arterial tension is very strong. Full doses of bromid, opium, and chloral in combination may be given at intervals of two hours, by mouth or rectum, and inhalation of ether or chloroform be tried. Combat exhaustion and collapse, and treat all complications promptly, especially supporting the heart.

Treatment directed to the *causes* of epilepsy is not promising in insanity, as the disease has been of too long duration. Hence head operations are usually contra-indicated. The time to operate for trauma, etc., is when the lesion occurs, or immediately thereafter. The *prevention* of epilepsy can only be secured by preventing marriages of the epileptic, insane, defective, and alcoholics.

Finally, in view of the liability to assaults and injuries to self or others, every epileptic should be under constant surveillance at all times, night and day.

XII. THE PSYCHOGENIC NEUROSES

Neuroses are commonly designated as a group of diseases characterized by changing and transitory nervous disturbances, to be distinguished from psychoses by the fact that the symptoms do not involve the mental field. But in practice psychoses without nervous symptoms or neuroses without mental symptoms are not encountered. Among the neuroses there is a distinctive group of cases, the individual symptoms of which are of a purely psychogenic ori-

gin. This group, which comprises *hysterical insanity, traumatic neurosis,* and *dread neurosis,* is in general characterized by a more or less marked *hysterical constitution,* the numerous manifestations of which are seen on every side. While traumatic neurosis and dread neurosis are closely related to hysterical insanity, they are, however, characterized by a different method of development, by different clinical symptoms, and a different course.

A. Hysterical Insanity

Although it is difficult to give a perfectly satisfactory definition of hysterical insanity, it may be described as *a* Moebius, Schmidt's Jahrbucher, 199, 2,185 (Literatur); Neurologische Beitrage, I; Monatsschr. f. Geburtshilfe und Gynkaologie, I, 12; Pitres, Lecons cliniques sur lTiysterie et lliypnotisme, 1891; Gilles de la Tourette, Traits clinique et therapeutique de l'hystene, 1891; Janet, Der Geisteszustand der Hysterischen (die psychischen Stigmata), deutsch von Kahane, 1894; Sollier, Genese et nature de l'hysteie, 1897; L'Hyste'rie et son traitement, 1901; Ziehen, Eulenburgs Realencyclopaedie, 3. Auflage; Krehl, Ueber die Entstehung hysterischer Erscheinungen; Volkmanna klinische Vortrage, Neue Folge, 330, 1902; Fuerstner, Deutsche Klinik, VI, 2, 155, 1901; Jolly in Ebstein u. Schwalbe, Handbuch der praktischen Medizin.

i *neurosis in which mental states produce manifold physical symptoms with extraordinary ease and facility.*

Etiology. — Hysteria develops upon a morbid constitutional basis. Defective heredity occurs in seventy to eighty per cent. of cases. An equally important factor is the influence of defective education and training. Other factors are trauma, shock, acute and chronic diseases. Mental stigmata are of ten recognized in early life; as, irritability, waywardness, indolence, talkativeness, undue piety, and sudden and rapid changes of emotional attitude. Sometimes such physical disturbances as chorea, headache, and loss of speech have been noted. More than two-thirds of the patients are women.

In children, in whom the disease is more prevalent among males, special symptoms are more prominent, as mutism, reflex convulsions, paralyses, and attacks of screaming, convulsive coughing, and silly befogged states (Chorea Magna). These symptoms are easily produced by physical injuries, but more especially by emotional disturbances, and not infrequently result from psychical infection (school epidemics). Poverty, seclusion, and faulty physique favor their development.

Hysteria does not often develop in adult life, although the symptoms may become more prominent during the climacterium. The role played by the disturbance of the female sexual organs in the production of the disease is not clear. On the one hand, it has been observed that disturbances of these organs may produce severe physical and mental disorders without creating hysterical symptoms, that the disease sometimes appears long before puberty, and finally that it develops in individuals with normal sexual organs. On the other hand, it is known that uterine disturbances frequently exist and are a source of complaint, and that the relief of even minor uterine disorders leads to a marked improvement. It seems probable, therefore, that disorders of the female sexual organs act only as prominent exciting causes.

Bruns, Die Hysterie im Kindesalter, 1897; Sfinger, Monatsschr. f. Psy., IX, 321.

Pathology. — The true nature of the disease is still unknown. A short and satisfactory explanation is that hysteria is a congenital morbid mental state whose chief characteristic lies in the fact that, as Moebius expresses it, physical symptoms are produced " by ideas." To this might be added that these ideas are strongly emotional, and, indeed, also indefinite. This would account for the fact that the physical symptoms do not always correspond to the character of the stimulus or to the content of the ideas, that they can appear in fields not accessible to the influences of the will, and sometimes are not even noticed by the patients. The internal relation between sadness and tears is no better understood than that between fright and hemianaesthesia. Terror can cause a movement of the bowels and whitened hair, just as hysteria can produce edema and disturbances of the heart's action. Even clouding of consciousness may be brought about by states of feeling. While it must be confessed that this is not an entirely satisfactory explanation of the nature of hysteria, yet it seems probable that increased emotional excitement and the morbid prominence and duration of the involuntary expressions that accompany it play an important rAle in the production of the disease.

There is no known anatomical pathological basis for the disease.

Symptomatology. — *Apprehension* presents no striking disturbance. On the contrary, many patients exhibit an uncommon sensitiveness; they are very keen in the perception of details in the environment, and especially any defects. A few patients are gifted along certain lines, while others are dwarfed mentally. Although the patients appear vivacious and bright, close observation discloses distractibility and lack of sound judgment. They are easily attracted by anything new or striking, are deeply impressed by show, become the clients and champions of the most recent physician, and adopt peculiarities in dress and ornament. This weakness is observed especially in the field of religion. They are eager for sensation, and take pleasure in gossip and in all sensuous enjoyments.

Memory is generally accurate, yet it is often not well balanced. Furthermore, what is perceived is not always correctly interpreted. In some cases there is a marked tendency not only to amplify events of the past, but even to distort them by pure fabrications. Patients will rehearse startling personal experiences and, in order to make thentales all the more credible, will present marks of violence, which they themselves have made. In such cases there is no doubt that the patients consciously deceive in order to arouse sympathy or to cause a sensation. But in the minor variations

from the truth shown by the average hysterical patient it is difficult to say how much is intentional deception and how much is due to the subjugation of memory by a lively imagination. In some cases, no doubt, the imagination dominates entirely all thought and action without creating the picture of a real delusion.

Disturbances in the *emotional attitude* are very important symptoms. The fluctuation of the feelings determines to a large extent the whole mental life of the patient. Their influence is stronger than rational deliberation or moral principles. Patients are excitable, and take an active personal interest in everything around them, are extraordinarily sensitive, and exhibit a tendency to outbursts of feeling on slight provocation. Occasionally there is heightened sexual excitement, but, on the other hand, there may be an absence of all sexual feeling. Frequent and abrupt changes in the emotional attitude are also characteristic. One never knows where to find the patients; they pass abruptly from a state of merriment into passionate anger; at one moment they may be distastefully sentimental, at the next crotchety and antagonistic.

This increase in the emotional irritability is perhaps a cause of the concentration of thought upon self. Some patients even seem to take pleasure in meditating upon and busying themselves over their ill-health. Thus numerous *hypochondriacal ideas* originate and dominate thought. Moreover, emotional depression has a more powerful influence than in the normal person in producing all sorts of physical ailments. The ease with which this influence is excited and the variety of the symptoms are especially characteristic of the hysterical constitution. Insignificant feelings of discomfort receive undue attention, and may even create sensations of injury. Real complaints are greatly exaggerated by the lively imagination of the patient until hypochondriacal ideas are evolved. Genuine pain arising from a definite lesion fails to disappear with the removal of the cause, but continues indefinitely, and may even become

more widespread. The headache and backache coincident with menstruation may be the foci from which there arises a grievous and agonizing condition, the symptoms of which the patients rehearse in all detail on every possible occasion.

Patients develop a most remarkable attitude toward their disease. They believe that it is an object of distinction, and even become proud of their invalidism. This is also evident in their failure to cooperate in treatment. Although complaining bitterly, they lack all feeling of personal responsibility in carrying out treatment, and may even stubbornly refuse to assist. However, any new or striking method of treatment, although it may entail some suffering, often will be undertaken for the sake of notoriety. Many refuse to deny themselves the pleasures of life, and continue to attend entertainments, to visit and receive company, in spite of the claim that their suffering is even enhanced by such endeavors.

Many patients complain particularly of *mental suffering:* terrible thoughts that constantly torture them, ungrounded fears, the memory of the failures of their lives, etc. These are repeated over and over at every opportunity with great show of emotion, but.not without emphasizing their own heroic struggle or martyrlike submission. Occasionally they wish they were dead and utter threats of suicide; sometimes they make melodramatic and even absurd attempts, such as tying a ribbon about the neck or jumping into shallow water.

The numerous hypochondriacal complaints necessitate constant medical attendance. Some patients develop a state of absolute dependence upon one physician. On the other hand, it is not unusual for patients to change physicians frequently, to visit celebrities and ask for many consultations. They often fall into the hands of quacks who gratify them by offering some wonderful cure. These cures, if effected, are usually as transitory as they are striking.

An exaggerated *self-consciousness* is a common symptom. Hysterical patients are markedly self-conscious, and display a corresponding lack of regard for the interests of others. They perceive with morbid acuteness any encroachment upon their own comfort, but accept the most extreme sacrifice on the part of others as a mere matter of course. They are always exacting beyond reason, dissatisfied with the best efforts of others, and deeply grieved over neglect or lack of sympathy. The *insatiable cravings* of many hysterical patients develop out of this heightened self-consciousness. Dissatisfied with what they have, they are constantly asking for something new, usually objects difficult to obtain, — new furniture, new quarters, new clothing, different food, etc. It is often surprising to see how undeserving patients successfully establish intimate relations with churches, societies, and well-meaning philanthropists, who gratify the most unreasonable demands. These patients regularly tyrannize the family.

In the *volitional field* the most pronounced symptom is an increased susceptibility to external influences. Patients yield readily to all sorts of influences, quickly become enthusiastic in any cause and just as quickly lose interest. In contrast to this extraordinary pliancy of the will to the most varied and insignificant conditions there is frequently observed the apparent opposite state of *vrilfulness*. When patients "get something into their head," they are most obstinate and headstrong in their purpose. Some subject themselves to great discomfort and pain, even torture themselves, and refuse to eat or speak without any apparent reason. In reality these apparently contradictory states of the will arise out of the pliancy of the will to accidental influences, whether they are external impressions or personal fancies. The unreasonable and impulsive conduct of the hysterical patient arises from the same source.

Consequently, in *conduct* the patients are unstable and erratic, and change rapidly from one act to another without sufficient reason. Because they lack uniformity and persistency, there develops more or less restlessness, which stands out in strong contrast to their

physical weakness and helplessness. They have a pressure to do something, to take part in something, to distinguish themselves, to do some mischief, and they long for adventure. In *manner* they are at times vivacious and frank, at others reserved and bashful, or, again, silly and sentimental. They are demonstrative and often express themselves in the most exaggerated terms. Their vehemence of expression by no means always corresponds to the intensity of their feelings, as the latter often fluctuate rapidly from one state to another. Patients characterize their own condition by such expressions as "Mosthorrible!" "Excruciating 1" "Inexpressible!" and in depicting their suffering it is not unusual for them to add color to the description by copious weeping or even fainting. In spite of their intense misery, the thought of self-enjoyment usually remains in evidence. One patient, after filling several sheets of her home letter with the most horrible selfexecrations, closed with the request for macaroons.

The capacity for employment is impaired; the patients have no disposition for earnest and strenuous occupation, lack perseverance, are weak and easily exhausted, and always feel that they must spare themselves. On the other hand, they pass much time with trifles, arranging and rearranging pretty ornaments in the rooms, and dillydallying with their toilet and personal adornment.

Physical Symptoms. — The physical symptoms of hysterical insanity are wholly functional and are often referred to as " stigmata." They consist chiefly of different degrees of paralyses of a single limb, astasia abasia, choreiform movements, contractures, localized and general convulsions, aphonia, impairment of speech, numerous sensory disturbances, including paresthesia, anaesthesia, hyperaesthesia, and visual disturbance; globus clavus, singultus, fainting fits, loss of appetite, obstinate vomiting, disturbance of respiration, and anomalies of secretion. Anaesthesia of the mucous membrane of the mouth and of the cornea is regarded as a characteristic symptom of hysteria. Finally, disorders

of sleep are very frequent. It is characteristic of all these symptoms that they do not follow anatomical and physiological rules, but are dependent in their appearance, persistence, and departure upon psychic influences. Hemicrania or convulsive movements can often be made to disappear by pressure upon the eyeballs. Contractures or paralyses may be made to vanish by firm pressure over the ovaries or in the hypogastric region, or by an unexpected dash of cold water upon the face or body. Patients who for years have been bedridden, reduced to a skeleton by fasting, and secretly inflicting wounds upon themselves to incite sympathy, may be immediately transformed into entirely different individuals by a sharp command, new environment, or some sudden freak. But such transformations are usually short-lived, and the patients relapse either into their former, or a still more distressing, condition. Furthermore, the symptoms sometimes disappear when the patients believe themselves unobserved or are left alone, only to reappear as soon as their illness is referred to, or when confronted by the physician.

Thesevarious mental and physical symptoms just described are characteristic of the *hysterical personality and constitute the groundwork upon which there develop other characteristic transitory hysterical states.*

Of these transitory hysterical conditions, the befogged states are the most prominent. They are characterized by *a marked clouding of consciousness, of varying duration, and either follow, take the place of, terminate in, or are interrupted by, a convulsion.* In the simple hysterical attack there is, throughout its entire course, only a clouding and not a complete abolition of consciousness. The patients usually sink to the floor without injuring themselves, and during the attack often show in one way or another that they are influenced by external stimuli. The attack may consist of simple fainting, or may be accompanied by pronounced convulsive movements. The convulsive movements do not show fixed rigidity or uniform trembling, but seem more complicated and at times even appear purposeful. The patients twist themselves about, groaning and screaming, they roll over and straighten out, strike their feet on the floor, or roll themselves up like a ball; at the same time there is a spasm of the diaphragm, marked slowing of the pulse, flushing of the face, and rolling of the eyes. Very often the back is so strongly bent that the patient's body rests on the bed only at the back of the head and at the heels, forming the arc of a circle. At intervals the patients may turn somersaults, or suddenly leap up, clutch at various articles, or cling to something; they may also make grimaces. Occasionally they exhibit *delirious states,* in which they imagine that they are passing through some exciting experiences and make all sorts of active movements. Often the patients repeat some actual occurrence in all its details, but usually in a theatrical manner. Sometimes the content of the delirium is wholly fictitious, when the patients find themselves in some fearful predicament or a state of ecstasy with heavenly visions and feelings of joy.

All of these different symptoms of the hysterical attack may succeed each other in various ways. Frequently, they are repeated over and over in a regular order. The delirium may be interrupted by fainting spells or convulsions. Sometimes the physical and mental symptoms of the attack occur separately, and at other times combined in various ways.

Following the attack, the patients lie quietly with relaxed limbs, occasionally showing a slight tonic rigidity, breathing quietly, and with a slow pulse rate, the eyes turned upward or rotated laterally. They are irresponsive, except to a powerful stimulus, such as an electric shock or sudden terror, which sometimes entirely arouses them. Such a condition, interrupted by occasional convulsions and short lucid intervals, during which food can be taken, may last from a few hours to three weeks. This condition has been termed *hysterical lethargy.*

Sometimes the befogged state simulates ordinary sleep. The patients become drowsy, the eyes close, the limbs become relaxed, as in a profound sleep, and the respiration deep and regular. This state is usually of short duration, and the patients awaken gradually with no recollection of the interval, although it is possible to arouse them by means of a strong stimulus, when they rub their sleepy eyes and look about as if surprised.

This last form borders closely upon *somnambulism,* which occurs during the natural sleep of hysterical patients. The patients leave their beds, wander about the room, open the window, and perform many peculiar acts, all of which are well coordinated. Sometimes they destroy clothing, hide objects, or set fire to furniture; later they return to their beds, and arise the next morning with only a confused recollection of what has happened. Similar attacks may occur during the daytime, either independently or in connection with a convulsive attack, a fit of laughing or crying. The patients then walk about, muttering unintelligibly to themselves, are oblivious to the environment, and not the least distractible, although able to avoid obstacles. It is very difficult to arouse them from this state, even by the application of powerful electrical currents.

This last condition is perhaps related to those *befogged states with inconsequential speech,* which have been described by Ganser. It occurs mostly among prisoners awaiting trial, who suddenly become dazed, suffer from active hallucinations, and when questioned give inconsequential answers in spite of the fact that they apparently comprehend the questions, although with some difficulty. At the same time there exist extensive and variable areas of anaesthesia to pain. After a duration of a few days, the symptoms disappear, and the patients have no memory of the psychosis. In a few cases a series of these befogged states may extend through several months.

Befogged states with silly excitement are encountered in young patients in whom the clouding of consciousness is moderate, and does not prevent a recognition of their environment. Patients usually exhibit a happy, unrestrained mood, sometimes with marked silly behavior. They perform all sorts of foolish, wanton pranks, scream, imitate the cries and behavior of animals, and scramble about. The real morbidity of this apparently conscious behavior becomes evident when, as occasionally happens, it is suddenly terminated by a light convulsive seizure, and then, without memory of the foregoing behavior, the patients pass into a short period of depression.

The *memory* of the events during the befogged states, as well as occasionally for events just prior to the onset, is always much disordered, and sometimes completely abolished. In some cases there are encountered examples of a sort of dual personality, in which the recollection of previous attacks occurs only during subsequent attacks, being completely lost in the interval. It occasionally happens during an attack that some definite period of the patient's life is lived over again, similar to what occurs in hypnotic states. Such alterations in personality arise only under the influence of autosuggestion.

Nissl finds that twelve per cent. of female insane patients suffering from various psychoses present some hysterical symptoms. These occur especially in manic-depressive insanity, and also in the early stages of dementia. But in addition to this there occur during the course of hysterical insanity well-defined mental disturbances, which are a part of the hysterical personality. These include *sad and anxious states* of varying duration which appear independently of any sufficient cause and are accompanied by indefinite delusions of self-accusation and persecution. The patients may also speak of seeing forms and hearing threats, but it is doubtful if these are genuine hallucinations or are really connected with dreams. Conditions of *excitement,* arising as the result of jealousy, spite, and the like, more frequently appear in the form of passionate outbreaks with violent abuse, and sometimes a tendency to destroy objects, or even to smear their bodies. These usually pass off in a few hours or at the most a few weeks. Sometimes they recur in connection with the menses.

Course. — The course of the disease is usually protracted, sometimes extending over many years. In women especially the onset of the disease is early, frequently appearing at the age of puberty, but it may occur even earlier. The individual symptoms may show the greatest variation in thenappearance and prominence; indeed, the rapidity and abruptness with which the symptoms change is distinctly characteristic of hysterical insanity. In a way the disease may be regarded as a series of attacks which recur on the basis of the hysterical personality. These attacks rarely last longer than a few months, and usually do not exist more than a few days or even hours. But the different depressed, excited, and befogged states, together with the physical disturbances, may produce a variegated and incongruous picture extending over considerable time. The course of the disease in children is characterized by less variety of symptoms and a shorter duration, while in males there is a far more uniform picture with little variation of the individual symptoms, which may persist unchanged for years.

Diagnosis. — The diagnosis of hysterical insanity is most difficult in men. The *constitutional psychopathic states* present a more uniform course, while hysterical befogged states and various physical symptoms are not encountered. In *traumatic neurosis* there is a far more uniform development. The differentiation from *epilepsy* has received sufficient consideration under that disease. Finally there may be some difficulty in differentiating the hysterical befogged states with inconsequential speech from *catatonia,* in which inconsequential speech is frequently encountered, and in which the areas of analgesia may be mistaken because of the presence of negativism. In catatonia there is practically no clouding of consciousness.

The differentiation of hysterical insanity from those psychoses in which individual hysterical symptoms sometimes appear, such as manic-depressive insanity, dementia praecox, paresis, etc.

, must depend wholly upon the presence of the symptoms which are characteristic of those forms of disease.

Prognosis. — The prognosis of hysterical insanity, as regards the befogged states, is, in general, good; sooner or later, either with or without treatment, there is an improvement or at least a considerable change. The disease in itself does not progress. The improvement or aggravation of the symptoms depends very materially upon the peculiar conditions in which the patients find themselves. At any rate dementia never develops. The prognosis is less favorable where there is an increasing tendency to relapses into the varied forms of the disease. Hysteria in children is decidedly more hopeful, as the symptoms usually disappear with the development of the child. Occasionally, remarkable cures are effected by the removal of prominent exciting causes; as, diseases of the sexual organs, injurious environment, and improper hygiene. In male patients there is a severe form of hysterical insanity with pronounced hypochondriacal complaints which is resistive to all modes of treatment.

Treatment. — The disease, developing as it does upon a psychopathic basis, demands prophylaxis in the way of care of the pregnant mother, and careful supervision of the education and training of psychopathic children. The pregnant neurotic mother should avoid all forms of excitement and sources of fear and worry, and conform as closely as possible to a life of mental equanimity. The child, especially if it shows a tendency to insomnia, with night terrors or restlessness and evidences of unnatural excitability and precocity, must be removed from the presence of a hysterical mother, who is naturally least fitted for its training. Such pernicious environment, where the child must witness emotional outbursts and fits of temper and other hysterical symptoms, has an indelible effect, particularly in the formative period between the fifth and twelfth years.

Relieved of such surroundings, the main object in the education should be the development of physical strength

and vigor, and the maintenance of an effective state of nutrition. For this purpose, plenty of out-of-door exercise, with an abundance of sleep and wholesome diet, must be prescribed in connection with a discouragement of all elements of precocity in the mental, moral, and sexual life, and inculcation of self-control and the nobler sentiments. The same care must be continued during the period of puberty and youth, but should include advice in relation to sexual matters, sentimental love affairs, and later relative to the assumption of the duties of early married life, especially sexual relations.

In the treatment of the disease itself the element mo?. essential to success lies in the personality of the physician, who must inspire the patient with confidence and secure the cooperation of the family. Except in the light-: cases, it is of first importance to isolate the patients ani establish a suitable routine in the mental and physicvlife, thereby removing from the environment the disturbing factors which have always been a source of annoyana and have acted as exciting causes. This isolation, although best carried out in a small, well-selected sanitarium, under the direct supervision of a physician, can be accomplished, with the aid of an efficient nurse, at the home. At all event the patient must be given over entirely into the hands oi the physician, who establishes confidence and control, noby harsh and dogmatic opposition, but by gentle persistence in which he must combine firmness and even boldness. Tbs accomplished, he is in a position to bring about great in provement, and often recovery, by simple remedies. Attention should be directed to any possible organic disturbance in the stomach, intestines, kidneys, heart, lungs, and sexut organs. Iron should be prescribed in anemia, and restoratives employed in conditions of emaciation, as well as bitW tonics for anorexia.

On the other hand, *mechanical therapy* can be reliet upon to produce excellent results. Of the mechanic measures the most important are hydrotherapy, electricity massage, exercise, and employment. In the use of hydrotherapy Collins regards the tonic bath the best, in which the water, at a temperature varying from fifty-five to sixty degrees, is applied under from fifteen to twenty pounds' pressure for from four to five seconds, followed by a Fleury spray of eighty degrees and similar pressure for one to two seconds. In the use of the bath hysterogenic zones must be protected. The reaction should be facilitated by passive movements, walking, or gymnastics, for one halfhour following the bath. Where this bath fails to produce the desired effect or is not well borne, he suggests the use of the Scottish spray. It is always desirable, when possible, to avail oneself of a hydriatic institution for these purposes. The treatment can be accomplished, however, in a house supplied with water under sufficiently high pressure by the simple use of a detachable hose and a tube. This should always be under the direct supervision of the physician, who will find it necessary to vary the details of the treatment according to individual cases. When the bath is not accessible, the drip sheet may be used, the description of which may be found under the treatment of acquired neurasthenia.

In the application of electricity the faradic current is of most service in improving the nutrition and in relieving anaesthesia and hyperaesthesia.

The daily routine of the hysterical patient should be one of activity, alternating with rest and relaxation, including massage, gymnastics, and out-of-door exercise, combined with some sport which tends to increase self-reliance.

There are a few cases which require *surgical treatment* for the alleviation of organic disturbances in the sexual organs, especially where the symptoms of the disease seem to bear a definite relation to the menstruation. Removal of slightly diseased or even normal ovaries has produced improvement in a few cases, but it is the general verdict of to-day that this drastic procedure has more often been of detriment than benefit, and should be discarded. *Hypnotism* is of limited value, because those susceptible to hypnotic suggestion are apt to be in-

fluenced by any powerful suggestion that happens to be presented. Furthermore, hypnotic experience brings about an undesirable dependency of the patient upon the physician, which makes impossible an effective subjugation of their own wills in the strife with the morbid influences. The greater the influence exerted, the more easily autosuggestions arise, and the quicker the efficacy of the hypnotic suggestion is nullified by other and opposing ideas. In mild cases, and especially in children, suggestive therapy is of considerable importance in overcoming individual hysterical symptoms, such as paralyses, sensory disturbances, and tremor. On the other hand, *simple suggestion* is a therapeutic measure of great value in every case, and often suffices for the complete disappearance of paralyses, contractures, aphonia, etc.

In the treatment of the hysterical attacks, the patient can often be restored to clear consciousness by a brisk command, or, if this fails, by a dash of cold water upon the face, by the electric brush, or pressure over the ovaries or upon the hysterogenic zones. In very severe cases inhalations of chloroform may be necessary.

Angelucci, e Pieracini, Rivista sperimentale di freniatria, XXIII, 290. *B.* Traumatic Neurosis
(Traumatic Hysteria)
Traumatic neurosis arises as the result of trauma and is characterized by the *gradual appearance of a prolonged period of mental depression accompanied by numerous motor and sensory nervous symptoms.* The trauma may occur in the form of sudden fright, intense anxiety, great misfortune, or an injury in connection with a fire, railroad accident, explosion, earthquake, sunstroke, or electrical shock.

Cases of this sort were first recognized and well described by Erichsen in 1886, but it was not until the investigation of Oppenheim and Striimpell in 1889 that the disease was clearly differentiated and received its present name. The recognition of such a disease has always met with more or less opposition, especially by French writers, and

more recently from Schultze, Hoffman, and Mendel, who maintain that the disease is either hysteria or neurasthenia of traumatic origin.

Etiology. — At present there is no adequate explanation of the pathology of the disease. Westphal and his school consider that there is an organic basis to be found in changes of the central nervous system. Charcot regards the disease as closely related to the hypnotic condition, because the disease picture wholly resembles the picture of a firmly rooted autosuggestion. The psychical origin of the disease is the generally accepted view. This theory is substantiated by the facts that the neurosis sometimes appears without known injury, as when it follows fright or slight injury to other parts of the body than upon the head; and that the manifestations of the disease are not necessarily limited to the part where the injury occurs, but may be general. In cases following head injury it is held that delicate pathological changes occur in the cortical neurones. Experimentation upon test animals, in which definite pathological lesions in the neurones can be produced by concussion without severe injury, would seem to verify this supposition.

Oppenheim, Die traumatischen Neurosen, 2. Auflage, 1892; Schultze, Sammlung klinischer Vortrage, N. F., 14 (Innere Medicin, No. 6); Deutsche Zeitschr. f. Nervenheilkunde, I, 5. u. 6, 445; Striimpell, Miinchner Medicinische Wochenschrift, 1895, 49 u. 50; Sanger, Die Beurteilung der Nervenerkrankungen nach Unfall, 1896; Ffirstner, Monatsschr. f. Unfallheilkunde, 1896, 10; Schuster, Die Untersuchung und Begutachtung bei traumatischen Erkrankungen des Nervensystems, 1899; Sachs und Freund, Die Erkrankungen des Nervensystems nach Unfallen mit besonderer Bcruchsichtigung der Untersuchung und Begutachtung, 1899; Bruns, Die traumatischen Neurosen. Unfallsneurosen, Nothnagels Handbuch, XII, 1, 4, 1901.
It is doubtful whether the emotional disturbance at the time of the accident should be regarded as the cause of the disease, as very frequently weeks and

even months elapse before the first symptoms appear. An important factor, undoubtedly, is the psychical influence of membership in accident insurance societies, of possible indemnities, and of suits for damages. At any rate, in cases where these factors exist, the neurosis seems to run a more unfavorable course. The symptoms regularly worsen until settlement is reached, when they are apt to improve rapidly and often entirely disappear. Another element of importance is the defective constitutional basis, in which alcoholic intemperance plays a considerable role.

Symptomatology. — The symptoms develop gradually in the course of a few weeks or months following the shock, and consist chiefly of *despondency wtik anxious fears and loss of the power of physical and mental resistance, and an incapacity for any earnest employment.*

Patients seem quiet and low spirited. *Apprehension* is slow, and they take less and less interest in the environment. The *association of ideas* becomes unusually uniform and sluggish, and centers mostly about the accident, to which the patients refer over and over and often describe in detail, laying stress upon their " hard luck," present deplorable condition, and hopeless future. Sometimes *compulsive ideas* and *phobias* appear. *Hypochondriacal ideas* become very prominent. Patients cannot rid themselves of thoughts of the accident and fear that they have been severely injured, because they are not the same, are always tired, exhausted, and unable to work. They observe carefully everything about their physical condition connected with the injury.

In *emotional attitude* patients are very irritable, sensitive, and easily thrown into a state of perplexity or confusion, are unable to express themselves with perfect coherence, and are conscious that their thoughts and actions are constantly hindered by feelings of inward oppression and anxiety. This anxiety may lead to passionate outbursts and even suicidal attempts. *Memory,* in spite of complaints to the contrary, is good, if one makes allowance for the lack of interest in the environ-

ment and the faulty attention. When agitated, the patients may not be able to solve even simple problems. Their capacity for work is greatly hampered by hypochondriacal notions and numerous nervous complaints. Whenever they attempt to do something, headache, palpitation of the heart, excessive perspiration, etc., develop.

The mental symptoms usually do not progress. Occasionally befogged states or an acute hallucinatory excitement appears. If mental impairment develops, it is usually due to a cerebral lesion.

Physical Symptoms. — Sleep is disturbed by anxious dreams, the appetite is poor, and nutrition becomes impaired. Patients complain of various sensations in the head and back, especially paraesthesias and pains in parts of the body injured at the time of the accident. Pain, which is usually the most prominent symptom, is persistent and troublesome and may lead to immobility of the parts involved. In addition, patients complain of ringing in the ears, loss of strength, palpitation of the heart, difficulty of urination, and occasionally obstinate vomiting. Some cases present objective symptoms, such as areas of analgesia and of hyperaesthesia, constriction of the field of vision, difficulty of hearing, increased tendon reflexes, paralyses, slowness and uncertainty of movement, and disturbance of gait and speech. Tremor, especially of the fibrillary type, is often present, being either general in character or involving only muscles of the paralyzed part. Paralysis may occur in the form of hemiplegia or paraplegia, but the facial and hypoglossal nerves are seldom included. The *paralysis almost always occurs on the same side as the accident,* and is frequently accompanied by contractures. There is often an acceleration of pulse and sometimes of respiration following emotional disturbance, pressure on painful points, or muscular exertion. Occasionally, also, vertigo or even epileptiform attacks may be produced in the same way. Localized muscular spasms and convulsions are common. Vasomotor disturbances occur, as localized blushing, cyanosis, and dermogra-

phy. Sensory disturbances, both subjective and objective, of which hyperaesthesia is most prominent, usually involve the injured side of the body.

All of the motor and sensory nervous disturbances are to be distinguished from those accompanying organic brain and cord lesions by their location, their broad extent, changing condition, and the fact that they worsen under the influence of emotional and physical disturbances. Friedmann adds that these patients have little power of resistance to alcohol, galvanization of the head, and compression of the carotids. Diagnosis. — The diagnosis is often very difficult. *Hysterical insanity* is distinguished by the lack of uniformity of the symptoms in a given case; the hysterical patients present a variegated and transitory alteration of symptoms, capriciousness, pronounced changes of disposition, desire for undertaking something new, and great pliancy. Furthermore, traumatic neurosis does not present befogged states. The *constitutional psychopathic states* are differentiated by the fact that the onset is not sudden, does not depend upon an injury, and has a less favorable course.

Simulation should always be taken into consideration. Unfortunately the various objective symptoms, constricted field of vision, acceleration of pulse, increased tendon reflexes, and absence of galvanic excitability, are of little value in establishing a positive knowledge of the existence of a mental disorder. Deception cannot be unmasked by the presence or absence of any one symptom or group of symptoms, but must depend upon *the conformity of the whole clinical picture to one of the known disease-symptom groups.* Recently psychological tests have been successfully employed to prove the mental symptoms; as, for example, psychological tests of the power of apperception, test of diminution of the ability to figure, the susceptibility to training, and especially fatigue. Thus it has been shown that in traumatic neurosis there should be a marked loss in the capacity for work and a very great increase in the susceptibility to fatigue.

Prognosis. — The lighter cases of traumatic neurosis appearing soon after the accident may improve rapidly, but even some of these run a long course and have an unfavorable outcome. Yet, after a duration of many months or even a few years, the disease may terminate in recovery or great improvement. The prognosis is less favorable in the presence of pronounced focal symptoms or general arteriosclerosis.

Treatment. — The first indication is to dispel as far as possible all ideas of litigation. Next to this, employment is of the greatest value. It often happens that the symptoms of the disease disappear rapidly as soon as litigation is settled or patients are compelled to go to work again. A residence in an institution with the opportunity for employment and distraction frequently serves to bring about great improvement or recovery. In all cases hydrotherapy, massage, exercise, electricity, and hypnotic suggestion, as well as dietetic regimen, are of value.

C. Dread Neurosis

The dread neurosis comprises a small group of neurotic cases in which the patients suffer from a *more or ka constant feeling of anxious suspense which dominates tk entire life.*

The conditions about which the anxiety develop are usually processes that normally take place without conscious interference, such as walking, standing, drinking, writing, etc. The anxiety almost always appears for the first time immediately following some real but trifling condition, such as an experience during which the eyes have been subjected to fatigue or a dazzling light, moderate overexertion, fatigue after a long walk, etc. Anxiety about sleep may follow periods of emotional stress. Frequently some physical disease initiates some of the symptoms: a feelin: of weakness follows a mild rheumatic attack, or pain in the leg follows a fall. In addition to feelings of anxiety then regularly develop uncomfortable and even painful sensations, as well as a sort of paralytic weakness which interferes with the movements. The painful sensations, especially, accompany the

process of apprehension, while the muscular weakness appears during exertion of the will, though both occur together. The anxiety and the accompanying sensations usually occur first in connection with some simple act, such as eating certain kinds of food, reading in bright sunlight, or sleeping in a certain place. But they gradually become more extensive and may finally render some particular acts wholly impossible. In one patient insomnia first developed whenever she anticipated doing something unusual the next day, such as going to the city, but later the most trifling affairs would cause it to appear.

The clinical picture is variegated; while patients are reading, letters will disappear, then there is a feeling of heat, a sensation of tension, photophobia, and pains that streak across the forehead, which ultimately compel them to cease reading altogether. Similar disturbances develop in connection with hearing. In writing the fingers soon stiffen, or there is great weakness. Swallowing can be rendered difficult by the appearance of a cramp in the throat. Walking is hindered by weakness in the legs, pains, etc. Sleep may be impaired by an increasing restlessness, twitching of the limbs, and palpitation. Some cases of psychical impotency belong here.

Patients mistake the true origin of the disorder and begin to refer it to real diseases of the eyes, ears, muscles, and nerves. This causes them still greater anxiety, and undermines their self-confidence. Attention is directed more and more to these supposed physical disorders, and thus there develops a vicious circle, each factor adding fuel to the other and making it impossible for the patients to free themselves. Increasing sensitiveness of the eyes causes the patients to systematically avoid light, therefore they do not venture out 2i save at twilight or on cloudy days. Pain and weakness, which interfere with walking and standing, cause the patients to gradually limit their movements and ultimately to remain in bed altogether. In this state both active and passive movements may produce excruciating pain. Speech and movements of the head are

singularly free. Furthermore. the disorder ordinarily does not extend into other fields, but confines itself to the particular process which was originally involved, as, for instance, to sight or to walking.

Consciousness remains clear; patients are oriented, orderly. and do not exhibit emotional deterioration. They complacently endure the severe suffering which they regard as purely physical. Hysterical symptoms are never a part of the disease picture.

Course. — The course of the disease is usually protracted though there are frequent remissions. Efforts upon the part of the patients to overcome their symptoms only aggravate the condition. Strenuous efforts to relieve tk patients by various mechanical and medicinal device usually effect only a transitory improvement. On the other hand, many of the patients get well of their own accord.

Diagnosis. — There is some question as to the clinical position of the dread neurosis; indeed, the lighter forms have often been considered as cases of *nervousness* or *neurasthenia,* while Janet describes many such cases under *psychasthenic,.*

Against the former view may be cited the fact that the patients need not at any time exhibit any other nervous symptoms, while there is at no time any evidence of nervous exhaustion. Although the symptoms may originate in some physical ailment, they do not disappear with the recovery from that condition and restoration of strength. The differentiation of *hysterical insanity* depends upon the presence of the unconscious influencing of the physical processes through emotional excitation, while in the dread neurosis it is alone the condition of weakness and instability which deprives the patients of their ability to withstand the supposed physical affliction. In hysteria the symptoms frequently alternate from one field to another, but in the dread neurosis the symptoms are uniform and progressive.

The *phobias* are distinguished from this disease by the fact that the fears are more general in character, while in this disease there is some definite personal experience which forms the starting-point. In the phobias the fears frequently change in several different directions, but in the dread neurosis fear is uniform, always hypochondriacal, and has to do only with the patients' own bodies. Furthermore, in the phobias there are real states of anxiety which embarrass the patients or force them to secure protective measures, but in this disease the patients are not conscious of the origin of their difficulties, which appear to them as real pain, actual weakness, or genuine ataxia.

Treatment. — Many patients recover of themselves, without any treatment. In some way or other, frequently through the influence of some one whom they trust, they regain self-confidence and with it the strength to conquer the disease. On the other hand there are many cases in which failure at the first trial destroys all hope of recovery. Patients at first seem to react well to new methods of treatment, but in reality from the very beginning they are apt to cherish a vague fear that they cannot recover. Simple *hypnotic treatment* often effects a rapid and permanent recovery. Cases of even ten years' standing have been restored in this way. This form of treatment, however, is often difficult, and demands that one should thoroughly understand the technique, in order to gain the confidence of the patient, without which success is impossible. In sever? cases it is often necessary to begin by giving only quieting suggestions, because premature suggestions as to the cure might prove disastrous. This method rarely fails. In case it does, one may employ waking suggestion, but its influence is not as effective. Failing in this, there is no hope for cure.

XIII. CONSTITUTIONAL PYSCHOPATHIC STATES (Insanity of Degeneracy)

The fundamental symptom in the constitutional psychopathic states is the continuous morbid elaboration of normal stimuli as manifested in a morbid misdirection of thought, feeling, and will throughout life. These states develop on a morbid constitutional basis. The commonest type of psychopathic degeneracy is characterized by those little imperfections of the individual constitution which we ordinarily designate as *nervousness*. These symptoms form the groundwork upon which the more marked forms of the insanity of degeneracy develop. These various forms of the insanity of degeneracy are hard to group, because there are so many combinations and border-line states. In the present state of our knowledge the best arrangement seems to be *constitutional despondency, constitutional excitement, compulsive insanity, impulsive insanity,* and *contrary sexual instincts. A.* Nervousness' *Nervousness comprises several congenital morbid mental states which are characterized in general by an inability to withstand the misfortunes of life, together with a lack of symmetry in the development of the entire psychical personality.* Saury, Etude clinique sur la folie he're'ditaire (les de'ge'ne'res), 1886; Koch, Die psychopathischen Minderwertigkeiten, 1893; Binswanger, Die Pathologic und Therapie der Neurasthenie, 1896; v. Krafft-Ebing, Nervositat und neurasthenische Zustande, 2. Auflage, 1900; Gilles de la Tourette, Les Stats neurasthe'niques, 1898; Janet, Les obsessions et la psychasthe'nie, 2. Bande, 1903.

Intellectual endowment usually is not equal to the average, although occasionally it may be excellent. Some particular faculty may be unusually well developed; as, for instance, the sense of form, of color, or memory for numbers. Some patients may be able to perceive keenly, but yet lack insight into character, or may possess profound knowledge without any practical bent. Some patients are remarkably precocious. *Increased susceptibility to fatigue* is a prominent symptom. Hence patients tire quickly and have little endurance. Occasionally they learn with difficulty and quickly forget what they have learned. Attention shows an increased distractibility. Patients are very sensitive to interruption, and are easily distracted from their customary ideas and plans by anything new. These symptoms give rise to *flightiness* and *superficiality.* An unusual activity of the imagination is often present. Ideas possess a great sensory vividness and are easily united. Consequently there develops a strong tendency to revery, which is also favored by the distractibility of the attention.

While egotism usually prevails, on the other hand, selfdepreciation and a lack of self-confidence may be present. Most patients lack the *sense of reality.* To them the daily occurrences of the immediate environment seem distant; they have a " far-away feeling "; indeed, things do not concern them any more than if they lived in another world. *Deceitfulness* is also a common symptom, arising in part from the tendency of patients to busy themselves with the products of their own imagination. Superficial recollections are easily falsified by the addition of fictitious facts, even without the patients being conscious of it. Furthermore, the emotional states exert a great influence over the ideas; hopes and fears guide the thoughts, while vivid impressions as well as accidental ideas dominate intuition and recollections.

In the *emotional field* there is a tendency to asymmetrical development. Great sensitiveness, eagerness, and excessive enthusiasm may predominate, while the more natural feelings are arrested. In connection with an artistic sense of appreciation there may be a lack of tact or a moral obtuseness. Unnatural affections arise; for instance, a fanatic affection for one of the animals, an idolatrous adoration of some person, also numerous idiosyncrasies, or a senseless abhorrence or fear of certain persons, objects, or disease symptoms. There are many striking peculiarities of the emotional attitude,— morbid tender-heartedness, extravagances, or persistent timidity and cowardice. Rapid and sudden changes of the emotional attitude are frequent: exuberant happiness suddenly changes to seclusiveness or outbursts of fury; patients become excessively angry and just as quickly placid.

In accord with the feeling of *egoism,* the patients attend chiefly to their own thoughts and busy themselves with their own welfare. Thus they observe in a most painstaking manner the minor physical changes, which then rapidly multiply and cause apprehension. Constant thought of self and superficiality of the feelings gradually leads to selfishness. Patients are cold, unapproachable, associate with no one, and are most inconsiderate of nearest relatives. They degrade themselves in numerous ways in an effort to arouse special recognition and sympathy.

The *actions* of the patients show constant constraint. Voluntary impulses do not arise from established principles, but from momentary feelings and impulses, as well as through accidental impressions. Fears and passionate impulses interfere with a harmonious development and release of voluntary action. Hence patients are never able to follow anything to its conclusion, as is clearly indicated in their occasional foolish and weak attempts at suicide, showing an inability to transform their desperate feelings into resolute acts.

The patients themselves usually feel their inability to do satisfactory and uniform work. If at the outset they seek to become masters of their own imperfections by means of a strong exertion of the will, they gradually lose ground. A constant struggle regularly leads to weariness and enervation. Many patients gradually withdraw from any serious activity and let things go as they will. Impulsive acts, foolish journeys, precipitate betrothals, changes of location and profession, and attempts at suicide are constantly occurring.

Impulsiveness becomes more and more prominent, and certain habits of will often develop which are exceedingly difficult to break up. Patients must conduct their business always in a certain way, and at once become embarrassed and ill at ease as soon as a change takes place. They are apt to fall an easy prey to the misuse of drugs, become drunkards, drink strong tea and coffee, and are frequently given to excessive dosing with quack remedies.

The *sexual* life is usually an important factor. Sexual impulses develop early and to an abnormal degree, often leading to masturbation, which usually be-

comes deeply rooted and is often practised in addition to regular sexual intercourse. Occasionally the sexual impulse becomes the central point about which the entire life revolves, producing the picture of *sexual neurasthenia.* The sexual desire may be accompanied by an intense feeling of discomfort, even incapacitating the individual, and disappears only with gratification. On the other hand, intense feelings of anxiety may accompany the sexual act, frustrating its accomplishment and leading to mental impotence. Increased sexual excitement induces reckless masturbation, resulting in a constant overexcitation, premature ejaculation, and spermatorrhoea, associated with hypochondriacal fears. Ultimately all kinds of morbid sensations and ideas may develop around this central point.

The weakened power of resistance may manifest itself in the most varied ways. Nervous individuals often develop a high temperature upon slight provocation, easily become delirious, or faint during excitement. Furthermore, there is great susceptibility to alcohol, as well as to tea and coffee, rapid collapse under stress, inability to withstand hunger or thirst, and a great dependency upon weather and temperature. There is also a tendency to pressure in the head, headache, false sensations of all kinds, and increased irritability of the heart. The taking of food is also involved in the general disturbance; voracious appetite alternates with loss of appetite, nervous dyspepsia often develops, as well as sensations of pressure or fulness in the stomach, etc. Sleep is frequently disturbed. In some cases there is an extraordinary demand for sleep, so that even after eight or nine hours of sleep the patients can hardly be aroused. Many patients feel a great weariness upon awakening, and their sleep is disturbed by restless dreams.

Degeneracy is often apparent in various physical defects; such as, a lack of development of the body beyond a puerile stage, either a very youthful or a senile countenance, localized or general cessation of development of the brain and skull, abnormal position of the

teeth, malformation of the ears, palate, sexual organs, and hands. Occasionally there are residuals of an old cerebral disease.

Course. — Since nervousness according to our conception is a congenital morbid state, one cannot speak of the disease as having a characteristic course. Usually the morbid constitution first shows itself in childhood by great restlessness, by irritability, sensitiveness to injuries, minor nervous disturbances, convulsions, enuresis, night horrors, stuttering, etc. Later, difficulties are encountered in teaching the children; on the one hand, great irritability, passion, and rebelliousness, and on the other, susceptibility to seduction and sexual influences, fickleness, anxiety, irresolution, great sense of fatigue, and distractibility. Occasionally there develops a tendency to lying, thieving, and truancy. Many of these symptoms may improve under favorable circumstances. There is often observed an increase of the morbid symptoms during the period of development, in spite of all possible corrective measures. This may be due in part to the unfavorable influence of the general physical and mental evolution at this period, and in part to the gradually increasing demands of life. Furthermore, persistent masturbation, alcoholic excesses, exhausting diseases, pregnancy in women, and, under some conditions, intense emotional excitement are pernicious influences which regularly aid in bringing the disease to its full development.

Diagnosis. — Nervousness is often mistaken for *neurasthenia.* In neurasthenia the symptoms of fatigue only are present, except in marked conditions, while in nervousness there are signs of degeneracy. The more marked these signs are in a given disease picture, the more cautious one should be in considering as a cause for the condition an alleged nervous exhaustion. The symptoms of simple nervous exhaustion rapidly mend under the influence of rest, but the symptoms of nervousness, when once aroused, run an independent and, under certain conditions, a progressive course, even if the immediate exciting factors have been corrected. In addition to this, nervousness develops at any time from youth up without any appreciable external cause and assumes varied forms, while nervous exhaustion never attacks healthy nervous systems without some powerful injury.

Treatment. — Prophylaxis is of greatest importance. Defective persons should be dissuaded from marrying each other. Of the particular injurious influences to be combated, alcoholism is the most prominent. During childhood patients need special attention paid to their education and training, which should be proportionately divided between the body and the brain. The mental development should be retarded if there are any evidences of precocity. Particular stress should be laid on the amount of sleep received, and the patients should be permitted all the sleep they desire. At the time of the awakening of the sexual impulses, the children must be carefully watched and instructed. Very often it is best that the childhood should be passed in the country, in order to give the body as much opportunity as possible to develop, to eliminate confinement in school, and to avoid the pernicious influences of bad associations in cities. If the disorder is very pronounced, manual training under the supervision of a physician is desirable. Psychopathic children, on account of their faulty constitution, do not tolerate routine training well. The training should be adapted to personal peculiarities. In the choice of an occupation one must take into consideration their imperfections. Uncongenial and annoying employment makes the symptoms worse, while simple, regular, and uniform work often does much good. Patients should avoid all excesses. Alcohol in any form must be forbidden. Furthermore, morphin and hypnotics can be prescribed only with the greatest care.

The individual symptoms themselves are best combated by means of an intelligent training under medical supervision, regulation of the entire life, with due regard to a proportionate amount of work and recreation, sufficient sleep and nourishment. Long-drawn-out "cures" are usually unsatisfactory, especially in institutions, as the complaints and hypochondriacal fears tend to increase under such conditions, and should be resorted to only for very definite reasons. On the other hand, the necessity of meeting some regular obligations serves as an important remedy. If relaxation is necessary, it is usually best accomplished by a short journey or a sojourn at the sea or in the mountains. These patients, in general, demand frequent but short periods of relaxation. Where there is despondency, diversion is best obtained by means of social intercourse, distractions, artistic efforts, and amusements.

B. Constitutional Despondency

Constitutional despondency is characterized by a *persistent feeling of sadness which pervades att of life's experiences. Intellect* shows no striking disturbances. Some patients are well endowed, while others from youth are somewhat backward in mental development. The *susceptibility to fatigue* is greatly increased; while patients are capable of taking up a piece of work with intelligence and skill, they tire quickly, demand frequent rests, and are wholly unfit for steady application to mental or physical work, because of resulting headache, insomnia, or general malaise. Under stress of circumstances they are often able to temporarily overcome these hindrances. Distractibility of the *attention* is greatly increased, so that even the most trifling affairs in the surroundings may greatly interfere with systematic work. Hence their work is uncertain, and sometimes has to be done over several times. There is a tendency to display *hypochondriacal* complaints. Consciousness remains unclouded, and thought is coherent. Patients often appreciate their unfortunate condition.

In *emotional attitude* they are oppressed and sorrowful. They may have always been especially susceptible to the cares, sorrows, and misfortunes of life. Present pleasure is always clouded by past sorrow or troubled fears for the future. Many patients to all external appearances seem normal and only disclose their sadness to their families or the physician. Under the influence of some excitement they may temporarily become happy and cheerful, but soon relapse again into their misery. Any undertaking dismays them, and they take little or no pleasure in any occupation. They lack self-confidence, are easily discouraged, feel that they are of little use in the world, are nervous, sick, and fear the outbreak of some awful disease, especially insanity. Some are always troubled with the feeling that they have done something wrong, or that some ill will befall them. They are especially apt to worry about their sexual life. The sexual impulses are usually awakened early and lead to excesses, especially masturbation, the consequences of which the patients always paint in the darkest colors. Sometimes the patients are sentimental.

Conduct is greatly influenced. If anxiety predominates, patients shrink from every obligation, dread the most remote possibilities, and avoid everything to which they are unaccustomed. Many patients are deliberate, find it difficult to arrive at a decision, and tend to exhibit great precision and punctuality in little things. They use an endless amount of time without accomplishing anything. They stick so tenaciously to every task that they are gradually reduced to a smaller and smaller sphere of activity. They excuse themselves for not going out into society because they have not time, and they cannot travel because it is too difficult to get ready. Ultimately their whole activity may be confined to keeping the house clean and preparing meals on time. Some patients are constantly thinking of death and are always making preparations to die. Though they may not seem in earnest about it, yet it not infrequently happens that they make attempts at suicide. Very often all sorts of nervous complaints interfere with their ability to work, such as pressure and pain in the head and peculiar sensations in all parts of the body. Occasionally some peculiar motor symptoms are observed, as grimacing, choreiform movements, clucking with the tongue, snuffling, and twitching of muscles. These " tics " accompany all the different forms of degeneracy. Sleep is usually much disturbed.

Course. — The course of the disease is prolonged, with irregular remissions; but within certain limits it runs a very uniform course, lasting for years. The condition regularly becomes worse after emotional shocks and physical disease and even without any apparent cause. Gradually the patients may become better, but it rarely happens that they are entirely free from symptoms. At first remissions may occur, but later there is a tendency for the symptoms to persist, until finally there is a continuous morbid condition with little variation. Even during the remissions, patients always display some evidence of mental peculiarities: they are quiet, dull, shy, or unfriendly.

Treatment. — The patients can be made very comfortable by a well-regulated life in a favorable environment, but family strife and increased responsibilities always diminish chances of recovery. On the other hand, absolute freedom tends to make the patients worse. Suitable employment is necessary, which must be so adjusted as to gradually increase the responsibility and the exercise of strength. While the special therapeutic agencies, as massage, hydrotherapy, electricity, etc., are of importance, their chief value lies in the psychical influence which can be exerted through them in creating new energy for work and in establishing self-confidence. Hypnotic suggestion is often helpful in cases with insomnia and pain.

0. Constitutional Excitement

Constitutional excitement constitutes a small group of cases characterized by *permanent moderate psychomotor excitement.*

The *intellect* of these patients is fairly good, but they are hindered in acquiring full and complete knowledge, because they are not persistent at their studies and are extremely distractible. Perception is usually unimpaired, knowledge of life and the world is superficial, mental elaboration of experiences is hazy and scanty, and *memory* of early experiences is fleeting, one-sided, and often colored and falsified with many additions. *Thought* is flighty and aimless, and *judgment* is hasty and superficial.

In *emotional attitude* the patients are happy and thoughtless. They possess a marked feeling of egotism and are boastful of their own capabilities and accomplishments. They do not appreciate their imperfections. Toward others they are apt to be lofty, irritable, dogmatic, and unsympathetic. They usually deride, torment, and abuse those who do not agree with them, but on the other hand, they do not become mortified when reproached and insulted. They devote much time to amusements and diversions of all kinds and are given to making fun of themselves and others and playing tricks. They readily adapt themselves to new conditions and are always longing for a change. Occasionally transitory, anxious, or despondent emotional conditions develop.

In *actions* and *manner* the patients are restless and unstable. They are easily approachable, often loquacious, but wholly untrustworthy and vacillating in their judgment. Consequently their lives are one series of thoughtless, venturesome, and often foolish acts. Even in school they are rebellious and disorderly. They react badly under military discipline, neglect the rules of cleanliness and order, misuse furloughs, neglect their duties, and frequently need to be punished. Sexual impulses often develop early and lead to excesses. They frequently become addicted to the use of alcohol. They are constantly moving and changing employment without sufficient reason, always beginning something new and devising great schemes which are soon forgotten. They often make propositions which they cannot live up to, assume lofty titles, and secure recognition by boasting. The lack of plan in their undertakings is most characteristic and clearly shows how little their pressure of activity is held in check by careful reasoning. They soon exhaust their resources, and then they begin to borrow, to cheat, and to swindle. In trying to maintain their credit they always refer to some great "deal" which they are about to put through, a position which awaits them, their intimacy with prominent individuals, betrothals to heiresses, etc. When thwarted they maintain that they are in the right, that they had no idea of fraud, and that they will shortly be in a position to meet all of their obligations. Following punishment, they again return to their old tricks, until finally the morbid character of their conduct is recognized.

Diagnosis. — The similarity of constitutional excitement to *hypomania* is very striking. The differentiation depends upon the fact that in constitutional excitement the excitement is less pronounced, does not recur in definite attacks, but is a fixed personal peculiarity. Nevertheless some cases of constitutional excitement develop transitory exacerbations and even delirious states, while others show periodical vacillations together with irritability and rebelliousness, and, finally, occasional anxious states with indefinite delusions of persecution. These cases are only another indication that we really have to do with a permanent disorder of the mental equilibrium which constitutes the first step toward true manic excitement. These cases also remind one of those cases of manic-depressive insanity, in the lucid intervals of which moderate excitement of the same character occurs. Some refer to both conditions as a *chronic* or *constitutional mania.*

The mildest forms of constitutional excitement approach very closely to certain defective constitutions which are ordinarily regarded as belonging within the realm of normal man. These are usually encountered in families some of whose members have suffered from forms of manic-depressive insanity. They comprise certain brilliant but nevertheless one-sided personalities which charm one by their versatility, their enthusiasm, their artistic abilities, and happy, sunny dispositions, but who at the same time astonish one by their restlessness, volubility, lack of steadiness and persistency in employment, and their tendency to evolve numerous schemes. Occasionally they exhibit periods of unreasonable despondency, which sometimes follow overwork and disappointments. The frequent history of despondency ending in suicides occurring in the parents, brothers, sisters, and their children, or of genuine manicdepressive insanity, leads to a strong presumption that sanguine temperaments of this sort are nothing more than initial psychopathic stages of manic excitement.

Treatment. — The treatment is difficult because the patients lack insight into their condition and, therefore. will not submit to medical advice. In many cases it is necessary to occasionally restrict the freedom of the patients, because otherwise they get into serious difficulties. By means of firm and friendly guidance and especially by sufficient protection against sexual and alcoholic excesses these patients can sometimes be made to follow some useful employment, but in spite of all advice and regulation they always remain fickle and unreliable and a source of constant care and anxiety to their friends.

D. Compulsive Insanity

In this psychopathic state *compulsive ideas and compulsix fears are the predominant symptoms.*

The intellect is not only undisturbed, but may be unusually good. Patients exhibit throughout a pronounced feeling of mental illness and frequently a clear insight into the morbidity of the individual symptoms. Many present symptoms of constitutional despondency before the compulsive ideas and fears appear. Moreover, the initial symptoms usually develop during conditions of despondency.

The compulsive symptoms may be grouped under three heads: the *tormenting ideas* (manies mentales), the *phobva.* and the *impulsions.*

Tormenting Ideas. The feeling of *anxious uneasiness* which accompanies all of these symptoms produces a series of psychogenic disturbances. It is not improbable that the sensation of strangeness referred to in nervousness is nothing more than a peculiar expression of a concealed anxiety, which impairs the patients' sensations and influences the perception of the outer world. Con-

sequently the feeling frequently arises in the patients that they cannot comprehend anything more, cannot follow conversation, or cannot get the sense of that which is read. Thus there develops an endless repetition of the same tormenting thoughts which disturb the patients all the more if they attempt to dispel them. Associated with these feelings there develop peculiar physical sensations all over the body; such as, weariness, palpitation of the heart, blushing, blanching, nausea, and sometimes even vomiting. Furthermore, the anxiety leads to a mixture of voluntary and involuntary impulses, which are thus altered in various ways. Finally the patients evolve peculiar methods of self-relief.

The simplest form of compulsive insanity is represented by the simple compulsive ideas which force themselves upon the patients against their will, and in this way influence the freedom of thought. Sometimes the compulsive idea is very simple or at least not irritating. It is only the frequent repetition of the idea that causes annoyance. Sometimes the idea is accompanied by an hallucinatory picture of great vividness. Odors and melodies may similarly haunt patients. Such ideas are especially annoying when they are disgusting or create horror. Many patients complain because they are compelled to contemplate the sexual organs of those about them. Others when at stool have to dwell upon all sorts of disgusting scenes.

In another group of cases there is a compulsion to ponder over certain definite things; for example, the names of persons (onomatomania), and particularly difficult names. Unable to recollect a name casually heard or seen, the patients immediately strain every nerve to recall it, think about it all day long, lie awake nights trying to recall it, and the tension cannot be relieved until they succeed. Some patients feel compelled to inquire the names of people whom they meet on the street; others feel that they must form a definite picture of the face, form, or color of the hair of strangers. Other patients dwell on fig-

ures (arithmomania), and are compelled to busy themselves with the number of the house, the street, the number of guests about the table, the number of forks, knives, and glasses, the number of designs in the carpet or wall paper.
Magnan, Psychiatrische Vorlesungen, 1893.
Compulsive ideas sometimes take the form of questions; as, "Who is God?" "How was the universe created?" etc. Sometimes these questions refer to objects in the surroundings, when such questions arise as, "Why does that chair stand thus and not so?" "Why does it have four legs and no more or less?" "Why is that house painted green and not brown?" This has been been called *Grubelsucht* — a passion for pondering over things.

Some patients are in doubt as to the accuracy of their memory; still others have the feeling that they may not recognize their acquaintances when they meet them again, or will not remember what they last said to them. Sometimes these feelings of uncertainty seem like ideas of selfaccusation. Patients feel that they have neglected something or have not done something right. When urinating or defecating, the patients may have the feeling that the discharge is incomplete, and therefore they must make further efforts. After every conversation the idea arises that they may not have made themselves clearly understood. After leaving a friend, they sit down and write a letter in order to be sure that they are understood, but the letter is barely off before they are in doubt as to whether they made themselves clear in it. These patients weigh every word before they express themselves, trying to avoid false interpretations. Some patients always have the idea that they have taken some other person's hat, umbrella, or overcoat. In counting money they carefully scrutinize every coin for fear that they might have made a mistake, or that they had not paid out enough, and hence would be accused of fraud. Many patients accuse themselves of not having confessed everything at the confessional or of not being "contrite of heart."

Very often the patients have the fear of destroying or misplacing something of value. In many cases their fears are quite silly; they feel that they are guilty of crime, of homicide, have committed a theft, or have poisoned a relative. In the lighter forms these doubts exist only in one field of activity; in the severer forms they influence all the actions of the patients. "Perhaps it would have been better if I had not drunk that glass of water," or " I have harmed myself by taking that piece of cake." "Had I not gone out of doors, it would have been better; that accident would not have happened or that fire would not have broken out." It is actually impossible for these patients to remain at rest because of the uncertainty as to whether they have closed a door or have sealed a letter that they have mailed. Consequently they manifest an ever increasing painstaking in all the little details of daily life. They are always turning back to see if they have locked the door, or tearing open letters to see if they have enclosed the right one. It is often characteristic of these patients to make use of some particular phrase or movement which they have discovered, such as " High Jinks," or to cough, upon which all doubt is dispelled. This whole group of cases has been designated by Legrand du Saulle as "folie du doute."

There is also a condition called *erythrophobia,* in which patients fear blushing. When any one enters the room or their name is spoken, they immediately blush, which causes great discomfort for fear that they may be thought guilty of some misdeed. It may even create so much annoyanct that they are compelled to give up business. There is also the fear of wearing new clothing because of the newness and accompanying physical discomforts.

The strongest feelings are connected with the welfare of the body. Many patients perceive all kinds of sensation.' in their bodies which cause them anxiety. When droppin? off to sleep, the body seems to increase to an enormous size. Some patients have the uncomfortable feeling that the urine is trickling. They fear that they are going to lose their

minds or become paralyzed. Others have the idea they will suffer from syphilis. Some fear a sunstroke, and in consequence are taking all possible precautions; still others have the foolish fear of snakes, of cats, or that a beetle will crawl into their ears. Some avoid going into the street for fear that a stone or a man may fall upon them from a building. The sexual relations also offer a fruitful field for compulsive fears. Such fears often frustrate the sexual act.

Phobias. In the "*phobias*" fear arises in connection with certain definite conditions. It is impossible to draw a sharp distinction between the states described above and those of phobia, as they are often intimately associated But the phobias are always characterized by the sudden appearance of pronounced anxiety in connection with the general idea of fear. When subjected to them, patients may suffer from palpitation of the heart, become pale, tremble, have a cold sweat, nausea, faintness, polyuria, weakness of the legs, and finally may even lose control of themselves and collapse. The conditions in connection with which such attacks of fear arise are varied, yet there are some forms which recur with notable regularity. Sometimes the same patient may suffer from a whole series of phobias. The best known of these is *agoraphobia,* in which there is great fear of public places. Patients are unable to walk down a long, broad street or in a place where they are alone. When they attempt this, they are so overcome that they cannot proceed. When the condition is extreme, they are afraid to go out on the street at all, some even remaining in bed. Closely related to this is the fear of height which prevents patients from standing near a railing, on the brink of a precipice, going over bridges, or of being in a theatre. Among other morbid fears might be mentioned that of being alone in the dark, riding on trains, and going through tunnels. These patients find no pleasure in travelling, do not enjoy going to church, and always sit near the door, ready to fly at the first sign of danger. Various phobias may develop in connection with the occupation of

the patients; for instance, barbers sometimes suffer these attacks whenever they see a razor, or telegraphers when they catch sight of their instruments, etc., which finally necessitates giving up the occupation.

Among women, especially, there occurs the fear of *dirt* (mysophobia), contagion, or infection. The countless bacteria always present in the ah are one of the chief sources of annoyance. The patients are everywhere complaining of the bad air and throwing up windows; they are afraid of handling brass or copper, or are always taking things up by nails or pieces of glass. They notice in their food a shining bit which may possibly be a pin. Books, especially, are avoided as a possible source of contagion. Occasionally a patient has the fear of destroying something of value. One lady was always in fear of throwing some important letter into the fire or destroying it, and for this reason carefully avoided touching any paper and finally even printed books. Patients are constantly washing themselves, and are fearful of disease from touching money, books, or papers. In taking food they have to wipe the dishes frequently and inspect carefully every morsel.

As the result of fear of misplacing something or of soiling themselves there develops the fear of contact, *ddire du toucher.* Patients throw away all the needles in the house, and they give up sewing for fear that they may injure themselves. They no longer wash the windows, because the glass might break and cut them. They refuse to shake hands, but wear gloves and open windows with their elbows. They begin the habit of washing not only their hands, but also all of their clothing. Some patients spend the entire day in dressing, undressing, and washing.

A common characteristic of almost all phobias are the *crises.* As soon as one threatens to do that feared by the patients or to hinder them from carrying out their usual means of protection, they develop an anxious condition with excitement. It is quite astonishing to see how patients, until now hoping for relief of the disease, suddenly turn about and oppose any real attempt at combating it.

Impulsions. — In this last series of cases the compulsive fears apparently take the form of impulses. In reality, however, we still have to do only with fears which are directed against the dangers that the patients suppose are threatening them. Such questions as the following press themselves upon the patients: "What would happen if you should undertake to do this or that, if you should kill some one with that knife, or set that building on fire, or shout aloud in church?" Whenever they see sores or ulcers they feel impelled to touch them, and at the sight of filth must wallow in it. It seems to them they must smear everything with urine. Religious anxieties create the idea of fouling the communion bread, or of bringing it in contact with the genitals. Other patients think that they must bore nails into the heads of their children, cut off their heads, commit sexual assaults upon them, steal the silver from the table, or rip open their own abdomen or that of others. Usually these thoughts arise in connection with beloved ones. Sometimes illusions are associated with these ideas, when the patients see a bloody knife suspended before their eyes, are followed by a picture, feel as if their arms and hands are extending out to grasp a pile of filth, etc. Thus, there arises a fear of all objects, which can call up impulses of these kinds. The patients no longer venture to attend communion and show the greatest anxiety when coming in contact with dangerous weapons. Many patients permit themselves to be locked up or to be bound, in order that they may withstand these impulses. In reality, however, these patients never perform the dreaded acts; at most it only happens that they are unable to withstand the temptation to flee from some religious ceremony or during prayer to substitute some blasphemous or obscene expression.

The *consciousness* of all these patients is entirely clear. They have an insight into their condition, and the desire, but not the strength, to free themselves from it. They know well enough that no real harm threatens them, but that they are overwhelmed only by the "fear of the fear." Their *emotional attitude* shows anxiety which often is in marked contrast to their courage in real danger. They are usually of a weak, dependent nature. In their behavior and actions they frequently show nothing abnormal, and control themselves perfectly before strangers.

Course. — The course of the disease varies much. Complete disappearance of the symptoms seldom occurs, and then only for a short time, but rapid improvement is often noticed, usually during the period of development.

Prognosis. — The prognosis in general is unfavorable. Occasionally, especially in cases of simple compulsive ideas, agoraphobia, and the allied symptoms, the disturbance may disappear for longer or shorter periods, but there is great fear of relapses. There are many cases in which striking symptoms appear temporarily only under the influence of specially unfavorable conditions. In the *folie du doute* and the fear of contact there is little chance for improvement. On the other hand, compulsive insanity never develops into other psychoses, as the patients often fear.

Treatment. — The treatment is chiefly directed to combating the condition of degeneracy. In youth careful attention to the demands of physical development is necessary. Threatening peculiarities should be warded off by careful training, and all deleterious influences removed which tend to weaken the physical and mental powers of resistance. The symptoms of the disease can be combated by persistent and patient training with a view to strengthening and encouraging the patients to struggle step by step against the morbid compulsion. The significance of their condition should always be made clear to the patients, and they must be impressed with the fact that they will overcome it more by abstraction and diversion than by exercise of will power. Occasional interviews with the physician aid in quieting the patient and giving him additional courage. Hypnotic suggestion may be of value during crises in supporting the patients, but its influence is transitory.

E. Impulsive Insanity

Impulsive insanity is characterized by *the development of morbid tendencies and impulses which either dominate over volition continually or in recurring paroxysms.*

These acts, which appear without motive, are performed because of an irresistible impulse. The impulses do not arise as the result of a conscious plan, but appear suddenly, are quickly executed, and often quite indefinite, thereby causing the actions to appear unpremeditated, purposeless, and even absurd. In case the act is serious or dangerous, its accomplishment may be preceded by a conscious struggle. But yet the worst acts are often performed without delay, and as a matter of course. Neither the regret that follows the act nor the fear for the results suffices to suppress the recurrence of similar impulses.

Those so-called normal individuals who suffer from trifling and insignificant impulses, which appear only under certain circumstances, disappear rapidly, and lead to very simple acts, represent a sort of transition stage between normal health and impulsive insanity. Maudsley tells of a man who for weeks was annoyed by an impulse to overturn two stones which lay upon a wall, finally forcing him to sneak out at night in order to perform the absurd act. Such impulses become of more consequence to the patient when they are constantly involving the environment and interfering with comfort and occupation. The impulses that develop in certain definite directions are of far more importance. *These include the impulse to tramp, to set fire, to steal, and to destroy or kill.*

In the impulse to *ramble* the patients are suddenly seized with an intense desire to roam about, sometimes in connection with some sort of an adventurous purpose. So they wander about here and there until their means are exhausted. They have a clear memory of their experiences, and they do not see anything peculiar in their conduct. Occasionally during these periods they commit all sorts of frauds, assume false names, and are boastful.

The impulse to set fire *(pyromania)* is

exhibited especially by young females, most often during puberty. Sometimes the morbid pleasure of seeing things burn and at hearing the crackle dates from early childhood. Another common form of impulse is the tendency to skilful but foolish stealing *(kleptomania)*, encountered almost exclusively among women, and especially during menstruation and pregnancy. The stolen articles are frequently almost or quite worthless for the patients. In some cases there is a desire for some one definite thing which is accumulated in great quantities. Sexual impulses may accompany this condition. Further expressions of degeneracy of normal impulses are seen in silly fondness for animals, irresistible tendency to play, marked increase of sexual impulses, and many similar digressions.

Morbid impulses to *destroy and kitt* are other instances. There is a special group of young women who show a morbid impulse to beat little children intrusted to their care. Here there exists a close relationship to those sexual impulses which have been called sadism, masochism, and fetichism. The men who prod women, who snip hair, slash ladies' dresses, steal women's shoes or linen, and many exhibitionists belong to this class.

The *mental endowmerd* of these patients usually shows no marked defect, but in some severe cases there is a more or less high grade of mental weakness. In the emotional field the defect is more evident; the patients are apt to be childish, unstable, shy, seclusive, or vulgar.

Course. — The symptoms of the disease appear only during certain periods of life, and particularly during the period of development, at which time there is a condition of lessened resistance in both the physical and mental fields. In some cases there is improvement, with physical and mental development and the formation of a stable personality. Periodicity is noticed only occasionally.

Diagnosis. — One should not confound the ineradicable relapsing of *criminals* with the regular repetition of similar criminal acts in these patients. The criminal sets fire, kills, and steals,

but he does it from selfish motives, and for some definite purpose, perhaps to do some one injury, while the patient suffering from impulsive insanity is forced by the dominating impulse to the deed against his will. Frequently the patient has a feeling that the action is inconsistent, unnatural, and morbid. *Compulsive insanity* is distinguished by the fact that the patients do not commit deeds that are in their minds; they often have an abhorrence of them and fear that they may yield to something which really does not exist. In impulsive insanity there is apt to be associated with the idea of the morbid act a feeling of desire and eagerness for its performance, and the patients cannot remain quiet until it is done. The performance of the act is immediately followed by a feeling of relief, while failure brings disappointment.

Treatment. — The treatment of impulsive insanity naturally lies in the education of the patients, which must be adapted to individual cases and carefully conducted, with proper regard for the physical development. It is of greatest importance that the patients do not become addicted to the use of alcohol. There are some cases which, for the protection of society, need to be confined in an institution where they can be educated to lead a useful life.

F. Contrary Sexual Instincts 1
This psychopathic state, which received its name from Westphal, refers to those sexual propensities, appearing mostly in youth, exhibited by individuals of the same sex for each other, with an indifference or even an abhorrence of the opposite sex. The condition has also been well described by Krafft-Ebing, Moll, and Schrenk-Notzing.

Etiology. — The contrary sexual instincts are far more prevalent among men. It is an uncommon condition, the cases reported to date numbering but a few hundred, although homosexual patients maintain that it is by no means rare. Ulrichs, in his own morbid experience, claims to have encountered two hundred cases. It is more prevalent in certain employments, such as among decorators, waiters, ladies' tailors; also

among theatrical people. Moll claims that women comedians are regularly homosexual.

The condition develops from a state of degeneracy. It is a view of Krafft-Ebing, emphasized by the statements of the patients themselves, that the peculiar perversion of the sexual impulse is congenital. Schrenk-Notzing, on the other hand, lays some stress upon accidental factors which happen to exert an influence upon the sexual feelings long before the age of sexual development, such as the intercourse of naked boys while bathing, wrestling, etc. Sometimes passionate friendships exist among young children who are still ignorant of the sexual differences. But it is only with the abnormal child that such accidental influences upon the early sensual feelings can have any power in the later development of the sexual impulses. It seems most probable, then, that the morbidity of the condition depends not upon impulses which are perverted from the onset, but upon a characteristic tendency originating in a hereditary state of degeneracy.

Westphal, Archiv f. Psy., II, 1.
v. Krafft-Ebing, Psychopathia Scxualis, 1900.
Moll, Die eontrare Sexualempfindung, 1891.
Schrenk-Notzing, Die Suggestionstherapie bei krankhaften Erscheinungen des Geschlectssinnes, 1892.

Symptomatology. — Sexual impulses develop early and usually to a marked degree, sometimes leading to onanism. The natural heterosexual impulses may have developed first, being displaced later by stronger morbid tendencies. The patients, both in the waking and dream states, experience pleasurable sexual feelings only in connection with their own sex. Attempts at natural sexual intercourse are unsuccessful, or accomplished only with difficulty. Close associations are usually formed with some individuals of the same sex, which usually develop into passionate friendship, with extravagant display of affection, letter writing, sending gifts and flowers, and exhibitions of jealousy. This frequently extends to kissing, embracing, and occasionally to masturbation and other forms of sexual perversion, but rarely to pederasty. In these friendships the physical and mental superiority af one individual over another may aid in arousing the 3exual feelings. Usually both individuals are homosexual, but sometimes the patient desires intercourse only with i normal individual. Frequent changes of the affection, with disruption of these friendships, often occur, showing the fickleness of the patients, though in some cases such-elationships are maintained for years. Differences in social rank is of less importance than in normal individmls. A few patients of the better classes are attracted jy mechanics, and especially by soldiers.

The patients usually remain unmarried. Those who do marry, either in the hope of overcoming their perverse tendencies or from the desire to have children, are usually true to their marital duties, except in the matter of sexual intercourse. Some indulge occasionally, but most of them regularly, in homosexual intercourse.

Other symptoms indicative of a morbid constitutional basis are usually present, especially the physical stigmata. Judgment is usually unimpaired, as well as the ability to comprehend, but there is an increased sense of fatigue, lack of perseverance with mental work, and a tendency to dream. Imagination is prominent and interferes with the capacity for purely rational activity. Some are especially endowed in an artistic way, being good musicians and artists; but they also possess a keen sense of appreciation of their abilities. Mental weakness may exist. Many patients have an insight into the morbidness of their impulses, and defend themselves on the ground that the impulses are the natural and involuntary product of their constitution. In the emotional life they present irritability, are sensitive, moody, and impressionable, often timid, and given to passionate outbursts of feeling. In actions they appear effeminate, vain, pliable, unstable, and are sometimes sluggish. They are often careless about their work, easily dis-

tractible, and untrustworthy. The sexual impulses are apt to gain control over them, causing neglect of business. Fetichism and other perversities may also be present.

The condition of psychic hermaphroditism is occasionally present, when sexual feelings are exhibited toward both sexes, though usually stronger toward one sex than the other. Where homosexuality is very pronounced, the individual may experience a change of personality, a man becoming feminine in manner, gait, and countenance. He becomes affected in manner, vain, coquettish, takes great pains with his personal appearance, desires to be in fashion, wears flowers, and uses cosmetics. Some develop a fondness for women's employment, do needlework, arrange their rooms after the fashion of a woman's boudoir, and they may even dress in women's clothes, padding the hips and breast, talk in a falsetto voice, and in every possible way simulate feminine traits. Early evidences of such traits may make their appearance in childhood. A few patients present physical characteristics indicative of the opposite sex; men are beardless, possess high-pitched, light voices, have soft white skin, with a more marked pannicus adiposus and well-developed mammae; while the homosexual females have a deep, coarse voice and show a tendency to grow beards. The former are called by KrafftEbing androgyny, and the latter gynandry. Hermaphroditism has never been encountered in homosexual individuals.

The course of the disease, which usually reaches its full ievelopment between twenty-five to thirty-five years of ige, is always prolonged. In the acquired homosexuality;here is often a long struggle before the patient becomes i confirmed pervert. The homosexual tendencies may ippear periodically, with or without accompanying states)f general excitement.

Diagnosis. — It is not a difficult matter to identify lomosexual patients where there has been a marked trans»osition of the traits characteristic of the sexes. Yet lormal sexual instincts

may exist in spite of such a transition. Usually the condition becomes known to the hysician only through the communication of the patient. t is necessary to distinguish between contrary sexual in 2l stincts and mere practice of homosexual acts, the latter being pure perversity, as practised among prisoners, etc. , who return to normal sexual relations upon gaining freedom.

Prognosis. —The prognosis is more favorable than is usually thought. Very many cases improve, and some even recover under the influence of treatment.

Treatment. — The most successful method of treatment is through the use of hypnotic suggestion. This is directed first against the increased sexual excitability and masturbation which is frequently present; next it is applied to the insensibility of the patient toward his own sex, and finally in creating an excitability toward the opposite sex and a tendency to heterosexual intercourse. The hypnotic influence over the patient, dealing as it does with a deeply rooted habit, is acquired slowly and with difficulty. Schrenk-Notzing lays great stress upon regular natural intercourse, but excessive coitus must be avoided, because it may have an injurious effect upon the selfconfidence. Treatment directed at the general nervous condition is also of importance, and should include the establishment of a routine in the physical and mental life, with attention to the diet, exercise, and relaxation. One should remember that even though marked improvement or recovery takes place, the original defective basis still remains.

XIV. PSYCHOPATHIC PERSONALITIES

Those psychopathic conditions which develop on a morbid constitutional basis include an extensive borderland between pronounced morbid states and mere personal eccentricities which are wont to be regarded as normal. We consider personal deviations from the regular course of mental development as morbid only when they are of special consequence to the physical and mental life; but the distinction is one of degree and is to a certain extent arbitrary.'

There is a considerable group of such morbid conditions which may be properly regarded as mental deformities. They are not characterized by any definite disease process, but rather by a general deviation from the normal mental life. Our discussion of this group will be limited to conspicuous types which are of special interest to the psychiatrist.

A. Born Criminals

The French alienists were the first to call attention to the fact that there was a form of insanity in which the disorder was limited to the fields of the feelings and the conduct. In 1835, Pritchard grouped together, under the name of "Moral Insanity," those diseases in which there existed a perverse state of the feelings, temperaments, dispositions, habits, and actions, while the intellectual functions presented no apparent abnormalities. The possibility of a circumscribed impairment of the morals was combated by pointing out the correlation between the different phases of the mental life and the presence of concurrent intellectual abnormalities, hence " Moral Insanity" ceased to be regarded as a separate disease and came to be classed as one of the sub-forms of imbecility. One of the causes of this change of attitude was the supposedly demoralizing effects of the doctrine on criminal law.

Daily experience teaches us that the intellect and the emotions develop more or less independently of each other. There are, undoubtedly, men with conspicuous mental endowment who are morally bad and *vice versa*. We must admit, however, that the complete independence of the separate fields does not obtain. Even in congenital emotional indifference there is always present a certain impairment of intellectual capacity. But unquestionably there is a large number of individuals in whom the inadequate development of the moral feelings is more conspicuous than that of the intellect.

The doctrine of "Moral Insanity " has received new meaning through the activities of Lombroso and the Italian positivistic school in the attempt to describe and differentiate the born criminal — " Delinquente nato." According to Lombroso about twenty-five per cent. of

criminals, and a still higher percentage among the murderers, cany the marks of the born delinquent. It is a reasonable hypothesis that in these conditions we have to do with various grades of psychopathic degeneracy. The lighter forms may be scarcely distinguishable from the inadequate moral development of normal life. But on the other hand, there are persons whose shocking moral incapacity clearly indicates morbid degeneracy. At the present time there is a certain justification for calling the severest forms of criminal endowment "Moral Insanity" or "Moral Imbecility. " But more exact characterization of the various conditions which have hitherto been collectively designated by this term would help to clarify the matter; for instance, it would be advisable to differentiate between those who suffer from constitutional excitement, the unstable and the morbid swindler, and the group which we are here describing and which is characterized in general by moral stupidity.

Etiology. — The general causes of this type of degeneracy are practically the same as those which we have come to regard as the causes of degeneracy itself. *Alcoholism* in the parents easily stands first. Among two hundred inmates of a reform school seventy-eight had drunken fathers; five, drunken mothers; and in two cases both parents were drunkards. There were also twenty-four cases in which parents suffered from mental disturbances, twenty-six from epilepsy, and many more from other nervous diseases. The correlation between illegitimacy and born criminals is partially accounted for by the presence of defective heredity and of alcoholism in the parents.

These facts, together with the prevalence of stigmata and the unresponsiveness of the genuine criminal nature to all educational influences, indicates the existence of a certain group of cases with abnormal endowment gradually merging into disease. Moreover, some of these patients after a long criminal career develop severe psychoses which lead to deterioration, especially the paranoid forms of dementia praecox.

Symptomatology. — The *intellect* of these patients is tolerably developed within the limits of practical life. They comprehend well, acquire a certain amount of knowledge and experience, which they may exploit with some craftiness; they show no defect of memory and are fairly logical in their thought. But their views are narrow. They cannot perform exacting, intellectual work and are unable to develop any coherent conception of life. Experts on criminal natures have demonstrated a decided lack of comprehensive reflection and foresight. Born criminals do not feel the need of reflecting beyond the present and the more immediate future.

Even in early youth there are conspicuous *moral defects,* such as a lack of sympathy, shown by barbarous cruelty to animals, malicious teasing, illtreatment of their playmats, and general unresponsiveness to kindness. Later there develops pronounced selfishness without sense of honor or proper affection for parents, brothers, and sisters. Here belong those *monstrous* children who even at the tenderest age try to murder the members of their family for trivial reasons, and then report in a stupid, matter-of-fact way the details of their plans, and show obvious regret at their failure. Attempts at education are fruitless, since the most important incentives — love and ambition — are lacking. Force alone is able to suppress the manifestations of their unbridled selfishness, but it is soon met by duplicity, cunning, deceit, callousness, stubbornness, and a disposition to lie. Development throughout is selfish. Patients manifest affection toward parents, relatives, and companions only when they anticipate some advantage from it. The egotism expresses itself in vanity, braggadocio, peevishness, love of idleness, excesses, foolish prodigality, and often in weak sentimentality. Usually, there is little resistance to temptation and sudden impulses, and there is great emotional irritability, vindictiveness, unreliability, instability, and susceptibility to alcohol.

It is evident that such an endowment

will lead almost necessarily to a criminal career. It usually begins with truancy, loitering, begging, and petty larcenies, oftentimes in connections with gangs, and, in females, with prostitution. Often this leads to commitment to reform schools. Such children of the well-to-do classes shock their parents at an early age by vulgarity, lying, persistent laziness, petty larcenies, and peculations. They wander from one teacher to another, always with the same lack of success, until finally it becomes impossible to protect them from the results of their conduct.

The further life of these morally incapable personalities is a constant conflict with society. They soon find themselves thoroughly out of harmony with any social environment in which they are located. But they are wholly unable to appreciate that it is their own actions which necessitate their being condemned to pass their lives in prisons and penitentiaries. They rather consider themselves martyrs who are cruelly persecuted, while others, no better than they, live in honor and wealth. They regularly fail to comprehend the probable outcome of their lives. They are convinced that it will be possible for them to succeed, even when they are determined to return immediately to their old ways. Many submit with cringing docility to imprisonment, while others even in confinement continue their struggle against the regulations of society by insubordination, deceit, and treachery. But as a rule they are cowardly and less inclined to open violence than to passive opposition and to treachery. They are frequently hypochondriacal, and there is often an increased susceptibility to bodily pain. Their inaccessibility to friendly advances is quite noticeable.

From this class of morally defective individuals the majority of "professional criminals" originate. These criminals derive increasing pleasure from conflicts with the laws, pride themselves on their performances, and show a conscious effort to develop themselves for their art. Thus there develop criminal "specialists," who become exceedingly

cunning and skilful. But it is a notable fact that in their criminal acts they often show an astonishing degree of heedlessness and lack of foresight. Evidences of pronounced physical degeneracy often accompany the criminal natures. There are no definite and inevitable deviations, but there is a considerable group of signs of degeneracy, which show unmistakably that confirmed criminals often possess an inferior physical endowment. The number and variety of these signs are certainly more apparent in criminals than in the general population. This fact of itself naturally proves nothing in an individual case. A given person may, therefore, be mentally sound in spite of numerous signs of degeneracy. On the other hand, we would expect a larger percentage of mental deviations in men of that sort than in those who present no stigmata. To be sure they do not need to be criminals on that account. Rather, the born criminal is only one of the forms in which degeneracy expresses itself.

Diagnosis. — It is exceedingly difficult to draw a sharp line between health and disease. Hence, judges of the court especially combat the assumption of a "moral imbecility." But the existence of the moral incapacity extending back into early youth, in spite of satisfactory intellectual development and the complete unresponsiveness of the patient to all moral influences, justify the assumption of a morbid personality. Moreover, the existence of numerous and definite signs of physical degeneracy, as well as the history of injurious prenatal influences, such as alcoholism or mental disease in the parents, are significant, but in any individual case they are of value only as indicating the necessity of a careful scientific examination of the mental condition, and are not proof of disease. It is a notable fact that many of these patients fail to show any striking disturbances during imprisonment or while confined in institutions, but their great incapacity at once becomes evident as soon as they are released and exposed to the numerous vicissitudes of life.

Treatment. — The treatment of born

criminals unfortunately offers little opportunity and still less prospect of success. If a quiet, rigid, but at the same time kindly education in a limited sphere, preferably under psychiatric supervision, does not succeed, the individual cannot be prevented from entering a criminal career. Lombroso has advocated the view that many of these persons under favorable conditions need not come into conflict with the law, but may gratify their criminal tendencies in other and inconspicuous ways. This, however, is true only of the lighter forms, which closely approximate health. Baer reports that occasionally children who were originally emotionally deficient have later in life improved considerably. It is also a well-known fact that some of the criminal tendencies that appear early in life, such as the propensity to lie, to steal, and to cruelty, can almost completely disappear as the patient matures mentally. In later life the best that one can do is to compel the person to follow a regular occupation under proper control, to choose proper associates, and finally to abstain from alcohol and sexual excesses. Unfortunately, this can be carried out successfully only In the light cases.

B. The Unstable

The "unstable," as the French call them, constitute a 3econd large group of psychopathic personalities which are characterized by a *weakness of will in all their activities.*

Symptomatology.—The intellectual endowment may be very good, but is often only mediocre. Some patients astonish one by their rapidity of comprehension, their ease of committing things to memory, and their ability to express themselves. Patients are often keen observers, quickly recognizing the defects and peculiarities of their environment, are vivacious and understand thoroughly how to use their information to the best advantage. On the other hand, they lack altogether energy for continuous and satisfactory work. They start out zealously, but soon grow weary and are, therefore, unable to complete any course of education. They never probe to the bottom of things and their knowledge is superficial and fragmentary. Knowledge is often readily acquired but is not elaborated and, therefore, is quickly forgotten. At school their talents sometimes arouse great expectations, which are never fulfilled because of their inconstancy and unreliability. It is often said of such children, " They could do much better if they only would," but unfortunately they lack the power to will.

Higher intellectual development is always defective. Conception is confused and indistinct, judgment is immature and onesided, and the understanding of life undeveloped and short-sighted. Their interests center on sports and on frivolous pleasures, and they do not respond to more serious matters. They often show a propensity to dream, to poetical or dramatic efforts, etc., but they are never earnest or thorough.

In *emotional attitude* the patients show abrupt changes, at times being elated and confident, and at others spiritless, sensitive, or pessimistic. They are very easily aroused to enthusiasm, and as readily disheartened. There is usually an increased irritability, sensitiveness, and peevishness. They are offended and dispirited upon slight provocation, are suspicious and prejudiced, but one can easily put them into good humor again. Very often their relations with their relatives become strained. The patients often become dissatisfied and embittered, the cause of which in their opinion never lies in their own behavior, but in the unkindness of their people. Although they are generally harmless and good natured, they are dominated by the most pronounced *selfishness*. Their own welfare is their chief concern, while they show little interest in their environment and even less sympathy. They are not inclined to submit to privation, but demand comfort and luxuries, and regard all restrictions as gratuitous insult. They often show vanity in the effeminate care of their personal appearance, their affected utterance, and tendency to braggadocio. The patients' lack of perseverance, of power of resistance, and energy usually becomes evident as soon as they are deprived of home influences. At school they are considered pliable, unstable, and easily led off into foolish pranks, but they are susceptible to education, which, however, does not last. As soon as they have to stand on their own feet, they are helpless. Since work is not agreeable, they often change, hoping to find an easier occupation. They lack punctuality, neglect their business, do not work full hours, and allow little things to interfere with fulfilling their obligations. They excuse their unproductiveness in various ways. In one place the work is stultifying, in another too strenuous, the shop is unsanitary, the foremen are too severe, etc. Conditions of emotional excitement are aroused by ridiculously trifling occurrences and prevent the patients from working; under no circumstances can they continue work, they must cool down, and must Beek diversion by going to the theatre. They are often hypochondriacal, are deeply concerned for their health, feel exhausted, have headaches, or a feeling of faintness as soon as they are set to work. Hence, they are frequently discharged as useless, or at most are tolerated as unpaid assistants, and are wholly incapable of obtaining an independent livelihood.

They are usually not ashamed of this state of affairs. They see no impropriety in being supported by others, and believe circumstances justify their conduct. Even though they earn nothing, they are careless with their money, buying useless articles in large amounts without thought of the future.

They readily yield to temptation. If placed under guardianship, they become slack, indolent, and unproductive, but they lead their useless lives without gross disturbances, tend to fill them with loafing and useless fads, take cures when not sick, and seek recreation when not weary. In bad company, they give themselves up to sexual extravagances, get diseased, and begin to drink and gamble. Under these influences they sometimes do very questionable things and even perform criminal acts. Such patients sometimes develop the picture of *"pseudo-dipsomania."* They may abstain for months and then upon some occasion when their weak will is overpowered, they begin to drink and continue drinking until thoroughly intoxicated and their money is all gone. It is not their emotional condition that impels the patients to drink, but mere incidents, such as an intimate friend or a farewell banquet. The debauches are not periodical, but are determined by external circumstances. Moreover, the patients are not excited by the alcohol, but are simply intoxicated.

Lighter grades of this weakness of will are very common. A very large proportion of those whom Aschaffenburg calls "habitual criminals," and particularly a large number of tramps, mendicants, and even prostitutes belong to this ;roup. The instability first becomes evident as soon as ihese individuals encounter some difficulty in their lives, investigation shows that a large number of vagabonds are orced into their life by their congenital instability and not »y unusual circumstances. The same condition is clearly hown to exist in the offspring of well-to-do parents, who, lotwithstanding an apparently good endowment and good ducation, continue wholly unstable. One rarely fails to ind in these families traces of degeneracy.

Diagnosis. — The gradual appearance of the symptoms if *instability,* as the patients attempt to undertake the luties of life, resembles somewhat the picture of *dementia rrmcox.* But without question they are two totally different onditions. Instability often leads to idleness and abanlonment of certain lines of work, but never to dementia, he condition of the patients remains essentially the same s it was in youth; they are not dull and apathetic, but inly afraid of work. They retain their hobbies and always eel the necessity of passing the time in some agreeable ray. Notwithstanding their perverted and onesided apprehension, they develop neither delusions nor hallucinaions. Finally, the patients are natural in their manners; heir will is weak and yielding, but never shows eccenricities.

Other forms of the insanity of degeneracy sometimes esemble the unstable; for instance, the increased suggesibility reminds one of *hysteria*. The unstable do not show he extensive influence of the emotional states upon the 'hysical processes, although there are occasional hysterical ymptoms. Like the *born criminals* the unstable present reat susceptibility to temptations, distaste for work, uperficial intellectual work, lack of foresight, selfishness, nd are often enough impelled to criminal careers. Never theless, it is better to distinguish the two forms of psychopathic personalities. The unstable lack the passion and persistency characteristic of the born criminal; there is no trace of the independent criminal will and of professional warfare against social order. When the unstable commit crimes, they are the result of opportunity and temptation, and are limited to actions which demand neither resolution nor energy.

Treatment. — Since this disease represents a form of degeneracy, the treatment is limited. The value of educational measures in individual cases, such as afforded by a strict regimen in the performance of duties and development of physical capacity for work, depends on the severity of the disturbance. In later years sanitarium life may be helpful, where it is possible to remove all sorts of morbid inhibitions and to direct employment. Unfortunately, the patients rarely possess sufficient determination to submit to compulsion for any length of time. In some cases total abstinence from alcohol causes great improvement. Under favorable circumstances it is sufficient if one is able to protect the patients against relapses for some time.

0. The Morbid Liar And Swindler
The morbid liar and swindler — the "pseudologia phantastica" — has been described by Delbrueck. This disorder consists of a *morbid hyperactivity of the imagination, inaccuracy of memory, and a certain instability of the emotions and volitions*.

Symptomatology. — At first glance these patients often appear specially gifted. They apprehend quickly, easily comprehend new situations, and readily acquire special information, such as geographical and historical data, citations from poets, and even foreign languages. They can converse fluently on the most varied subjects, have heard of almost everything, and are sure in their judgments. They thus give the impression of being cultured and well read, but in reality their knowledge is very superficial and made up of isolated, incoherent scraps, and a mixture of details, which are insufficiently comprehended and elaborated and at times even falsified. Their thought lacks system, order, and coherence; their judgment is immature and their conception of life shallow and insincere.

There is associated with the susceptibility to new impressions an extraordinary *mobility of the content of memory.* But both of these symptoms are an expression of one and the same fundamental disturbance; namely, an increased lability of the psychic processes. Recollections, moods, wishes, and accidental impulses alter and color the experiences of life in various ways, so that before long there appears an inextricable mixture of truth and fiction. In morbid liars these fabrications and falsifications of memory appear on a large scale. At first there may be an indistinct feeling of uncertainty as to their statements, but very soon the actual and invented details become so mixed that the patients themselves are no longer able to account for their real origin.

The specially characteristic feature of morbid lying is the *satisfaction which the patients derive from wilful falsifications of memory — the "joy of lying."* They are very apt to embellish the most unimportant statements with alterations and additions; indeed, they often cannot tell a story twice alike. The activity of their imagination enables them to fancy unreal occurrences in a dreamlike fashion; they think of themselves as participating in them, and finally they recount them as actual facts, clothed in varying forms.

In this way patients come to involve themselves in a maze of statements and narrations from which there is no other escape except by new falsehoods. The most extraordinary experiences are related in a most matter-of-fact way, with a cautious secrecy or with outbursts of emotion; such as their descent from royal families, dangerous experiences, powerful enemies, unheard-of incidents like those encountered in dime novels, etc. Indeed, many details may be borrowed directly from their reading. The content of these fabrications can change according to need or fancy. Yet some elements tend to recur. In spite of appearances the patients do not present genuine delusions. They know well enough that they are fabricating, but allow themselves to be carried away by their material, and keep on spinning it out. They are soon forced by the contradictions with their earlier utterances to new fabrications, but even without this they are unable to withstand the impulse to give full sway to their imagination on every occasion. For the time being they completely forget the distinction between reality and fiction. When confronted with their lies, they are either contrite and promise to do better, only to justify their conduct by a new tissue of fantastic lies; or they disavow outright their early statements, assuming the attitude of injured innocence and declining further discussion. If they can gain a little time in this way, they very soon astonish one by further disclosures.

In *emotional attitude* the patients are usually high spirited and self-conscious. They live from one day to another in a wholly indifferent manner, have no care for anything, trust their star, are thoughtless, and are always devising jokes and pastimes. At intervals there are occasional dramatic outbreaks of despair or of angry irritability. Any criticism of their pretensions is apt to be met with real excitement, but such emotional fluctuations are usuaDy superficial and soon give way to the usual self-complacency. Patients show absolutely no insight, but, on the other hand, consider themselves specially gifted, clever, and boast most impressively of their family connections, liberal education, brilliant attainments, and prospects. They lay the blame for any apparent lack of success upon adverse circumstances, nadequate support, or the hostility of relatives, etc. Even xi their simplest narratives, they are easily led into apparent exaggerations.

In *conduct* patients are clever, confident, and presumptuous. They are uncommonly curious, like to participate in everything, and understand how to make an impression, md to inspire common people with confidence and respect. rhey have a tendency to gossip, to read much,, and to busy themselves, but not persistently, and they are fond of pleasjres, dissipations, entertainments, and gay society. Left;o themselves they are prone to live an irregular, extravagant, md prodigal life, are exceedingly polite, dress in the latest ashion, and lavish their money on trifles.

With this sort of an endowment these morbid patients are mturally impelled to the career of *swindlers* and *tramps.* The tendency to swindling of all kinds appears even in early routh. Thirst for adventures leads patients to undertake idventurous journeys, during which they employ their gift or lying to make credulous people believe their fabulous ales concerning themselves, their past history, and their uture prospects, and to lure money from their pockets.?hey know how to conceal their real personality so that it 3 often impossible to expose them. They are especially,pt to pose as scions of a famous family, who have been lompelled by various circumstances to flee and to conceal hemselves, but they have the prospect of securing great iches. They know how to establish the probability of all 2m this by all sorts of dodges, such as forged letters and papers. They swindle every one possible by relating to them pathetic stories. They present themselves as col leagues, turn up under different names, and use high-sounding titles to order merchandise of all kinds. Their procedures resemble those of the ordinary swindler, but it is noteworthy that these patients swindle in reference to things of little consequence and often get no advantage out of their representation?. Many patients simply wander about acquiring a livelihood by irregular but respectable occupations, boast and lie for no other purpose than the mere pleasure derived from their falsehoods and im-

pressions which they make on their surroundings.

Morbid swindling and lying are also forms of degeneracy. They are very often accompanied by definite hysterical symptoms. However, they should not be regarded simply as a type of hysteria, because they often occur without hysterical symptoms. Moreover, they are in some respects related to the group of the *unstable;* indeed, there are even transition forms into that group. There is really some question as to whether these patients should not be included in *constitutional excitement.* While it is probably as difficult to draw sharp lines here as for other forms of degeneracy, still prominent psychomotor excitement may be the cue. It is lacking in morbid swindling and lying. Great distractibility, marked irritability, loquacity, fondness for new undertakings, great instability, and restlessness indicate constitutional excitement, in which fabrications often occur but are not necessarily concomitant symptoms. On the other hand, fondness for invention of details, dignified manners, a great gift for fabrications unaccompanied by excitement, and the clever ability to take advantage of credulous persons, are rather the charac teristics of the born swindler. It seems of special importance that in constitutional excitement the tendency to swindle appears at a certain time and may show definite exacerbations, while in born swindlers it is a permanent personal peculiarity. Also, the occurrence of frequent and sudden changes of disposition, especially periods of causeless dejection and despair, favors the diagnosis of constitutional excitement.

The prognosis and treatment of the morbid swindler and liar are the same as that indicated in the related forms of the insanity of degeneracy. Many of these patients cause so much trouble that they require permanent custody.

D. THE PSEUDOQUERULANTS

The pseudoquerulants comprise a group of morbid personalities whose conduct resembles somewhat that of genuine querulants (see p. 432), but who never develop genuine delusions. Whether these pseudoquerulants com-

prise a uniform group is undecided.

The intellectual capacity of the patients is usually mediocre, but is sometimes very good. As a rule they possess a certain craftiness, which enables them to utilize any advantage and to correctly comprehend the weaknesses of their opponents; some show a tendency to quibbling and hairsplitting. Memory is generally good, however; its accuracy often suffers because of personal coloring. The memory of earlier events is unconsciously modified in accord with their emotional needs. Judgment is also biassed, irrelevant, tends to exaggerations, is in many ways perverse and influenced by intense feelings. Hence persons and conditions are often incorrectly judged. Patients themselves are often uncommonly credulous; that is, ideas and communications which correspond to their tendencies and views are considered correct without further proof, but if they do not conform to their desires, the patients oppose them with the most extreme and obstinate distrust.

This marked personal influence over apprehension, memory, and judgment arises from an increased *emotional irritability.* The patients are very passionate and become greatly excited over trifles. They regard every real or apparent infringement upon their rights as gross injustice, which they believe themselves justified in combating with the keenest weapons. They are, therefore, revengeful and persistent in their hostility, regard every opposition as a personal matter, are always ready to impute to their adversaries dishonorable motives, and to carry on their fight in every possible way. Associated with their passion there is a marked egotism. Patients regard themselves as especially intelligent and superior to then-environment, and are also disposed to consider their own affairs as matters of public importance — that they themselves are champions of an important cause. Hence even trifling affairs lead to longdrawn-out litigations, because they feel under obligation to fight to the finish for their rights. The combination of sensitiveness with recklessness and arrogance inevitably involves patients in many difficulties and conflicts with their environment. There arise innumerable misunderstandings and provocations which gradually involve them in a perfect maze of complications. Patients follow up, as far as they possibly can, each affair with bitter determination. They do not rest with the judgments which are handed down, reject favorable settlements, appeal to higher courts, and seek to interest the public in their suits. They do not give up the fight until every possibility of success has disappeared; however, they sometimes renounce beforehand the most extreme measures, if the disproportion between the prospect of triumph and the probable cost is very great. Then they attempt to obtain satisfaction in other ways, by charges of forgery against the witnesses, who have not agreed with them, or by petty denunciations, false dealings, slanderings, etc. These give rise to new controversies, which only increase the embitterment and develop other elements of discord. Meanwhile there develop, in one way or another, petty misdemeanors which, in their minds, soon grow to be occurrences of the gravest import. Thus, then, it fairly rains complaints and counter complaints of insults, claims for damages, warrants, examination of witnesses, trials, legal expenses, attachments without number, so that patients are constantly busy in one court or another. Thenmeans of natural livelihood become more and more depleted. In addition to their vexations and constant excitement the demands of a livelihood come in to increase the irritability and embitterment of the patients.

The development of this condition of affairs may require ten years or more. There is progress in the disease only in so far as the relations of the patients to their environment gradually become more and more strained. They not only feel that upon every occasion they are treated in an unfair and hostile manner, but they also think their neighbors and acquaintances are angry and retaliating. Thus, there are continuous warfares which, because of their contrary dispositions, are being constantly incited by every little incident, but they never go

as far as to form true delusions. The patients regard their opponents, without exception, as blockheads, trash, and scoundrels. They are not always at strife with the same persons, sometimes this one and sometimes that one, although the hostility toward certain ones may be held for many years. The same occasion does not always serve as the starting-point for all the controversies that arise later, but there are numerous individual occurrences, which are not necessarily related, although they may have all arisen from the same source of personal animosity. In other words they lack the subjective bonds which unite and draw together all the individual experiences into a continuous chain.

Diagnosis. — The pseudoquerulants are distinguished from the *genuine querulants* by the absence of genuine delusion formation. The controversies of querulants arise only from an endeavor to obtain expiation for an injustice originally inflicted on them, and which appears to them as the outcome of hostile persecution. This is the reason why they are dissatisfied with the court's verdict, regard later failures as a further continuance of that persecution, and resort to the most desperate measures in order to win. In pseudoquerulants there is nothing of this kind. The patients usually give up when they see they can obtain nothing more, rarely doubt the impartiality of the courts, and come to regard them as accomplices of their enemies and slander them. They forget the old quarrels, or at least do not revive them, and are not always striving to renew investigations. The circle of their enemies also becomes enlarged as a result of some particular personal friction, which, however, has no delusional connection with the central point of their struggle. Not infrequently the rights of the pseudoquerulants are maintained by the courts on many points. This also is an indication that their contact with the courts is not influenced by uniform delusions. Patients are usually much the worse for their incessant conflicts; they by no means carry them out with the grim satisfaction which is afforded the querulants in the fulfilment of their

delusional tasks. On the other hand, they are sometimes rather unhappy because of their everlasting troubles. Occasionally the removal of the chief source of trouble by some change in the manner of living may produce a marked improvement, if some other occasion does not arise to create new difficulties. As the patients grow older they become dull and indifferent, but on the other hand they are often stubborn. Pseudo-querulants never develop later into true querulants. One seems justified in spite of their external similarities in maintaining that they represent totally different conditions. Pseudoquerulancy is a form of constitutional endowment which exists from youth up and continues without essential change, while in true querulancy we have a disease process which begins at a definite time and runs its regular course. There is a sharp line between psychopathic pseudoquerulants and the ordinary manifestations of those persons who are irritable, litigious, and obstinate.

Treatment. — There is little opportunity for efficient treatment of the pseudoquerulant. A temporary residence in an institution, or a change to an environment which is free from the former difficulties, may be an advantage. In the same way the removal of the chief source of trouble or the friendly intervention of trusted persons is helpful. Patients do not do well without some restraint of their liberty.

XV. DEFECTIVE MENTAL DEVELOPMENT
Under this heading are described those mental states which are the result of an *incomplete* or *early interrupted* development of mental life. As distinguished from the process of mental deterioration, these states may be regarded as conditions of retarded mental development. It not infrequently happens that both conditions exist in the same individuals, as when a deterioration psychosis develops in an individual with defective development.

A defective hereditary endowment is almost always present. The pathological basis for defective mental development is the incomplete development of the cerebral cortex. This is often due to some disease occurring during fetal or infantile life which has an injurious influence upon the developing nervous elements. Our knowledge of the anatomical facts is as yet so incomplete that it is impossible, on a pathological basis, to differentiate between the different grades of defective mental development. In a general way the lighter forms are designated *imbecility,* and the severer *idiocy. A.* Imbecility

This form of defective mental development is characterized by a *moderate degree of mental incapacity which is usually of equal prominence on all sides of the mental life.* Clinically imbeciles may be divided into two groups, the *stupid* and the *active,* according to the degree of mental activity.

The fundamental symptoms in the stupid form are obtuseness and stupidity. There is an inability to receive many impressions, or to grasp and utilize the experiences of life; consequently the knowledge of the outside world confines itself to the immediate surroundings, while events without the patients' narrow mental horizon pass unnoticed. Probably the sensory presentations are retained, but there is an absence of an elaboration of individual experiences into general ideas. The individual and insignificant elements make up the fund of experience. Essential and fundamental relations and distinctions are not recognized. Thought is scanty, limited mostly to daily experiences, usually travels the same path, and, according to the research of Buccola, is really retarded.

Judgment is defective and uncertain, and often determined by chance ideas not the outcome of past experience. Patients also fail to consider the possible consequences of their actions, either in reference to themselves or others. *Memory* is accurate only for the most prominent events of life. Yet sometimes trifling incidents are firmly retained, while the more essential are forgotten. The narration of events, as remembered by them, is noticeably faulty because of numerous omissions and changes. The same events narrated at different times show many contradictions, though

sometimes they may be repeated parrot-like. *Consciousness* is unclouded. The patients recognize the surroundings and comprehend questions. They have no insight into their mental condition, but usually regard themselves as perfectly sound.

In the patients' actions and conversations their *ovm personality* always comes into prominence. The central point about which the whole life revolves is their own physical well-being, — eating and drinking and the possession of things desired, — while all else is indifferent. Occasionally they fail to show the natural affection for parents and relatives. The superficial sorrow at the loss of some relative is quickly lost in the pomp of the funeral procession and the joy over a new suit of mourning. The absence of sympathy for those who are in want and unfortunate may explain the cruelty which they sometimes display toward animals and in then combats with others.

In *emotional attitude* these patients are indifferent, apathetic, at times shy and anxious, but more often displaying a simple, childish happiness. Occasionally patients exhibit sudden outbreaks of passion, especially if irritated or if they believe themselves misused. In *conduct* they are usually harmless and tractable, but under evil influences they become ill-humored, sometimes stubborn and peevish. The sexual impulses often remain wholly undeveloped, or they are perverted. Attempts to rape, especially children and even animals, are sometimes observed. Patients are incapable of independent activity, yet they are able to do things under supervision. An occasional patient shows a striking technical ability, some knowledge of music or a certain knack in drawing, — but even this knowledge does not aid them in producing valuable work.

Lighter grades of this type of imbecility often fail of recognition because of the absence of sharp border lines between them and the stupidity sometimes present in normal individuals. Imbecilic defects, however, become more and more apparent as the individual advances in age and is compelled to take

up some responsibility in life. Yet these defects may not be recognized, because of the patients' ability to utilize a certain amount of experience and to engage regularly in a simple occupation. But just as soon as anything extraordinary occurs,—a mental shock or a temptation which demands discretion and decision of action, —the mental and moral incapacity becomes evident. Unfortunately at this time their actions are judged from a legal and not from a medical standpoint. Rigid military discipline brings to the light many such cases, especially in those countries where military service is required. It becomes most apparent in stubbornness, insubordination, desertion, and attacks upon officers. Lack of judgment in handling these cases sometimes results in suicidal attempts.

Imbecility is usually recognized at an early date. In Infancy it may be noticed that patients are tardy in learning low to laugh, to imitate, and to speak. Later, at school,;hey are backward in studies, are sluggish, indolent, show joverty of thought and inability to comprehend, and soon become the sport of their playmates. They find difficulty n learning to read, write, and reckon, and the few facts in geography or grammar which are committed to memory ire soon forgotten, since they are not essential to their imited experiences of life. A fairly good memory may con:eal their incapacity for a long time.

The patients are very often refractory, hard to train, and tave a tendency to develop bad traits, such as stealing, nnoying dumb animals, and indulging in sexual improirieties, which often necessitates their commitment to indusrial schools. During youth and puberty their mental inapacity becomes still more evident, because of the marked ontrast to the rapid mental development of their playlates. At this time their own development comes to a tandstill or may even retrograde, presenting resemblances D the progressive deterioration of dementia praecox.

In the active or energetic type of imbecility *there is a lorbid activity of the attention and imagination,* in contrast to hie general sluggishness of the stupid form. Patients are ttracted by every new impression, and unable to direct their attention permanently to any one object; hence their observations are hasty and superficial. They are always ready to pass judgment without deliberation. This susceptibility to new and accidental impressions renders their view of the outside world very incomplete and fragmentary. Such vague pictures lead to faulty conceptions and form the basis for incorrect judgment. Circumstances existing only in their imagination are of far more importance in their deliberations than absolute facts. Thought, therefore, becomes unsteady and shows many inconsistencies; patients vacillate in their plans from day to day, draw inconsistent conclusions from the same premises, and thus their views of life and the outer world lack reality.

Their flighty conversation contains a frequent repetition of certain high-sounding remarks and commonplaces which often have little bearing upon the sense. They are very apt to lose the thread of conversation, refer to the most diverse subjects, but usually finish with some very striking remark. Such a bombastic style very often conceals from the inexperienced the actual mental enfeeblement, and leads to their being regarded as unusually bright individuals. It is quite in accord with these mental peculiarities that patients not only embellish and distort their recollections with many fanciful ideas, but also fabricate extensively. In spite of evident contradictions in their statements they reassert them tenaciously and refuse further discussion. Accusations of the patients against relatives and fellow-patients should, therefore, be accepted with the greatest caution. These energetic patients possess a better memory than the apathetic, are able to acquire some new knowledge, and to adapt themselves to new environment to a certain extent.

The *emotional attitude* presents a mobility equal to that encountered in the attention and the imagination. Every impression is accompanied by an accentuated but rapidly vanishing tone of feeling, and the moods vacillate from one extreme to another, showing de-spondency and exuberance, despair and enthusiasm, which appear upon little provocation. Violent likes and dislikes change from day to day; the dearest blessed doctor of to-day becomes the vilest scoundrel to-morrow. While extravagant in their emotional expressions, with a tendency to emotional outbursts, they are readily diverted and pacified. Irritability and sensitiveness are always present to a greater or less degree, especially when patients believe themselves interfered with; often they are docile and good-natured. An exaggerated feeling of self-importance regularly accompanies this form, some patients even believing themselves specially endowed and often boasting of their prospects, while at the same time showing a lack of insight into their diseased condition. Any shortcomings on their part are explained by the hostility of relatives or lack of support.

In *conduct* the patients are odd, freakish, sometimes loquacious, forward, pretentious, and silly; sometimes quiet, docile, and reticent. They are apt to dress in a peculiar manner or to be slovenly in appearance. They work with varying zeal. In youth they are frequently considered bright, especially by the parents, but later become fickle, unable to employ themselves at all, leave home, wander aimlessly about, drink, and indulge in all sorts of excesses. Many prostitutes belong to this class. In many of these cases, where there seems to be only a light grade of imbecility, there may be some question whether we are not really dealing with conditions of degeneracy, but the presence of profound mental deficiency, in spite of a certain amount of superficial activity, should leave no doubt. Gudden designated such patients as " high-grade imbeciles."

Imbecility may form the basis for the development of other psychoses; as, manic-depressive insanity, the psychoses of involution and dementia praecox, the last of which in seven per cent. of cases appears on an imbecile basis. Furthermore, it often happens that imbeciles present at times some of the symptoms characteristic of other psychoses; such as, periods of excitement and depression,— not of the manic-depressive type,— single transitory expansive or persecutory delusions, occasional hallucinations, and especially the attacks characteristic of the constitutional psychopathic states. Signs of physical degeneration are often found in anomalies of the skull, malformation of the palate, misshapen ears, puerile expression, chorea, etc.

Course. — The course of imbecility is quite uniform; some patients, unsuccessful in their attempts to enter a profession or to become employed in mechanical arts, engage in simple labor, and failing in this, they become a burden to the family. It is not infrequent for them to develop some psychosis later in life,—forms of the insanity of degeneracy, manic-depressive insanity, and senile dementia. Others show irregular periods of excitement, with aggressiveness, great irritability, and variable emotional moods. Also, the various symptoms of epilepsy not infrequently develop, which may also lead to further dementia. In some of these cases the signs of epileptic dementia predominate, and in others the epileptic attacks. Usually it becomes necessary at some time during their life to confine them in almshouses or hospitals for the insane.

Diagnosis. — There are some cases of *dementia prcecvx* which are difficult to differentiate from the lighter active forms of imbecility. The character of the onset, dating from childhood, the absence of hallucinations and pronounced delusions, and of any evidence of earlier acquired knowledge, speak for imbecility. Furthermore, in dementia praecox patients may show some improvement, while imbeciles present no change.

There are a few cases of *hysteria* with a moderate degree of deterioration which might be confounded with imbecility, but in them the course of the disease is not as uniform and the mental weakness is not as evident on all sides of the psychical life; while in imbecility but few patients present hysterical symptoms. There are all possible transition stages between imbecility and the normal state, among which should be classed those weakminded individuals who are overcredulous and superficial in knowledge, getting a smattering of everything, but knowing nothing thoroughly, who take hold of everything new with enthusiasm, are easily led astray and indulge in excesses, and who are always in doubt as to their real motives for action.

Treatment. — The treatment of congenital imbecility consists principally in providing an appropriate education, with a view to developing any capacity that may exist. This is best accomplished in the hands of some competent tutor or in a private or state institution established for that purpose. The training should by no means be directed simply toward mental education, but should include manual training. The use of alcohol should be strenuously avoided. The removal of adenoids, if present, even though they may not appear to impair the health of the child, is highly essential. Furthermore, all diseases of eyes and ears should be corrected. If, in spite of training, the patients develop dangerous tendencies, hospital care is necessary.

B. Idiocy1

Idiocy is characterized by *a more profound degree of mental incapacity than imbecility.*

Etiology. — Defective heredity is one of the most important etiological factors. Idiocy may be regarded as the final stage of hereditary degeneration. Wildermuth finds defective heredity in seventy per cent. of cases, mostly in the form of alcoholism in the parents. Possibly, also, intoxication of one or both parents at the time of copulation predisposes to idiocy. Severe illness or mental shock during pregnancy and hereditary tendency to tuberculosis (Piper) have been noted as causes. Injuries at the time of birth, prolonged asphyxia, but especially compression by narrow pelves or forceps are probably important factors. In idiocy developing after birth (one-fourth to one-third of cases) the most important causes are infectious diseases, — typhoid fever, measles, scarlet fever, and diphtheria; also head

injuries, congenital syphilis, and rachitis.

Premature ossification of the cranial sutures is no longer regarded as a cause of idiocy, but rather as an accompaniment, recent investigation showing that the growth of the calvarium is determined by the proportional growth of the brain and not *vice versa.* Malformation of the cranium occurs in at least one-half of the cases, in which anomaly macrocephaly is far more prominent than microcephaly. An extreme grade of the former of these conditions is represented by Plate 10, Figure 1, while Figure 2 represents the condition of microcephaly. Furthermore, the early closure of the suture has nothing to do with the malformation of the brain. Narrowness of the base of the cranium accompanies more often the profoundly stupid forms of idiocy, and smallness of the vertex the excited forms. More than one-half of idiots are first-born, and four to five per cent. are twins. The male sex predominates.

Emminghaus, Die psychischen Storungen des Kindesalters, 243 f.; Sollier, Der Idiot und der Imbecille, deutsch von Brie, 1891; J. Voisin, L'idiotie, 1893; Pellizzi, Studii clinici ed anatomo-patologici sulT idiowa, 1901; Bourneville, Recherches cliniques et the'rapeutiques sur I'e'pilepsie, ITiystene et l'idiotie (Regelmassige Jahresberichte ttber die Idiotenabtetlung des Bicetre). Piper, Zur Aetiologie der Idiotie, 1893.

Pathology.—Some cases present defective development of the central nervous system, either smallness or increased size of the entire encephalon or malformation of some of its parts; absence of corpus callosum, of cerebellum, inequality of hemispheres, sparsity or anomalies of convolutions, and aaicrogyri, which conditions represent cessation of development, or a reversion to structures characteristic of lower inimals. In many cases evidences of genuine disease)rocesses are found, particularly encephalitis, meningitis, lydrocephaly, and tumor formation, causing extensive lestruction of the cortex (porencephaly) or a general atrophy,

iimilar conditions may be due to vascular changes, of which he most important are endarteritis, thrombosis, and emolism; also occlusion of vessels caused by traumatic hemrrhage at the time of birth or later. Syphilitic disease, either leningo-encephalitis or endo-arteritis, may lead to idiocy, upillary disturbances in idiocy are usually associated with rphilis. Bourneville has described a series of cases of Hammarberg, Studien und Klinik und Pathologie der Idiotie, Deutsch,n W. Berger, 1895; Pfleger und Pilcz in Obersteiner's Arbeiten, eft V, 1897; Pilcz, Jahrb. f. Psy. , XVIII, 526; Mingazzini, Monatsschr. Psy., VII, 429; Kotschetkowa, Archiv f. Psy., XXXIV, 39; Kttppen,-chiv f. Psy., XXX, 896; Konig, Deutsche Zeitschr. f. Nervenheilinde, 1897, XI; Anton, Handbuch der patholog., Anatomie des srvensystems von Flatau-Jacobsohn-Minor, 416, 1904; Weber, Ibid., 40.

2n tuberous hypertrophic sclerosis, which are characterized by an excessive tumorlike development of glia following an extensive destruction of the cortical tissues.

The *amaurotic family idiocy* described by Sachs and Tay occurs almost exclusively among Jews. The disease develops during the first two or three years of life in healthy children, is accompanied by general paralysis and atrophy of the optic nerve, and always terminates fatally in a few months or years. While the real nature of the disease is still unknown, it is probably not due to arrested development, but to an extensive disease process.

Microscopically we may find either an insufficient development of the neurones or evidences of former disease processes. In underdevelopment the nerve cells do not develop beyond an embryonic stage (Hammarberg). The cortex is much thinner, the number of cells is reduced, and they stand closer together in regular rows with much less gray matter between them, so that the different layers cannot be clearly distinguished (a characteristic of lower animals). The cells themselves are embryonic in structure, being mostly of the same size and globular in form. The degree of underdevelopment may vary in different parts of the cortex. (See Figure 1, Plate 5.)

In other cases there may be normal development, with the usual number and arrangement of cells, but in areas the cells have entirely disappeared, as the result of a disease process, and the glia has increased. In the few cases of hypertrophic sclerosis, the increase in the size of the brain is due to the great increase of glia, either as an accompaniment or as a result of a degenerative process in the cortex. The nature of the causes which produce such lesions in fetal and early life is still unknown. They may be due to intoxication or infection.

Fig..'i. Fig. 4.

Figs. 3 and 4. —Representing asymmetries of cranium ami face. Plate 12

Symptomatology. —The symptoms of the disease are best considered in two groups, the *severe* and the *light* forms. The symptoms of the former correspond to the mental state presented by an infant during the first days following birth, while the symptoms of the latter correspond to the mental states of later infancy.

In the severe cases of idiocy patients are wholly unable to comprehend external impressions, to gather experience, or become acquainted with the environment, to form clear ideas or judgments, and indeed they do not possess self-consciousness. The emotional life is limited to mere fluctuations of the general feelings. Consequently the impulses arising from these feelings lead only to simple actions, such as the taking of food. The patients have no choice of food and eat anything placed before them, even to pieces of clothing and rubbish. Idiots are'not excitable; they show very little, if any, fear or pleasure, at the most manifesting some pleasure in kicking or swaying movements; while hunger or physical pain may be expressed in monotonous or shrill cries. If repeatedly pricked in the same place, causing them to cry out with pain, they do not try to protect themselves. Some even pound themselves and inflict severe wounds, but immediately repeat the act. One girl would impulsively bite deeply into the flesh of her arm, unless prevented.

Teething is delayed, and the whole physical development retarded. The countenance is usually stupid and vacuous. The movements are clumsy and awkward; patients do not walk until late, and some never even learn to stand, but are absolutely helpless. Some restlessness may develop, with a tendency to move aimlessly about, to sway the head or body back and forth rhythmically for a long time, to clap the hands, or to grunt. Convulsive attacks are of frequent occurrence. These patients are so utterly helpless that without constant attention they would quickly perish.

In *thelight* cases it is possible to fix the attention momentarily by the aid of some striking object, but the patients themselves are quite unable to direct the attention. A few clear sensory impressions may enter consciousness, and a limited number of ideas may be formed, which are extremely simple, always incomplete, and without connection. Memory is very poor; there is no ability to make a selection from different impressions in order to establish a basis for the formation of concepts; indeed, a psychic personality is never developed. Speech, and therefore intercourse with the environment, is poorly developed. Unable to form sentences, idiots present a mixture of incomplete words or syllables similar to the early efforts of an infant. They do not imitate, play, or busy themselves, and are very susceptible to fatigue.

The lower sensory or selfish feelings dominate the emotional attitude, and liberate only those impulses for action which gratify momentary pleasure. Idiots never feel attracted toward any special individual, never express gratitude, nor show grief. When irritated by rough treatment or opposed, they may show sudden outbursts of rage, attempting to destroy something or to injure some one. Sexual desires may either remain undeveloped or appear early and lead to reckless masturbation and sexual assaults. Often the appetite for food is abnormally developed, patients eating ravenously and feeding themselves with their hands. A few show some one-sided capabilities, such as a good memory for numbers or words or some very simple technical skill. Many idiots are fond of music.

In the lighter grades of idiocy two types may be distinguished, the *stupid* or anergic, and the *excited* or active, depending upon the distractibility of the attention. The anergic patients are torpid, thought is sluggish and very limited, and there is pronounced emotional indifference. In the active patients the attention wanders aimlessly, filling consciousness with a variegated, incoherent jumble. The emotions change rapidly. At one time patients are stubborn, at another show purposeless activity, running about, laughing, crying, and clapping the hands. Between these two groups there are numerous transition stages.

In idiocy transitory periods of excitement or depression may occur which present some similarity to epileptic excitement, attacks of manic-depressive insanity, and the excitement which occurs in the end stages of dementia praecox. Compulsive ideas, morbid impulses, periods of anxiety, sometimes with suicidal tendencies, may appear, and occasionally there may be simple, childish, expansive, or persecutory ideas.

Physical Symptoms. — There is a stunting of the whole physical development; the stature is undersized or even dwarfish. Countenance is childish. Hair is often absent from the face and pubes. The genitals are undeveloped; menstruation absent, late, or irregular. Teeth are late in developing and often faulty in arrangement, and the palate is usually asymmetrical. The special senses, especially hearing, are blunted. In eighty per cent. of cases the socalled stigmata of degeneration are present (Wildermuth), viz. malformation of the eyes, ears, mouth, nose, and especially the bones of the face. Other frequent symptoms are increase or loss of the reflexes, incoordination of the lower extremities and of the eye muscles, and difficulty of speech, with elision of the end syllables, stuttering, halting, and faulty articulation of some or most of the consonants.

All idiots are awkward and often show associated movements. Mirror-writing is found, especially among the girls. Evidences of focal cerebral lesions are manifested by hemiplegia, paresis, contractures, convulsions, choreic and athetoid movements, aphasia, and in thirty per cent. of the cases, especially in boys, epilepsy (Wildermuth).

Diagnosis. — The recognition of the disease, which is difficult only in infancy and in very early childhood, depends upon the insensibility of the children to external influences. They do not manifest a feeling of hunger, even when lying upon the breast or at the approach of the mother, are not attentive, do not smile or cry, and may be continually restless; many give evidence of some cerebral disturbance, as paralysis or hemiplegia. The limbs may remain in a fetal condition; they do not learn how to walk or talk, and are unable to understand speech.

Prognosis. — The prognosis is unfavorable. While idiots can never reach the rank of normal men, the question of how much they can develop is of great importance. In general it can be said that if their attention can be held for some time, and they give evidence of memory, *i.e.* recognize articles and resist what they have once experienced as disagreeable and appear to understand speech, the prognosis is more favorable. The appearance of epilepsy in early childhood is very unfavorable. During puberty idiots often lose what little knowledge they may have acquired, and some even present the hebephrenic or catatonic picture of dementia praecox. Their life is usually short, because of their lessened powers of resistance to intercurrent diseases.

Treatment. — Temperance in parents should be encouraged as an important prophylactic measure. The condition of faulty nutrition, which is frequently present, improves with the relief of insomnia, the prevention of masturbation, removal of sources of focal irritation, and strict cleanliness. Epileptic attacks should be combated with bromids, atropin, or other suitable measures, with the hope of preventing profound deterioration. Craniectomy in some cases of microcephaly is an irrational procedure and is fast disappearing from practice.

Besides treatment of the physical condition, the patients should receive training in institutions for the feeble-minded. Idiots left to themselves or in a poor environment rapidly go to the bad. Harmless patients in the care of sisters or brothers may become threatening or aggressive and attempt sexual assaults. Such patients are somewhat susceptible to training. This, however, requires a greater amount of kindliness and-patience, and more experience than can be obtained in the ordinary home. An effort should first be made to teach them to walk and use their hands, also to employ their different senses, to direct their attention and to speak, followed by special instruction in the perception of objects, in distinguishing them, and in forming simple judgments. As a result of such training, many patients yearly leave institutions well enough trained to be of use in a limited field. They, however, continue to need some care and supervision throughout life, as their inability to get along in the world and to utilize knowledge stands in striking disproportion to knowledge taught them.

PUBLISHED BY THE MACMELLAN COMPANY 66 FIFTH AVENUE, NEW YORE ALLBUTT
A System of Medicine. By Many Writers. Edited by ThoMaS ClIFFOrd Allbutt, M.A., M.D., LL.D., F.R.C.P., F.R.S., F.L.S., F.S.A. Regius Professor of Physic in the University of Cambridge, etc. In nine volumes.
Vol. I. Prolegomena and Fevers.
Vol. II. Infective Diseases and Toxicology.
Vol. III. General Diseases of Obscure Causation and Alimentation.
Vol. IV. Diseases of Alimentation (continued) and Excretion of the Ductless
Glands and the Respiratory Organs.

Vol. V. Diseases of the Respiratory Organs,
Diseases of the Pleura Diseases of the Circulatory System.

Vol. VI. Diseases of the Circulatory and
Nervous Systems.

Vol. VII. Diseases of the Nervous System.

Vol. VIII. Nervous Diseases (continued).
Mental Diseases, Skin Diseases.

Vol. IX. Gynaecology, Medical and Surgical.
8vo. Cloth. Price $ 45.00 net.
Sheep. Price $ 54.00 net.

Half morocco. Price $ 58.50 net. ALL-BUTT and PLAYFAIR

A System of Gynaecology. By Many Writers. Edited by Thomas Clif-
Ford Allbutt and W. S. Playfair.
This volume is supplied as Vol. IX. of Allbutt's " System of Medicine," or may be had separately at the following prices: 8vo. Cloth, $ 6.00 net.

Half morocco. $ 7.00 net. ALLCHTN

A Manual of Medicine. Edited by W. H. Allchin, M.D., (Lond.).
F.R.C.P., F.R.S.E., Senior Physician and Lecturer on Clinical Medicine, Westminster Hospital, Examiner in Medicine in the University of London, and to the Medical Department of the Royal Navy. In five volumes.

Vol. I. General Diseases. Diseases excited by atmospheric influences, the Infections. l2mo. Cloth. Colored Plates, pp. x + 442. Price $ 2.00 net.

Vol. II. General Diseases (continued). Diseases caused by Parasites, Diseases determined by Poisons, introduced into the Body, Primary Perversions of General Nutrition, Diseases of the Blood, l2mo. Cloth. Colored Plates and 2i other illustrations, pp. vill + 380.

Price j! 2.00 net.

Vol. III. Diseases of the Nervous System. Organic Disease of the Brain and its Membranes, Diseases of the Spinal Cord, Functional Diseases of the Nervous System. l2mo. Cloth. Colored Plates and 27 other illustrations. pp. x + 417. Price $ 2.00 net.

Vols. IV and V. *In preparation.* BAL-FOUR

The Senile Heart: Its Symptoms, Sequels and Treatment. By George William Balfour, M.D. (St. And.), LL.D. (Ed.), F.R.C.P.E., F.R.S.E., Consulting Physician to the Royal Infirmary, etc. Cloth, i2mo. 11 Illustrations. pp. ix + 300. Price J 1.50.

By the Same Author
Clinical Lectures on Diseases of the Heart and Aorta. By George WillIam Balfour. Third Edition. 8vo. Cloth. 35 Illustrations, pp. xxi + 479. Price $ 4.00 net. BARR

Manual of Diseases of the Ear. Including those of the Nose and Throat in relation to the Ear. For the Use of Students and Practitioners of Medicine. By Thomas Barr, M.D.. Lecturer on Diseases of the Ear, Glasgow University; Senior Surgeon to Glasgow Hospital for Diseases of the Ear, etc. Third Edition, Revised and Partially Rewritten. 8vo. Cloth. 236 Illustrations. pp. xxiii + 429. Price $ 4.00 net. BRONX

Dissections Illustrated. A Graphic Handbook for Students of Human Anatomy. By C. Gordon Brodie.
Price $ 9.00 net. BRUNTON

On Disorders of Digestion: Their Consequences and Treatment. By Sir T. Lauder Brunton. 8vo.
Cloth. Illustrated, pp. xvi + 389.
Price $ 2.50.

By the Same Author
An Introduction to Modern Therapeutics. Being the Croonian Lectures on the relationship between Chemical Structure and Physiological Actions in relation to the Prevention, Control, and Cure of Disease. Delivered before the Royal College of Physicians in London. By Sir T. Lauder BRuNTon. 8vo. Cloth. Illustrated. pp. vii +195. Price $ 1.50.
Lectures on the Action of Medicines. Being the Course of Lectures on Pharmacology and Therapeutics delivered at St. Bartholomew's Hospital during the Summer Session of 1896. By Sir T. Lauder Brunton, M.D., D.Sc. (Edin.), LL.D. (Hon.) (Aberd.). F.R.S., etc. 8vo. Cloth. 144 Illustrations. pp. xv + 673. Price $ 4.00 net. Sheep binding, Price 5.00 net. On Disorders of Assimilation, Digestion, etc. By Sir T. Lauder BrunTon. 8vo. Cloth, pp. xx + 495.

Price $ 4.00 net. CATON
The Prevention of Valvular Disease of the Heart. A proposal to Check Rheumatic Endocarditis in its early stage and thus prevent the Development of Permanent Organic Disease of the Valves. By Richard Caton, M.D., F.R.C.P., Hon. Physician Liverpool Royal Infirmary; Emeritus Professor of Physiology, University College, Liverpool. 8vo. Cloth. 6 Illustrations. pp. x + 92. Price $ 1.75 net. CHESTER

A Manual of Determinative Bacteriology. By Frederick D. Chester, Bacteriologist of the Delaware College Agricultural Experiment Station, and Director of the Laboratory of the State Board of Health of Delaware; Member of the Society of American Bacteriologists; of the Society for the Promotion of Agricultural Science, and of the American Public Health Association. 8vo. Cloth. Illustrated, pp. vi + 401. Price $2.60 net. CLELAND and MACKAY

Human Anatomy, General and Descriptive. For the Use of Students. By John Cleland, M.D., LLD., D.Sc., F.R.S., Professor of Anatomy in the University of Glasgow, and John Yule Mackay, M.D., CM., Professor of Anatomy in University College, Dundee; late Senior Demonstrator in the University of Glasgow. 630 Illustrations. 8vo. Cloth, pp. xx + 833. Price $ 6.50 net.

Sheep binding, Price 7.50 net. By the *Same Authors*

A Directory for the Dissection of the Human Body. Bv John Cleland, M.D., LL.D., F.R.S., Professor of Anatomy in the University of Glasgow, and John Yule Mackay, M.D., Principal and Professor of Anatomy, University College, Dundee, the University of St. Andrews. Fourth Edition. Revised and furnished with copious References to the Work " Human Anatomy, General and Descriptive." by the same Authors. i6mo. Cloth, pp. viii + 198. Price $ 1.00 net. COLLINS

The Genesis and Dissolution of the Faculty of Speech. A Clinical and Psychological Study of Aphasia. By Joseph Collins, M.D., Professor of Diseases of the Mind and Nervous System in the New York Post-Graduate Medical School, Neurologist to the New

York City Hospital, etc. Awarded the Alvarenga Prize of the College of Physicians of Philadelphia, 1897. 8vo. Cloth. Illustrated, pp. viii-f 432.

Price J 3.50 *net.* COPEMAN

Vaccination: With Special Reference to Its Natural History and Pathology. The Milroy Lectures. By S. Monckton Copeman, M.A., M.D., M.R.C.P. i2mo. Cloth. Illustrated. pp. x + 257. Price $ 2. co *net.* DAVIS

The Refraction of the Eye. Including a
Complete Treatise on Ophthalmometry. A Clinical Text-Book for Students and Practitioners. By A. Edward Davis, A.M., M.D., Adjunct Professor of Diseases of the Eye in the New York Post-Graduate Medical School and Hospital, etc. 8vo. Cloth. 119 Illustrations. pp. xii + 431.

Price $ 3.00 *net.* DOWN IE

Clinical Manual for the Study of Diseases of the Throat. By James Wallser Downie, M.B., Fellow and Examiner in Aural Surgery for the Fellowship of the Faculty of Physicians and Surgeons; Hon. Aurist, Royal Hospital for Sick Children. Glasgow. 121110. Cloth. 34 Illustrations. pp. xiv + 268. Price $ 2.50.

DRINKWATER

First Aid to the Injured and Ambulance Drill. By H. Drinkwater, M.D. l6mo. Cloth. Illustrated. pp. vii + 104. Price 40 cents *net.* ECCLES

Sciatica: A Record of Clinical Observations on the Causes, Nature, and Treatment of Sixty-Eight Cases. By A. Symons Eccles, M.B. (Aberd.). Member Royal College Surgeons, England, etc. 8vo. Cloth, pp. viii + 88. Price $ 1. 00 *net.* EHRLICH and LAZARUS

Histology of the Blood: Normal And Pathological. By P. Ehrlich and A. Lazarus. Edited and Translated by W. Meyers, M.A., M.B., B.Sc., with a Preface by G. Slms woodheaD, M.D., Professor of Pathology in the University of Cambridge. 121110. Cloth, pp. xiii + 216. Price $ 1.50 *net.*

ELLIS

The Human Ear: Its Identification and Physiognomy. By Miriam Anne Ellis. With Illustrations from Pho-

tographs, chiefly from Nature-Prints. i2mo. Cloth, pp. x + 225.

Price f 1.75. ESMARCH and KOWALZIG *WORKS ON MEDICINE AND SURGERY*

Surgical Technic: A Text-Book on Operative Surgery. By Fr. Von EsMarch, M.D., Professor of Surgery at the University of Kiel, and SurgeonGeneral of the German Army, and E. Kowalzig, M.D., late First Assistant at the Surgical Clinic of the University of Kiel. Translated by Professor Ludwig H. Grau, Ph.D., formerly of Leland Stanford Junior University, and William N. Sullivan, M.D., formerly Surgeon of U. S. S. "Corwin," Assistant ofthe Surgical Clinicat Cooper Medical College, San Francisco. Edited by Nicholas Senn, M.D., Professor of Surgery at Rush Medical College, Chicago. With 1497 Illustrations and 15 Colored Plates. 8vo. Cloth, pp. xi-(-866. Price $ 7.00 *net.* Half morocco. Price $ 8.00 *net.* FOSTER

A Text-Book of Physiology. By M. Foster, M.A., M.D., LL.D., F.R.S., Professor of Physiology in the University of Cambridge, etc. Revised and abridged from the Author's Text-Book of Physiology in Five Volumes. With an Appendix on the Chemical Basis of the Animal Body, by A. Sheridan Lea, M. A., D.Sc., F.R.S., University Lecturer in Physiology in the University of Cambridge. 8vo. Cloth. 234 Illustrations. pp. xlix +1351.

Price $ 5.00 *net.* Sheep binding. Price $ 6.00 *net. By the Same Author*

A Text-Book of Physiology. In Five Volumes.

Part I. Blood; The Tissues of Movement;
Vascular Mechanism. Price $ 2.60 *net.*

Part II. The Tissues of Chemical Action; Nutrition. Price $ 2.60 *net.*

Part III. The Central Nervous System. Price $ 2.50

Part IV. The Central Nervous System (concluded): the Tissues and Mechanism of Reproduction. Price $ 2.00 *net.*

Part V. The Chemical Basis of the Animal Body. By Lea. Price $ 1.75 *net.*

Lectures on the History of Physiology during the Sixteenth, Seventeenth,

and Eighteenth Centuries. By Sir M. Foster, K.C.B. M.P., M.D., D.C.L., Sec. R.S., Professor of Physiology in the University of Cambridge, and Fellow of Trinity College, Cambridge. 8vo. Cloth. pp. 310.

Price $ 2.25 *net.*
P0THERG1LL

The Practitioner's Handbook of Treatment; or, The Principles of Therapeutics. By the late J. Milner Fothergill, M.D., M.R.C.P., Physician to the City of London Hospital for Diseases of the Chest, Victoria Park; Foreign Associate Fellow of the College of Physicians of Philadelphia.

Fourth Edition. Edited, and in great part Re-written, by William Murrell, M.D., F.R.C.P., etc. 8vo. Cloth. pp. xvi-ii + 688.

Price $ 5.00 *net.* Sheep. Price $ 6.00 *net.* FOTHERGILL

Manual of Midwifery. For the Use of Students and Practitioners. By W. E. Fothergill, M.A., B.Sc., M.B., CM., etc. With Double Colored Plate and 69 Illustrations in the Text. i2mo. Cloth, pp. xviii + 484.

Price $ 2.25 *net.* FRIDENBERG

The Ophthalmic Patient: A Manual of Therapeutics and Nursing in Eye Disease. By Percy Fridenberg, M.D., Ophthalmic Surgeon to the Randall's Island and Infant's Hospitals; Assistant Surgeon, New York Eye and Ear Infirmary, nmo. Cloth. 95 Illustrations. pp. x + 312. Price $ 1.50 *net.* FROST

The Fundus Oculi. With an Ophthalmoscopic Atlas illustrating its Physiological and Pathological Conditions. By W. Adams Frost, F.R.C.S., Ophthalmic Surgeon, St. George's Hospital; Surgeon to the Royal Westminster Ophthalmic Hospital. 410. Half morocco, pp. xviii + 228 + Plates.

Price $ 20.00 *net.* FULLER

Diseases of the Genito-Urinary System. A Thorough Treatise on Urinary and Sexual Surgery. By Eugene Fuller, M.D., Professor of Genitourinary and Venereal Diseases in the New York Post-Graduate Medical School; Visiting Genito-Urinary Surgeon to the New York Post-Graduate Hospital. 8vo. Cloth. 137 Illustrations. pp. ix + 774.

Price $ 5.00 *net*. Sheep, Price $ 6.00 *net*.

Half morocco, Price $ 6.50 *net*. GIBSON

Diseases of the Heart and Aorta. By George Alexander Gibson, M.D., D.Sc, F.R.C.P. (Ed.), F.R.S.E., Senior Assistant Physician to the Royal Infirmary; Consulting Physician to the Deaconess Hospital; Lecturer on Medicine at Minto House, and on Clinical Medicine at the Royal Infirmary, Edinburgh. With 210 Illustrations. 8vo. Cloth. pp. xx + 932. Price $ 6.00 *net*. GILLIES

The Theory and Practice of Counter-Irritation. By H. Cameron Gillies, M.D. 8vo. Cloth, pp. xii + 236.

Price $ 2.50.

GRIFFITHS

Lessons on Prescriptions and the Art of Prescribing. By W. Handsel Griffiths. Ph.D., L.R.C.P.E., Licentiate of the Royal College of Surgeons, Edinburgh, etc. i6mo. Cloth. pp. x + 150. $ HALLECK *WORKS ON MEDICINE AND SURGERY*

The Education of the Central Nervous System. A Study of Foundations, especially of Sensory and Motor Training. By Reuben Post Halleck, M.A. (Yale), Author of "Psychology and Psychic Culture." ismo. Cloth. pp. xii + 258. Price $ 1.00 *net*. HAMILTON

A Text-Book of Pathology, Systematic and Practical. By D. J. Hamilton, M.B., F.R.C.S.E., F.R.S.E., Professor of Pathological Anatomy, University of Aberdeen. Copiously Illustrated.

Vol. I. pp. xix + 736. Price $ 6.25 *net*.

VoL II. Part I. pp. xxii + 514.

Price 5 5.00 *net*. Part II. pp. 515-1139. Price $5.00 *net*. HARE

The Cold-Bath Treatment of Typhoid Fever. The Experience of a Consecutive Series of Nineteen Hundred and Two Cases Treated at the Brisbane Hospital. By F. E. HARE, M.D., late Resident Medical Officer, Brisbane General Hospital, Queensland. With Illustrations. 8vo. Cloth. pp. xii-f-195. Price $ 2.00 *net*. HARRISON

Home Nursing. Modern Scientific Methods for the Care of the Sick. By Eveleen Harrison, I2mo. Half leather, pp. xi + 235. Price $ *uoo*.

HAWKINS

On Diseases of the Vermiform Appendix. With a Consideration of the Symptoms and Treatment of the Resulting Forms of Peritonitis. By Herbert P. Hawkins, M.A., M.D. (Oxon.), F.R.C.P., Assistant Physician to, and Lecturer on Pathology at, St. Thomas's Hospital; Assistant Physician to the London Fever Hospital; late Radcliffe Travelling Fellow of the University of Oxford. 8vo. Cloth.

Anaesthetics and their Administration. A Text-Book for Medical and Dental Practitioners and Students. By Frederic W. Hewitt, M.A., M.D. (Cantab.), Anaesthetist to His Majesty the King; Anaesthetist and Instructor in Anaesthetics at the London Hospital; late Anaesthetist at Charing Cross Hospital and at the Dental Hospital of London. With Illustrations. 8vo. Half leather, pp. xxiv + 528.

Price $ *400 net*. HILL

The Management and the Diseases of the Dog. By John Woodroffe Hill, Fellow of the Royal College of Veterinary Surgeons, etc. With Illustrations. Fifth Edition. To which are added the Standard of Points for Judg ing Dogs, and a Table of Medicines and Their Doses. 8vo. Cloth. pp. viii + 531. Price 3.50.

HILTON

Rest and Pain. A Course of Lectures on the Influence of Mechanical and Physiological Rest in the Treatment of Accidents and Surgical Diseases and the Diagnostic Value of Pain. By the late John Hilton, F.R.S., F.R.CS, etc. Edited by W. H. A. Jacobson. M.A., M.B., F.R.C.S., etc. 12010. Cloth. 105 Illustrations, pp. xv-(-514.

Price f 2.00.

HUGHES

Mediterranean, Malta or Undulant Fever. By M. Louis Hughes, Surgeon-Captain, Army Medical Staff. 8vo. Cloth. Illustrated, pp, xiv + 232. Price *$3JM*. ILLOWAY

Constipation in Adults and Children. With Special Reference to Habitual Constipation and Its Most Successful Treatment by the Mechanical Methods. By H. ILLOWAY, M.D., formerly Professor of the Diseases of Children. Cincinnati College of Medicine and

Surgery, etc. 8vo. Cloth. 96 Illustrations, pp. xv-r-495.

Price 14.00 *net*.

Sheep binding, Price J 5.00 *./*

JARDINE

Practical Text-Book of Midwifery for Nurses and Students. By Robert JARDINE, M.D. (Edin.), M.R.C.S. (Eng.), F.F.P. & S. (Glasg.), Physician to the Glasgow Maternity Hospital, Glasgow. With 36 Illustrations. i.mo. Cloth. pp. xv + 245.

Price *t* I.SO *net*. JENNER

Lectures and Essays on Fevers and Diphtheria. By Sir William Jenner, Bart., G.C.B., M.D., etc. evo. Cloth. pp. vii + 581.

Price $4.00.

By the Same Author

Clinical Lectures and Essays on Rickets, Tuberculosis, Abdominal Tumors, and Other Subjects. Sra. Cloth. pp. xii + 329. Price $4.00.

JORGENSEN

Micro-Organisms and Fermentatiom. By Alfred Jorgensen. Director of the Laboratory for the Physiology and Technology of Fermentation at Copenhagen. Translated by Alex. K. Miller, Ph.D., F.I.C., and A. E. Lennholm. Third Edition. Completely Revised. 8vo. Cloth. 83 Illustrations. pp. xhi + 318.

Price $ 3.25 *it!* KAHLDEN

Methods of Pathological Histology. By C. Von Kahluen, Assistant Professor of Pathology in the University of Freiburg. Translated and Edited Translated into English by HenrY M.

WORKS ON MEDICINE AND SURGERY by H. Morley Fletcher, M.A.,

M.D. (Cantab.), M.R.C.P., Casualty Physician to St. Bartholomew's Hospital, and Assistant Demonstrator of Physiology in the Medical School. With an Introduction by G. SIMS WOODhead, M.D., Director of the Laboratories of the Conjoint Board of the Royal Colleges of Physicians (Lond.) and Surgeons (Eng.), etc. 8vo. Cloth, pp. M-f-171.

Price $ 1.40 *net*. KANTHACK and DRYSDALE

A Course of Elementary Practical Bacteriology. Including Bacteriological Analysis and Chemistry. By A. A. Kanthack, M.D., M.R.C.P., and J. H. DrYSDalE. Price $ 1.10 *net.*

KEITH

Plea for a Simple Life and Fads of an Old Physician. By George S. Keith, M.D., LL.D., F.R.C.P.E. i2mo. Cloth. Price J 1.25.

KELYNACK

Renal Growths. Their Pathology, Diagnosis and Treatment. By T. N. Kelynack, M.D. (Vict.), M.R.C.P. (Lond.), Pathologist, Manchester Royal Infirmary; Demonstrator and Assistant Lecturer in Pathology, the Owens College, Manchester. With 96 Illustrations. 8vo. Cloth, pp. xiii + 269.

Price $ 4.00 *net.* KIMBER

Text-Book of Anatomy and Physiology for Nurses. Compiled by Diana Clifford Kimber, Graduate of Bellevue Training School; Assistant Superintendent New York City Training School, Blackwell's Island, N.Y., formerly Assistant Superintendent Illinois Training School, Chicago, 111. 8vo. Cloth. 137 Illustrations. pp. xvi + 268. Price $ 2.50 *net.*

KLEMPERER

The Elements of Clinical Diagnosis. By Professor Dr. G. Klemperer, Professor of Medicine at the University of Berlin. Second American from the Seventh (last) German Edition. Authorized Translation by NaThan E. Brill, A.M., M.D., Attending Physician, Mount Sinai Hospital, New York City, and Samuel M. Brickner, A.M., M.D., Assistant Gynaecologist, Mount Sinai Hospital, Out-Patient Department i2mo. Cloth. 61 Illustrations. pp. xvii + 292. Price $ 1.00 *net.*

LANG

Text-Book of Comparative Anatomy. By Dr. Arnold Lang, Professor of Zofilogy in the University of Zurich, formerly Ritter Professor of Phylogeny in the University of Jena. With Preface to the English Translation by Professor Dr. Ernst Haeckel, F.R.S., Director of the Zoological Institute in Jena.

Bernard, M.A. (Cantab.), and Matilda Bernard. 8vo. Cloth. Illustrated.

Part I. pp. xviii + 562.

Part II. pp. xvi + 618. LILIENTHAL
Price $ 5.50 *net.* I. Price $ 5.50 *net.*

Imperative Surgery. For the General Practitioner, the Specialist and the Recent Graduate. By Howard Lilienthal, M.D., Attending Surgeon to Mount Sinai Hospital, New York City. 8vo. Cloth. 153 Illustrations. pp. xvi + 412. Price $4.00 *net.* Half morocco. Price $5.00 *net.*

LOCKWOOD

Appendicitis: Its Pathology and Surgery. By Charles Barrett Lockwood, F.R.C.S., Assistant Surgeon and Lecturer on Descriptive and Surgical Anatomy in St. Bartholomew's Hospital. 8vo. Half leather. 52 Illustrations. pp. xii + 287.

Price $ 2.50 *net.* MACDONALD

A Treatise on Diseases of the Nose and Its Accessory Cavities. By GrevIll. e Macdonald, M.D. (Lond.), Physician to the Hospital for Diseases of the Throat. 8vo. Cloth. 69 Illustrations. pp. xix + 381. Price $ 2.50.

MACEWEN

Pyogenic Infective Diseases of the Brain and Spinal Cord. Meningitis; Abscess of Brain: Infective Sinus Thrombosis. By William MacEwen, M.D. 8vo. Cloth. Illustrated. pp. xxiv + 353. Price $ 6.00 *net. By the Same Author*

Atlas of Head Sections. Fifty-three engraved Copper-Plates of Frozen Sections of the Head, and Fifty-three Key Plates with Descriptive Text. By William Macewen, M.D. 410. Half leather. Price $ 21.00 *net.* MACLAGAN

Rheumatism: Its Nature, Its Pathology and Its Successful Treatment. By T. J. Maclagan, M.D., Physician in Ordinary to Their Royal Highnesses Prince and Princess Christian of Schleswig-Holstein. Second Edition. 8vo. Cloth, pp. xiii + 324.

Price $ 2.60 *net.* MACMILLAN'S Manuals of Medicine and Surgery. *See under AhlCHlti,* Smith *and* STonhaM. *The following Works will be added to the Series:*

A Manual of Diseases of the Skin. By Dr. Colcott Fox.

A Manual of Hygiene. By Dr. Leonard

Wii.de.

A Text-Book of Surgical Pathology. By G. Belungham Smith.

WORKS ON MEDICINE AND SURGERY

A Student's Guide to Surgical Diagnosis. By H. Betham Rodinson, M.D. The Application of Physiology to Medicine. By Prof. A. E. Wri.ht. The Application of Physiology to Surgery. By D'arcy Powhr, F.R.C.S. A Manual of Chemical Physiology and Pathology. By T. G. Brodik, M.D. A Manual of Surgical Anatomy. By Francis C. Abbott, M.S. Diseases of the Nose, Throat and Ear. By Dundas Grant, M.D., F.R.C.S. The Essentials of Morbid Anatomy. By B. Abrahams, M.D.

The Principles of Pathology. By B. Abrahams, M.D.

Medical Diseases of Childhood. By J. A. Coutts.

MACPHERSON

Mental Affections. An Introduction to the Study of Insanity. By JOhn MacpherSon, M.D., F.R.C.P.E. 8vo. Cloth. pp. x + 380. Price $ 4.00 *net.*

MAUDSLEY

The Pathology of Mind. A Study of Its Distempers, Deformities and Disorders. By Henry Maudsley, M.D. 8vo. Cloth, pp. xi + 571.

Price $ 5.00 *net.* MERCIER

The Nervous System and the Mind. A Treatise on the Dynamics of the Human Organism. By Charles Mercier, M.B. 8vo. Cloth, pp. xi + 374. Price $ 4.00.

MIGULA

An Introduction to Practical Bacteriology for Physicians, Chemists and Students. By Dr. W. Migula, Lecturer on Botany in the Grand-Ducal Technical High School of Karlsruhe. Translated by M. Campbell, and Edited by H. J. CaMpbell, M.D., M.R.C.P., Senior Demonstrator of Biology in the Medical School of Guy's Hospital, and Assistant Physician to the East London Hospital for Children. i2mo. Cloth. Illustrated. pp. viii + 247. Price $ 1.60 *net.* MILES

Muscle, Brain and Diet: A Plea for Simpler Foods. By Eustace H. Miles, M.A. (Camb.), Winner of the

Tennis Gold Prize, 1897, 1898, 1899, Amateur Champion, 1899, etc. 121110. Cloth, pp. xv + 345. Price $ 1.00.

MINOT

Human Embryology. By Charles Sedgwick Minot, Professor of Histology and Human Embryology, Harvard Medical School, Boston. 8vo. Cloth. 463 Illustrations. pp. xxiii + 815. Price $ 6.00 net. MTJIR and RITCHIE

Manual of Bacteriology. By Robert Mulr, M.A., M.D., F.R.C.P. (Ed.), Professor of Pathology, University of Glasgow, and James Ritchie. HA., M. D., B.Sc., Lecturer in Pathology, University of Oxford. Second Edition. 121110. Cloth. 126 Illustrations. pp. xviii + 564. Price $ 3.2s net. NEW-SHOLME

The Elements of Vital Statistics By Arthur Newsholme, MJ). (Lond.), F.R. C.P., Examiner in State Medicine to the University of London, etc. Third Edition. 8vo. Cloth, pp. xii-f 353. Price J 3x10.

OPPENHEIM

The Development of the Child. By Nathan Oppenheim. Attending Physician to the Children's Department of Mt. Sinai Hospital Dispensary. i2mo. Cloth. pp. viii. + 296. Price $ 1.25 net. *By the Same Author.*

The Care of the Child in Health. israo. Cloth, pp. vii + 308. Price S1..25.

The Medical Diseases of Childhood. By Nathan Oppenheim, A.B. (Harv.), M.D. (Coll. P. & S., N. Y.). 8vo. Cloth. 101 Illustrations and 19 Charts. pp. xx + 653. Price $ 5.00 net.

Sheep $ 6.00 net.

Half morocco $ 6.50 net. PALMBERG

A Treatise on Public Health. By A. Pai.mberg, Edited by Arthur Newsholme. 8vo. Cloth.

Price $ 5.00 net. PERCTVAL

Optics. A Manual for Students. By A. S. PercIval, MA., M.B., Trinity College, Cambridge. 121110. Cloth. pp. x + 399. Price $ 3.25 net.

RAMSAY

Atlas of External Diseases of the Eye By A. Maitland Ramsay, M.D., Fellow of Faculty of Physicians and Surgeons, Glasgow; Ophthalmic Surgeon, Glas-gow Royal Infirmary; Professor of Ophthalmology, St. Mingo's College, Glasgow; and Lecturer on Eye Diseases, Queen Margaret College, University of Glasgow. With 30 hill-page colored Plates, and 18 full-page Photogravures. 410. Half morocco, pp. xvi + 195. Price $ 20.00 net. REBMANN and SEILER

The Human Frame and the Laws of Health. By Drs. Redmann and Sf.ii.er. Translated from the German, by F. W. Keeble, M.A. i6ino. Cloth. Illustrated, pp. 148.

Price 40 cents net. REYNOLDS

Hygiene for Beginners. By Ernest Septimus Reynolds. M.D. (Ixmd.i. Fellow of the Royal College of Physicians of London, etc. i2mo. Clotb. 100 Illustrations. pp. xiv + 235.

Price 75 cents net. *By the Same Author*

A Primer of Hygiene. Illustrated.

Price 35 cents net. ROLLESTON and KANTHACK

Manual of Practical Morbid Anatomy.

Being a Handbook for the Post-Mortem Room. By H. D. Rolleston, M.A., M.D., and A. H. Kanthack, M.D., M.R.C.P. Price $ 1.60 net.

ROOSA

Defective Eyesight: The Principles of Its Relief by Glasses. By D. B. St. John Roosa, M.D., LL.D., Professor Emeritus of Diseases of the Eye, New York Post-Graduate Medical School and Hospital; Surgeon to Manhattan Eye and Ear Hospital; Consulting Surgeon to the Brooklyn Eye and Ear Hospital, etc. i2mo. Cloth. Illustrated, pp. ix + 193. Price $ 1.00 net. SCHAFER

Text-Book of Physiology. Edited by E. A. Schafer, LL.D., F.R.S., Professor of Physiology, University of Edinburgh. Cloth. Svo.

Vol. I. 27 Plates and 92 Text Illustrations, pp. xviii + 1036. Price $ 8.00 net.

Vol.11. 499 Illustrations. pp. xxiv + 1365. Price $ 10.00 net. SHEILD

A Clinical Treatise on Diseases of the Breast. By A. Marmaduke Sheild, M. B. (Cantab.), F.R.C.S., Senior Assistant Surgeon and Lecturer on Practical Surgery to St. George's Hospital; Late Assistant Surgeon, Aural Surgeon and Lecturer on Operative Surgery to Charing Cross Hospital; Assistant Surgeon to the Hospital for Women and Children, Waterloo Bridge Road. 8vo. Half leather. Illustrated, pp. xvi-f510. Price $ 5.00 net. SMITH

Introduction to the Outlines of the Principles of Differential Diagnosis, with Clinical Memoranda. By Fred J. Smith, M.A., M.D. (Oxon.), F.R.C.P. (Lond.), Physician and Senior Pathologist to the London Hospital. l2mo. Cloth. pp. ix + 353. Price $ 2.00 net.

8TARR

Atlas of Nerve-Cells. By M. Allen Starr, M.D., Ph.D., with the Co-operation of Oliver S. Strong, Ph.D., and Edward Leaming. With 53 Albertype plates and 13 diagrams. Royal 410. Cloth, pp. x + 78.

Price $ 10.00 net. STEPHENSON

Epidemic Ophthalmia, Its Symptoms, Diagnosis and Management; with Papers on Allied Subjects. By SydNey Stephenson, M.R, F.R.C.S. (Ed.), Surgeon to the Ophthalmic School, Hanwell, W. 8vo. Cloth. pp. 278. Price $ 3. 00 net. STONHAM

A Manual of Surgery. By Charles Stonham, F.R.C.S. (Eng.), Senior Surgeon to the Westminster Hospital; Lecturer on Surgery and on Clinical Surgery, and Teacher of Operative Surgery, Westminster Hospital, etc. In three volumes.

Vol. I. General Surgery. 115 Illustrations. pp. xiii + 343.

Vol. II. Injuries. 125 Illustrations. pp. xv + 383.

Vol. III. Regional Surgery. 206 Illustrations. pp. xxi + 725. i2mo. Cloth. Price $ 6.00 net. SUTER

Handbook of Optics. For Students of Ophthalmology. By William NorWood Suter, B.A., M.D., Professor of Ophthalmology, National University, and Assistant Surgeon, Episcopal Eye, Ear and Throat Hospital, Washington, D.C. i2mo. Cloth. 54 Illustrations. pp. viii + 209. Price $ 1.00 net. THOMA

Text-Book of General Pathology and Pathological Anatomy. By Richard Thoma, Professor of General Pathology and Pathological Anatomy in the

University of Dorpat. Translated by Alexander Bruce, M.A., M.D., F.R.C.P.E, F.R.C.S.E., Lecturer on Pathology, Surgeons' Hall, Edinburgh; Pathologist to the Royal Hospital for Sick Children; Assistant Physician and formerly Pathologist to the Royal Infirmary, Edinburgh. Volume I. With 436 Illustrations. 8vo. Cloth, pp. xiv + 624 + Plates. Price $ 7.00 net. THORNE

Diphtheria: Its Natural History and Prevention. By R. Thorne Thorne, M.B. (Lond.), F.R.C.P. (Lond.),F.R.S., etc. i2mo. Cloth, pp. vi + 266.

Price $ 2.00.

TUBBY

Deformities. A Treatise on Orthopaedic Surgery intended for Practitioners and advanced Students. By A. H. Tubby, M. S. (Lond.),F.R.C.S. (Eng.), Assistant Surgeon to, and in charge of, the Orthopaedic Department, Westminster Hospital; Surgeon to the National Orthopaedic Hospital, etc. Illustrated with 15 Plates and 302 Figures, and by Notes of 100 Cases. 8vo. Sheep, pp. xxii + 598. Price 15.50 net. TURNER

Hints and Remedies for the Treatment of Common Accidents and Diseases, and Rules of Simple Hygiene. Compiled by Dawson W. Turner, D.C. L. Revised, Corrected, and Enlarged by twelve Eminent Medical Men belonging 10 different Hospitals in London, and by one Right Rev. Bishop of the Established Church, formerly Surgeon to one of the London hospitals and F.R.C.S. i6mo. Cloth, pp. 106.

Price 50 cents. UNNA

The Hiatopathologv of the Diseases of the Skin. By DR. P. G. UNNA. Translated from the German, with the assistance of the Author, by NORMAN Walker, M.D.,F.R.C.P. (Ed.), Assistant Physician in Dermatology to the Royal Infirmary, Edinburgh. With double-colored Plate containing 19 Illustrations and 42 additional Illustrations in the text 8vo. Cloth. pp. xxvii + 1205. Price $ 10,50 net. VERWORN

General Physiology: An Outline of the Science of Life. By Max VerWORN, M.D., Ph.D., A.O., Professor of Physiology in the Medical Faculty of the University of Jena. Translated from the

Second German Edition and edited by Frederic S. Lee, Ph.D., Adjunct Professor of Physiology in Columbia University. With 285 Illustrations. 8vo. Cloth. pp. xvi + 6i5. Price S 4.00 net. WARING

Manual of Operative Surgery. By H. J. Waring, M.S., M.B., B.Sc. (Lond.), F.R.C.S., Demonstrator of Operative Surgery and Surgical Registrar, Late Senior Demonstrator of Anatomy St. Bartholomew's Hospital; Surgeontothe Metropolitan Hospital and Erasmus Wilson Lecturer to the Royal College of Surgeons, England. i2mo. Cloth. Illustrated, pp. xxvi + 661.

WARING

Diseases of the Liver, Gall Bladder, and Biliary System; Their Pathology, Diagnosis and Surgical Treatment. ByH. I. Waring, M.S., B.Sc. (Lond.), FiR.C.S., Demonstrator of Operative Surgery, and Senior Demonstrator of Anatomy St. Bartholomew's Hospital, etc. 8vo. Cloth. 58 Illustrations. pp. xiv + 385. Price J 3.75 net. WARNER

Three Lectures on the Anatomy of Movement. A Treatise on the Action of Nerve-Centres and Modes of Growth. Delivered at the Royal College of Surgeons of England. By FRANCIS WARNER, M.D. I2mo. Cloth. 18 Illustrations. pp. xiv + 135.

Price 75 cents net. By the Same Author

The Nervous System of the Child: Its Growth and Health in Education. By Francis Warner, M.D. (Lond.), F.R.C.P., F.R.C.S. (Eng.), Physician to and Lecturer at the London Hospital, etc. I2mo. Cloth. pp. xvii-f-233.

Price $ i.oo net.

The Study of Children and Their School Training. By Francis Warner, M.D. I2mo. Cloth. pp. xix-f-264. Price £ i.oo net.

WATSON

Practical Handbook of the Disease of the Eye. By D. Chalmers WatSon, M.B., C.M., Ophthalmic Surgeon, Marshall Street Dispensary, Edinburgh; late Clinical Assistant, Ophthalmological Department. Royal Infirmary, Edinburgh. With 9 colored Plates and 24 Illustrations in the text. I2mo. Cloth. pp. x-)-236.

Price S 1.60 met. WEBSTER

Diseases of Women. A Text-Book for Students and Practitioners. By J. C. Webster, B.A., M.D. (Edin.), F.R.C.P. (Ed.), Demonstrator of Gynaecology, McGill University; Assistant Gynaecologist, Royal Victoria Hospital. Montreal, etc. Illustrated with 241 Figures. I2mo. Cloth. pp. xxii-r-6S8. WHITE Price 13-5 «

A Text-Book of General Therapeutics By W. Hale White, M.D., F.R.C.P. Senior Assistant-Physician to and Lecturer on Materia Medica and Therapeutics at Guy's Hospital. i2mo. Cloth. pp. xi-)-371. Illustrated.

Price $ 2.50 net. WIEDERSHEIM

The Structure of Man: An Index to His Past History. By Dr. R. Wie-Dersheim, Professor in the University of Freiburg, Translated by H. and M. BERNARD. The Translation edited and annotated and a Preface written bv G. B. Howes, F.L.S., Professor ot ZoOlogy, Royal College of Science. London. 105 Illustrations. 8vo. Cloth. pp. xxi + 227. Price $ 2.60 net.

WILLIAMS

The Roentgen Rays in Medicine and Surgery as an Aid in Diagnosis, and as a Therapeutic Agent. By Francis H. Williams, M.D. 391 Illustrations. Svo. Cloth. pp. xxx-f-658.

Price 16.00 met.

Half morocco. Price , 7.00 met.

WILLIAMSON

Diabetes Mellitus and Its Treatment. By R. T.williamson. M.D. (Lond.). M.R.C.P., Medical Registrar, Manchester Royal Infirmary; Hon.Med.Officer, Pendleton Dispensary; Assistant to the Professor of Medicine, Owens College, Manchester. With 18 Illustrations. Svo. Cloth. pp. xi + 417.

Price 14.50 net. WILLOUGHBY

Handbook of Public Health and Demography. By Edward F. WilLoughby, M.D. (Lond.). Diploma in State Medicine of the London University and in Public Health of Cambridge University. i6mo. Cloth. pp. xvi-r-509. Price?:. 50 WILSON

The Cell in Development and Inheritance. By Edmund R Wilson, PtO)., Professor of ZoSlogy, Columbia

University. Second Edition, Revised and Enlarged. 8vo. Cloth. 194 Illustrations. pp. xxi + 483. Price $ 3.50 net.

WORKS ON MEDICINE AND SURGERY By the Same Author

An Atlas of tbe Fertilization and Karyokinesis of the Ovum. By Edmund B. Wilson, Ph.D., Professor in Invertebrate Zoology in Columbia University; with the co-operation of Edward Leaming, M.D., F.R.P.S., Instructor in Photography at the College of Physicians and Surgeons, Columbia University. Royal 4to. Cloth.

Price $ 4.00 *net* WILSON

Clinical Studies in Vice and in Insanity. By George R. Wilson, M.D., Medical Superintendent, Marisbank Asylum. 8vo. Cloth, pp. xi + 234. Price $ 3.00

net. WORSNOP

The Nurse's Handbook of Cookery; A Help in Sickness and Convalescence. By E. M. woRSnOp, First-Class Diplomee of THE MACMILLAN COMPANY the National Training School of Cookery, South Kensington, and for sixteen years Teacher of Cookery under the London School Board. Assisted by M. C. Blair. Second Edition. i2mo. Cloth. pp. 106. Price 75 cents.

ZIEQLER

A Text-Book of Special Pathological Anatomy. By Ernst Ziegler, Professor of Pathology in the University of Freiburg. Translated and Edited from the Eighth German Edition, by Donald Macalister. M.A., M.D., Linacre Lecturer of Physic and Tutor of St John's College, Cambridge, and Henry W. Cattell, M.A., M.D., Demonstrator of Morbid Anatomy in the University of Pennsylvania. 8vo. 562 Illustrations.

Sections I—VIII. pp. xix-f 575 + xxxii.

Cloth, Price $ 4.00 *net.*

Sheep, Price $ 5.00 *net.*

Sections IX-XV. pp. xv + 576-1221 + xxxi.

Cloth, Price $ 4.00 *net.*

Sheep, Price $ 5.00 *net.*

66 FIFTH AVENUE. NEW YORK LANE MEDICAL LIBRARY

Lightning Source UK Ltd.
Milton Keynes UK
UKOW07f1046211116

288165UK00012B/968/P